TROPICAL DISEASES - ETIOLOGY, PATHOGENESIS AND TREATMENTS

ANTIMALARIAL DRUGS: COSTS, SAFETY AND EFFICACY

TROPICAL DISEASES - ETIOLOGY, PATHOGENESIS AND TREATMENTS SERIES

Malaria Research Trends
Devin A. Flanigan (Editor)
2007. ISBN: 1-60021-589-0

Artemisinins in Malaria Therapy
Qigui Li, Wilbur K. Milhous and Peter J. Weina
2007. ISBN: 1-60021-781-8

Antimalarial Drugs: Costs, Safety and Efficacy
Emanuel Csizmadia and Istvan Kalnoky (Editors)
2009. ISBN: 978-1-60741-432-2

TROPICAL DISEASES - ETIOLOGY, PATHOGENESIS AND TREATMENTS

ANTIMALARIAL DRUGS: COSTS, SAFETY AND EFFICACY

EMANUEL CSIZMADIA
AND
ISTVAN KALNOKY
EDITORS

Nova Biomedical Books
New York

For permission to use material from this book please contact us:
Telephone 631-231-7269; Fax 631-231-8175
Web Site: http://www.novapublishers.com

Library of Congress Cataloging-in-Publication Data

Antimalarial drugs : costs, safety, and efficacy / [edited by] Emanuel Csizmadia and Istvan Kalnoky.
p. ; cm.
Includes bibliographical references and index.
ISBN 978-1-60741-432-2 (hardcover)
1. Antimalarials. 2. Antimalarials--Chemotherapy. I. Csizmadia, Emanuel. II. Kalnoky, Istvan.
[DNLM: 1. Antimalarials. 2. Drug Costs. 3. Drug Toxicity--prevention & control. 4. Treatment Outcome. QV 256 A6313 2009]
RC159.A5.A585 2009
362.196'9362--dc22 2009027047

Published by Nova Science Publishers, Inc. ✝ New York

Contents

Preface

Malaria is the leading parasitic infectious disease in sub-Saharan Africa (SSA) in terms of morbidity, hospitalization and mortality. Pregnant women and children under the age of five years, especially infants, are the most vulnerable. In SSA where 90% of the global burden of malaria is concentrated, at least one child dies of malaria every 40 seconds. Intermittent preventive treatment (IPT) describes the administration of a full course of antimalarial drugs to the population at risk at specified time intervals, irrespective of whether or not one is infected. Drug resistance, especially multidrug resistance, and difficulties in eradicating the mosquito vector have been the basis of malaria resurgence over the past 30 years. In addition, massive problems with logistics, planning, allocation of resources and a lack of operational research have contributed greatly to the failure of malaria eradication. This new and important book gathers the latest research from around the globe in this field.

Chapter I – Introduction: Intermittent presumptive treatment (IPT) for malaria during pregnancy (IPTp) is advocated against malaria. Yet, concerns prevail regarding safety, efficacy, and costs of the recommended anti-malarial interventions in economic, social and multi-faceted health contexts.

Objective: This chapter elucidates the views of frontline healthcare workers (HWs) and antenatal care (ANC) clients regarding feasibility of implementing anti-malarial drugs in formal healthcare settings of Tanzania, including the scaling-up IPTp delivery in attempt to attain higher population coverage. Emphasis is on efficacy, safety and cost issues related to SP for IPTp.

Methods: Semi-structured interviews with HWs and pregnant women at ANC clinics and investigators' observations in the fields were conducted. Content analysis was done on qualitative information whereas quantitative data were analyzed using computer software programs.

Results: The respondents expressed positive and negative attitudes towards IPTp currently in practice. The reported positives of IPTp were related to: sulfadoxine-pyrimethamine (SP) - a drug of choice being more efficacious than other anti-malarial drugs; easy deliverability in terms of users taking a full dose once; saving lives of women, fetuses and newborn babies; and un-bitter taste. The negatives include the: (i) perception about SP causing adverse treatment outcomes, this lowering users' adherence to treatment schedules, including directly observed treatment; (ii) perceived possible adverse reactions if SP is used by the users who take alcoholic drinks; (iii) increasing- parasites resistance to SP and HIV infections lowering public trust in SP; (iii) health facilities (HFs), especially the private ones facing SP shortages for free delivery, adding costs mainly to the service users and partly HWs who are forced to pay out of their pockets; (iv) HF-based IPTp services forcing pregnant women who reside far away to incur additional costs on re-visiting HFs, including the costs on transport, foods and/or drinks, besides purchasing SP elsewhere when the HFs concerned are out of stock of SP, and time lost for waiting for services. Moreover, user-fees for ANC services other than IPTp seemed to dissuade some potential clients to attend clinic. Additional findings and discussions are presented.

Conclusion: When institutionalizing policies, national and international authorities sometimes under-rate the operational barriers to the recommended interventions in local settings. This study reveals that the social perceptions on- and the real deficiencies of anti-malarial drug efficacy, safety and costs are a challenge for rolling back malaria in Tanzania, as elsewhere in Africa.

Chapter II - The resistance to antimalarial drugs, especially chloroquine, of *Plasmodium falciparum* has contributed to an increase in morbidity and mortality due to malaria in recent years. It has been well established that chloroquine-sensitive parasites accumulate more drug within *P. falciparum* food vacuoles than their resistant counterparts. Mechanisms underlying drug resistance in malaria remains unclear but three proteins have been implicated in quinoline resistance: Pgh-1 (P-glycoprotein homologue 1); PfCRT (*Plasmodium falciparum* chloroquine resistance transporter) and PfMRP (*Plasmodium falciparum* multidrug resistance protein). Whether these proteins act as channels or transporters of quinoline is still to be determined. Quinoline-reversing agents, a class of compounds unrelated to quinoline, are believed to act on these proteins. Although they do not have any intrinsic anti-malaria activity, they have the property of being able to reverse drug resistance. Recent advances in target orientated synthesis and structure activity relationship should be beneficial for the understanding of the mode of action of these agents and design of improved drugs for the control of malaria. Polymorphisms in the corresponding genes of the quinoline transporters (*pfcrt*, *pfmdr1* and *pfmrp*) have been detected and identified as potential molecular markers for parasite resistance to quinoline antimalarials. The integration of these molecular markers in surveillance program would be crucial for the monitoring of drug resistance and the management of strategies for the reversal of resistance. Resistance of *P. falciparum* to all the major drugs used for the treatment of malaria has evolved quickly after their introduction. The use of chemosensitisers could represent a potential therapeutic strategy to overcome failure treatments due to the increasing problem of drug resistance. This chapter discusses currently known quinoline transporters implicated in drug resistance, reversing agents and their potential as therapeutic strategy.

Chapter III - Although clinical trials on intermittent-preventive-treatment (IPT) for malaria in infants (IPTi) are underway in Africa following the notable benefit of IPT during pregnancy (IPTp) using sulfadoxine-pyrimethamine (SP), evidence on the socio-economic determinants of the acceptability and viability of IPTi within infant clinic settings is inadequate. This paper reports a study on the acceptability of IPTi in two Tanzanian districts implementing IPTp using SP. Data were collected from 24 focus-group-discussions (FGDs) with pregnant-women and infants' mothers; interviews with 823 antenatal clients, 78 antenatal workers and 14 district health-managers among whom some also participated in

FGDs. Qualitative findings indicated IPTi being appreciated among all the study population groups, considering the malaria situation. However, reservations were expressed about IPTi if SP is officially recommended. Skeptics pinpointed the side-effects, lack of antipyretic-effect and the general treatment failures of the SP drug. Another concern was that IPTi may face operational challenges such as those currently facing IPTp implementation, including the shortage of essential supplies, poor health facility infrastructural conditions, and low numbers, skills and motivation of human-resources. Based on a hypothetical question eliciting the pregnant women's willingness to allow (WTA) their babies to receive SP for IPTi if officially SP was the drug of choice, logistic regression analysis of the data obtained indicated variations among the respondents within and between the districts about in the WTA their babies to receive IPTi-SP. In conclusion, IPTi has limited potential acceptability in the healthcare system if SP is recommended, and despite some of the respondents having expressed speculative concerns, there is need for strong public sensitization before and during IPTi implementation towards enhancement of community and frontline health-workers' compliance.

Chapter IV – Introduction: Implementing Intermittent Preventive Treatment for malaria in Pregnancy (IPTp) with sulfadoxine-pyrimethamine (SP) through antenatal care (ANC) clinics is recommended for malaria endemic countries. The vast biomedical literature on malaria prevention focuses more on the epidemiological and cost-effectiveness analyses of the randomised controlled trials carried out in selected geographical settings. Such studies fail to elucidate the economic, psychosocial, managerial, organization and other contextual systemic factors influencing the operational effectiveness, compliance and coverage of the recommended interventions.

Objective: To review literature on policy advances, achievements, constraints and challenges to malaria IPTp implementation, emphasising its operational feasibility in the context of health-care financing, provision and uptake, resource constraints and psychosocial factors in Africa.

Results: The importance of IPTp in preventing unnecessary anaemia, morbidity and mortality in pregnancy and improving childbirth outcomes is highly acknowledged, although the following factors appear to be the main constraints to IPTp service delivery and uptake: cost of accessing ANC; myths and other discriminatory socio-cultural values on pregnancy; target users, perceptions and attitudes towards SP, malaria, and quality of ANC; supply and cost of SP at health facilities; understaffing and demoralised staff; ambiguity and impracticability of user-fee exemption policy guidelines on essential ANC services; implementing IPTp, bednets, HIV and syphilis screening programmes in the same clinic settings; and reports on increasing parasite resistant to SP. However, the noted increase in the coverage of the delivery of IPTp doses in several countries justify that IPTp implementation is possible and better than not.

Conclusion: IPTp for malaria is implemented in constrained conditions in Africa. This is a challenge for higher coverage of at least two doses and attainment of the Abuja targets. Yet, there are opportunities for addressing the existing challenges, and one of the useful options is the evaluation of the acceptability and viability of the existing intervention guidelines.

Chapter V - In the *Pharmacopoeias*, characterization of the toxic contaminant in primaquine is not described. The *Pharmacopoeias* require chromatographic separation Rs greater than 2 between the contaminant and API peak, based on separation using HPLC. The United States Pharmacopeia (USP) and The National Formulary (NF) seek submission of a monograph proposing an improvement of analysis of primaquine phosphate tablets.

In this study, resolution based on supercritical fluid chromatography (SFC) and supercritical fluid chromatography-mass spectrometry (SFC-MS) satisfy the *Pharmacopoeia* standards.

Primaquine diphosphate 7.5 mg tablets were analyzed. Separation Rs greater than 2 was achieved between the major contaminant peak and the peak of the API in less than 15 minutes. The novelty of this work is the determination of the main contaminant in medical form primaquine diphosphate tablets.

Chapter VI - It is well known that artemisinin-based combination therapy is the more effective way for fighting falciparum malaria, and this is the World Health Organization's recommended guideline for the treatment of malaria. However the modern antimalarial preparations made from semi-synthetic derivatives (arthemeter, artesunate) are not routinely available in remote rural areas, and they are still expensive and very frequently not easily affordable for poor families. Meanwhile many studies have confirmed the immediate efficacy of artemisinin, which may be a solution for resolving the tragedy of malaria in young children in endemic areas.

Tea preparations from *Artemisia Annua*, used in traditional Chinese medicine for centuries, have proved to be effective and safe in treatment of all human malaria parasites, and notably multidrug-resistant plasmodium falciparum. Artemisinin clears peripheral parasitaemia more quickly than other antimalarial drugs. It is active on early trophozoïte and ring blood-stages of the parasite cycle, with a rapid in vitro effect suggesting a high parasitocidal action. Administration of artemisinin prevents the development in the more mature trophozoïte stage with adherence of the parasite to the vascular endothelium, resulting in sequestration in the small blood vessels of vital organs: this sequestration stage is thought to be responsible for the complications of malaria or cerebral malaria.

The authors consider that, although not entirely satisfying, treatment of malaria by tea preparations from leaves of *Artemisia Annua* may be an alternative to modern antimalarial drugs. They have developed a program of cultivation of *Artemisia Annua*, the aim being to provide seeds to local populations in endemic areas of undeveloped countries, to favour local cultivation, to promote knowledge about *Artemisia Annua,* and to supply advice and documents. They have created an association entitled Artemisine Contre Paludisme, located in Longeville, Franche-Comté, East of France. The plant is cultivated there at 700 m above sea level, without fertilization.

Chapter VII - Quinine is a well-known antimalarial drug that is widely used in clinical practice. Although quinine is effective, it also poses a considerable toxicity. Quinine toxicity has been known for decades and the specific term "cinchonism" is used for describing the quinine toxicity. In this article, the author will review the cinchonism focusing on several aspects of this disorder. Important reports will be quoted and summarized in this chapter.

Chapter VIII - Malaria remains on of the most prevalent and deadly of the insect-borne communicable diseases. Since the parasite *Plasmodium* developed resistance to classical drugs of quinine type, artemisinin-based peroxides have become the most important antimalarial drugs. Various artemisinin derivatives have been developed to improve the antimalarial performance, while insights into its mechanism of action reveal that the pharmacophore unit in artemisinin is a peroxide group bound to the 1,2,4-trioxane skeleton. However, it is not economical to synthesize artemisinin directly and currently, the global demand for artemisinin cannot be met by the low yield obtained from the cultivation of herb *Artemisia annua*. Therefore, current research focuses on the development of easily accessible, cheap and effective antimalarial drugs based on synthetic peroxides. The main synthetic analogues of artemisinin belong to a 1,2,4-trioxane type of organic peroxides, that together with structurally related 1,2,4,5-tetraoxanes and 1,2,4-trioxolanes constitutes the core of antimalarial synthetic peroxides, while various endoperoxides, cyclic and acyclic perketals are also active antimalarial agents. Another interesting concept in antimalarial chemotherapy are chimeric compounds or hybrids; these are composed of two different antimalarial agents joined in one molecule. The following chapter discusses synthetic antimalarial peroxides with an emphasis on the development of synthetic compounds from 2000 onwards.

Chapter IX - The problem of drug resistance is the main problem affecting the success of malarial treatment worldwide. Southeast Asian countries including Thailand face up with the problem of antimalarial resistance at present. The details ranging from the molecular to social aspects of malarial resistance will be reviewed and presented. Also, the treatment of malaria in clinical practice in Thailand covering standard as well as alternative therapy for malaria to cope with the problem of high antimalarial resistance will be summarized in this chapter. New data were summarized and presented in this chapter.

Chapter X - Biochemoinformatics is a new science that can lead several advantages in medicine. New drug development can be easily performed with the new advancements in bioinformatics. Advanced biochemoinformatics technologies for drug search can be applied for new antimalarial drug search. This is useful in the case of antimalarial drug resistance.

In: Antimalarial Drugs: Costs, Safety and Efficacy
Editors: Emanuel Csizmadia and Istvan Kalnoky
ISBN: 978-1-60741-432-2

Chapter I

Efficacy, Safety and Costs of Intermittent Presumptive Treatment for Malaria in Tanzania: Beliefs, Attitudes, Experiences, and Views of Service Providers and Users

***Godfrey Martin Mubyazi*[ab], *Paul Bloch*[e], *Pascal Magnussen*[c], *Jens Byskov*[c], *Kristian Schultz Hansen*[d], *Øystein Evjen Olsen*[c], *Leonard E.G. Mboera and Ib Christian Bygbjerg*[e]**

[ab]National Institute for Medical Research (NIMR), P.O. Box 9653 Dar es Salaam, Tanzania; Amani Medical Research Centre, P.O Box 81 Muheza, Tanzania;
[c]University of Aarhus, Institute of Public Health, Department of Health Services Research, DK-8000 Aarhus C, Denmark;
[d]University of Copenhagen, DBL-Centre for Health Research and Development, Institute of Veterinary Pathobiology, Faculty of Life Sciences, Copenhagen, Denmark;
University of Copenhagen, Faculty of Health Sciences,
[e]Department of International Health, Immunology and Microbiology, Copenhagen, Denmark

Abstract

Introduction

Intermittent presumptive treatment (IPT) for malaria during pregnancy (IPTp) is advocated against malaria. Yet, concerns prevail regarding safety, efficacy, and costs of the recommended anti-malarial interventions in economic, social and multi-faceted health contexts.

Objective

This chapter elucidates the views of frontline healthcare workers (HWs) and antenatal care (ANC) clients regarding feasibility of implementing anti-malarial drugs in formal healthcare settings of Tanzania, including the scaling-up IPTp delivery in attempt to attain higher population coverage. Emphasis is on efficacy, safety and cost issues related to SP for IPTp.

Methods

Semi-structured interviews with HWs and pregnant women at ANC clinics and investigators' observations in the fields were conducted. Content analysis was done on qualitative information whereas quantitative data were analyzed using computer software programs.

Results

The respondents expressed positive and negative attitudes towards IPTp currently in practice. The reported positives of IPTp were related to: sulfadoxine-pyrimethamine (SP) - a drug of choice being more efficacious than other anti-malarial drugs; easy deliverability in terms of users taking a full dose once; saving lives of women, fetuses and newborn babies; and un-bitter taste. The negatives include the: (i) perception about SP causing adverse treatment outcomes, this lowering users' adherence to treatment schedules, including directly observed treatment; (ii) perceived possible adverse reactions if SP is used by the users who take alcoholic drinks; (iii) increasing- parasites resistance to SP and HIV infections lowering public trust in SP; (iii) health facilities (HFs), especially the private ones facing SP shortages for free delivery, adding costs mainly to the service users and partly HWs who are forced to pay out of their pockets; (iv) HF-based IPTp services forcing pregnant women who reside far away to incur additional costs on re-visiting HFs, including the costs on transport, foods and/or drinks, besides purchasing SP elsewhere when the HFs concerned are out of stock of SP, and time lost for waiting for services. Moreover, user-fees for ANC services other than IPTp seemed to dissuade some potential clients to attend clinic. Additional findings and discussions are presented.

Conclusion

When institutionalizing policies, national and international authorities sometimes under-rate the operational barriers to the recommended interventions in local settings. This study reveals that the social perceptions on- and the real deficiencies of anti-malarial drug efficacy, safety and costs are a challenge for rolling back malaria in Tanzania, as elsewhere in Africa.

Keywords: Cost, anti-malarial drugs, pregnancy, affordability, accessibility, healthcare

Introduction

The Malaria Burden

Malaria remains a retarding disease to socio-economic development of many tropical and some sub-tropical countries. Reports by the World Health Organization (WHO) and international and national organizations continue indicating 90% of the malaria cases in the world recorded each year as concentrated in sub-Saharan Africa (SSA). Each year, malaria kills 300-500 million cases, killing about 1 million people, and for every one minute it kills one child in SSA (Rugemalila et al., 2007). In Tanzania, malaria is so far the leading cause of hospitalization and mortalities, and contributes to 20% of all the maternal deaths (Mubyazi et al., 2008). The reports show that although all the community members in these countries are at risk, pregnant women and children aged below five years (i.e. the *underfives*, especially *infants*) are most vulnerable due to their low immunity capacities (Greenwood et al., 2007; Menendez et al., 1995; Snow 2004; Steketee et al., 2001; Mutabingwa et al., 1994; Brabin 1983).

Global Malaria Prevention Strategies

Malaria control methods in malaria endemic countries have taken various ways at varying degrees. High advocacy has been on public sensitization on environmental sanitation including bush clearing around residential houses to keeping mosquitoes away. Other key main traditional methods adopted in line with WHO's recommendations include use of: residual in-door or out-door sprays with appropriate chemicals that act as insecticides, (b) insecticide-treated nets, and anti-malarial drugs as a prophylaxis. The practice of each of these methods varies more or less from one country setting to another due to, among other contextual factors, the perceived or real conditions related to affordability, safety, efficacy and affordability of the recommended strategies in local settings (Goodman et al., 2003). The use of prophylaxis for malaria has been emphasized in favor of pregnant women and under-fives in malaria endemic countries and travelers from the rest of the world outside malaria endemic countries. Chloroquine (CQ) has for many years been the drug of choice used both as a prophylaxis (Greenwood 2004) and a first-line drug for the treatment of uncomplicated malaria. However, CQ has been replaced with sulfadoxine-pyrimethamine (SP) [Fansidar®] as the first line drug against uncomplicated malaria in Tanzania and several other countries of SSA after CQ had faced parasite resistance (Goodman et al., 2006; Mubyazi and Gonzalez-Block 2005; EANMAT 2001). SP has also been recommended for intermittent presumptive/preventive treatment for malaria during (IPT) during pregnancy (IPTp), as also considered for IPT in infant children (IPTi) (Vallely et al., 2007; Schellenberg et al., 2006; White 2005) and older children (IPTc) (Greenwood 2006) in the future. The IPTp strategy targets pregnant women attending antenatal care (ANC) clinics (WHO and UNICEF 2003). However, the scale at which malaria presumptive treatment strategy is implemented varies from within and between country settings, contributed by contextual factors, including those related to safety and essential supply conditions that have cost implications to the service providers and users (Worrall et al., 2007; Hill and Kazembe 2006).

Intermittent Presumptive Treatment (IPT) for Malaria

Responding to WHO advice, SSA countries officially instituted IPTp with SP. Besides curing possible infections, SP was found potential for preventing anaemia in pregnancy, low birth-weight, premature deliveries and improvement in other delivery outcomes (Vallely et al., 2007; Verhoeff et al., 2004). The initial policy target of SSA countries was to attain at least 60% coverage of IPTp and ITNs services for pregnant women registered for ANC by 2005 (WHO and UNICEF 2005; WHO and UNICEF 2000). Tanzania moved further by speculating that attainment of higher than 60% coverage of at least two doses was possible. However, this speculation appeared impossible due to operational constraints facing district healthcare systems (Mubyazi et al., 2008). The key operational barriers are related to: limited supply of SP and safe drinking water for the ANC clients to take IPTp doses under direct observation treatment procedure (DOT), inadequate skills of some frontline healthcare workers (HWs) and general low motivation of the frontline HWs to deliver the recommended/desired services, ambiguity of the guidelines regarding the timing of the IPTp doses, and amplified social perceptions about adverse effects of SP (Anders et al., 2008; Mubyazi et al., 2008; Worrall et al., 2007; Hill and Kazembe 2006; Nsimba 2006).

Efficacy of SP for Malaria IPT during Pregnancy

Concerns are high about the suitability of SP for IPTp everywhere in SSA. These are based on reports available in relation to: (*i*) the increasing treatment failure rates of SP in SSA, especially in Eastern Africa (EANMAT 2001). This has prompted several countries to recommend artemisinin-based combination therapies (ACTs) as the first-line drug for curing uncomplicated malaria, not for IPTp. This is a systemic challenge as SP may be considered by some of the service providers and many target service users as inappropriate for IPTp (Mubyazi et al., 2008); (*ii*) the apparent lack of regulatory mechanisms to enforce service providers and users especially in the private sector comply with the treatment guidelines (Malaria Consortium 2004); (*iii*) lack of evidence on whether SP works in similar or different ways in areas with different malaria transmission intensities (White 2007). Other concerns or challenges are highlighted by the authors of in the next chapter also published in this book.

Safety of SP for Malaria Treatment

It is widely evident that common self-medication practices in developing countries' community settings makes a considerable proportion of populations using pharmaceuticals, including anti-malarial drugs, fail to comply with the guidelines or instructions for drug use (Hanson et al., 2004; Goodman et al., 2003). This may contribute to the perceived- or really experienced- low safety of the drugs taken. Previous and ongoing studies depict that the use of drugs containing sulfar compounds by people who are infected with human immuno-deficiency virus (HIV) that causes acquired immune deficiency syndrome (AIDS), could be unsafe. This is a challenge to countries where HIV/AIDS pandemic is high while there is no drug recommended for IPTp alternative to SP (ter Kuile and Steketee 2006). Some people including pregnant women may still use SP while being aware or unaware that they are HIV positive (Filler et al., 2006; Holtz et al., 2004). Moreover, it is not safe to the mother and the fetus if SP is used by a pregnant woman during the first trimester of pregnancy and last stages of the third trimester (WHO and UNICEF 2000). Considering other possible, though rare side effects such as serious allergy or Steven-Johnson Syndrome (Phillip-Howard et al., 1989), one of the outstanding empirical questions in light of the last two points is 'to what degree the public including target drug administrators and users is informed of the warnings and what actions do they take?'

Costs Related to Accessibility of IPT for Malaria during Pregnancy

As in most other SSA countries (Worrall et al., 2007; Hill and Kazembe 2006), IPTp in Tanzania is still operated through health clinic settings along with other routine MCH services (Anders et al., 2008; Mubyazi et al., 2008; Mubyazi et al., 2005a; Nganda et al., 2004; MoH 2004). This service delivery strategy does not only add operation costs to the service providers, but also to the target clients/consumers in terms of inconveniences faced in for on traveling and time lost waiting for services at the clinic, even if the drug may be delivered free of charge (Ribera et al., 2007; Mubyazi et al., 2005b). Delivery of IPTp at local community levels is rarely practiced in SSA, although this could potentially help the foster efforts aimed to scaling up delivery and uptake by involving the local health service volunteers and even reduce the unnecessary costs and other inconvenience to the ANC clients in relation to travel time and financial expenditures (Mbonye et al., 2007; Mbonye 2006ab).

Pregnant women are advised to book early for ANC services and attend regularly in order to receive the basic services for better delivery outcomes (WHO 2005; Nigenda et al., 2003; WHO 1994). The effective implementation and coverage of malaria prevention during pregnancy in SSA requires accessible and affordable services (Menendez 1995). However, direct and indirect costs affect women's access to ANC services in many developing countries (Worrall et al., 2007; Borghi et al., 2006). The cost burden associated with seeking maternal and child health services (MCH) mostly affect women with low socio-economic status (Ribera et al., 2007; Worrall et al., 2007; Priya 2002). Economists look at costs in terms of direct or indirect dimensions (Drummond et al., 2005; Ensor and Cooper 2004). *Direct Costs for ANC services* faced by the ANC clients when contacting ANC clinics may be direct if they include user-fees/charges for the drugs or other services such as laboratory tests, ANC cards, or medical consultation. The costs may be indirect if associated with payment for transport e.g. bus fare or food and drinks while traveling or waiting for services, in addition to the time lost waiting time for services. The costs may also be categorized as *real* (i.e. actual) or just *perceived* if they do not really exist (Ribera et al., 2007; Kone-Pefoyo and Rivard 2006). Besides monetary costs, people often consider time spent on travel in rationing their need for medical care and type of medical care providers (Drummond et al., 2005; Hodgkin 1996; Dor et al., 1987). Shortage of literature on the existence and effect of the real or perceived user-fees for ANC services on attendances and utilization of ANC services (including IPTp) in SSA has called for more evidence and critical analysis based on systematic studies (Ribera et al., 2007; Worrall et al., 2007; Mubyazi et al., 2005ab).

The Scope of the Present Chapter

This chapter is about a study undertaken in two districts in Tanzania to explore the views of frontline HWs and ANC clients regarding implementation of IPTp for malaria in formal healthcare settings. The chapter emphasizes on drug efficacy, safety and cost implications of IPTp services to frontline HWs and target IPTp clients, and in light of these, pinpoints the contemporary challenges to efforts and prospects for scaling up and achieving a high coverage rate of IPTp services in malaria endemic local settings.

Study Methods

Design

This was a cross-sectional *exploratory case* study aimed to analyze data from multiple sources of informants and analyzing them in a triangulation fashion (Zach 2006; Scholz and Olaf 2002; Yin 1994; Fitzpatrick and Boulton 1994). The study was carried out in Mkuranga and Mufindi districts between November 2005 and January 2007, and was based on the experiences obtained from a baseline study previously undertaken in Korogwe and Muheza districts, in north-eastern Tanzania (Mubyazi et al., 2005a; CEEMI-GMP 2005, unpublished), and in The Gambia that involved the first and second authors of the present study (GMP, DBL 2005). The latter studies were followed by a pilot survey undertaken in two districts in Dar es Salaam and some localities of Mkuranga. The overall study looked at the economic and other contextual determinants of acceptability and viability of IPTp in Tanzania from the perspectives of healthcare managers, frontline HWs and target ANC users (Mubyazi et al., 2008; Mubyazi et al., 2005b). Case studies are useful in evaluation research, such as community-based preventive programs (Tellis 1997).

Study Districts and Selection Criteria: The two case study districts are located in different regions. *Mkuranga* is located in the Coast Region, near Dar es Salaam. Mufindi is located in Iringa Region, in the southern highland part of Tanzania. These districts being located in different geographical regions, they experience different malaria prevalence, ethnic/cultural characteristics, occupational and other economic opportunities, availability and distribution of different types of HFs, and previous MCH records.

►***Mkuranga*** district covers an area of 2,432km^2, and its capital is located at about 60km from the city of Dar es Salaam (Eriksen et al., 2007; Mubyazi et al., 2007), and is divided into 4 administrative divisions: *Mkuranga*, *Vikindu*, *Kisiju* and *Mkamba*. In 2002, it was estimated to have 186,927 residents mostly living in rural settings (NBS 2002). Rainfall ranges between 500–1000 mm per annum and mean daily temperate of 28^0C. The district faces a stable and perennial malaria transmission (MARA-MOH-TEHIP 2000). According to the district's Primary Health Care (PHC) Report, over 30% of outpatient and inpatient registrations in 2004 were related to malaria. It is predominantly inhabited by the *Zaramo, Ndegereko, Matumbi* and *Makonde* tribes (Mubyazi et al., 2004). It is one of the poorest districts in Tanzania (URT-MKUKUTA 2005), with an average mean annual income per head of 600,000 Tanzanian shillings (approximately US$600) or less than US1/person per day (IRA 2005). Most of the residents depend on seasonal cash, raised from the sale of coconuts, cashew-nuts, cassava, orange, pineapples and partly maize (Mubyazi et al., 2007). There was only one government hospital - *Mkuranga District Hospital*, 2 government health centers (HC) - *Kisiju-Kalole* and *Mkamba* (Mubyazi et al., 2007), 15 government dispensaries and 10 private dispensaries. By 2005 and 2006, about 50% of the private dispensaries operated on profit (or commercial) terms, as indicated in the district health plan of year 2006.

►***Mufindi*** district capital (*Mafinga*) is located at about 80 km south of the Regional capital (Iringa) in south-western Tanzania. It covers an area of 7,122km^2 and administratively is divided into 5 divisions (NBS 2002). There are two zones, a highland zone in the eastern side and lowland in the western side. Temperatures range between 15°C and 20°C (November-February). In 2002, there were 282,071 residents out of which 87.9% lived in rural areas (NBS 2002). It is predominantly resided by the *Hehe, Kinga* and *Bena* tribes. Most of the residents are engaged in farming maize, potatoes, beans, onions and rice both for food and cash. The District health plan of the year 2006-2007 indicated malaria accounting to 21-23% and 25-28% of outpatient and inpatient cases. By 2006, the district had 59 HFs, out of which 44 belonged to government, 10 to faith-based/mission organizations, and 5 to commercial runners. There were 2 hospitals - *Mafinga district government hospital* and *Lugoda Hospital* owned by the Unilever Tea Company. The district experiences unstable malaria transmission (MARA-MOH-TEHIP 2000), albeit malaria remains the number one cause of outpatient and inpatient cases registered (DMO and CHMT, per comm.).

Study Population

The target population include the frontline HWs and pregnant women attending ANC clinics. These were traced at HF levels, including the public (government) and private HFs since both of these participate in the delivery of ANC services in Tanzania (Mubyazi et al., 2005a; Boller et al., 2003). The HWs include those involved in day-to-day MCH services. Pregnant women were included as the current users of the ANC services who could give the most up-to-date experiences.

Sampling Approaches

Probability and non-probability sampling methods were applied. As for the non-probability methods, the ultimate number of the sample variables depended on the compromise between what was desirable and what was feasible (Hardon et al., 2001 p275), as clarified below:

►***Hospitals and Health Centers***: In Mkuranga, the only available 1 government hospital and 2 operating government health centers (HCs) namely *Mkamba* and *Kisiju-Kalole* were conveniently selected. In Mufindi, 2 hospitals namely Mafinga government hospital and Lugoda private Hospital were purposefully and conveniently selected. However, there were 5 HC that were included in the random sampling frame, out of which 2 and 1 government and private health centers, respectively were selected.

►***Dispensaries in both districts***: In total, 10 dispensaries were selected in each district. In Mkuranga, 5 dispensaries were government and 5 were private, including 3 private for profit and 2 faith-based. In Mufindi, only 3 dispensaries were private (both faith-based) and the rest 7 were government.

A list of HFs and district map indicating the locations and names of HFs available in each district was requested from the office of the district medical officer (DMO). Using a sampling frame, identification was made of the dispensaries that had ANC clinics. Although the original proposal/plan was to include equal number of government and private dispensaries, but it came to be noted that the number of government HFs in each district was generally larger than of the private facilities.

To allow a realistic selection of equal number of HFs representing the private and public sectors, the private dispensaries were listed separately from the list of the government dispensaries. However, this procedure was possible for Mkuranga district only. In the latter district, random selection was based on writing the names of the individual dispensaries on small pieces of papers that were put in two separate plastic jags, one jug representing government HFs and another one the private HFs. Then each jag was strongly shaken to mix the papers, after which one person outside the research team was invited to pick one paper after another randomly until the number of the papers required was reached. Fairly, each division in the study districts was represented by at least one HF.

In Mufindi, there were fewer commercial dispensaries reliably delivering ANC services. This could not allow an adequate number of such dispensaries for randomization. Therefore, the private and public dispensaries were all listed together for random selection of the study facilities.

►***Health Workers***: A convenient sampling method was applied in selecting at least two frontline HWs from the selected study HFs. The ultimate number of the HWs involved somehow depended on the convenience related to the availability of such workers at the HF targeted. It was initially targeted to cover at most four HWs at each study HF, based on the experience from previous surveys in districts of Korogwe, Muheza and Dar es Salaam and some localities of Mkuranga. In some situations even a single case study unit e.g. a HW, may be provide an acceptable data that can be replicated (Hamel et al., 1993), and generalization of results in case studies is scientifically based on theoretical proposition rather than necessarily on the sample sizes (Tellis 1997; Yin 1994). However, inferences drawn based on statistical analysis is also useful especially where comparison is made on specific study issues that could be quantified (Scholz and Olaf 2002). Until the end of the study, 78 HWs were covered, including medical and paramedical staff among which 35 and 43 HWs were from Mkuranga and Mufindi, respectively.

►***ANC clients***: These were involved in the exit interviews as described later. Likewise, the ultimate number of these participants depended on those who accepted for interview each study day, as several clients found it inconvenient to participate after they had spent a considerable time at the clinic waiting for services. In this regard, elements of convenient sampling were also unavoidable, although most of the HFs, particularly dispensaries in both districts and health centers in Mufindi district only were selected by using simple random sampling.

Using a template formula for calculating the sample size for cross-sectional kind of surveys was traced in EPI-Info version 6, asnd by applying a number of the parameters/indicators such as the estimated 80% of the pregnant women in Tanzania attending ANC at least once (WHO and UNICEF 2003) and the design effect of 3, the estimated number of the ANC clients to enrol in the study was 377 per district. References were also made to other text-books (Kirkwood and Sterne 2003). But, to cater for the possible drop-outs of some of the respondents and data recording errors (Smith and Morrow 1996), an addition of 10% of 377 was made. This added the overall sample size per district to reach 415. However, the ultimate numbers of the women actually covered in the field were 417 and 406 in Mkuranga and Mufindi, respectively. Inclination to participate in the study was shown by 31 and 18 women in the latter districts, respectively and this was due to the perceived inconvenience of the time they were approached for participation. They were replaced by approaching other clients.

Data Collection Techniques

The data were collected mainly using separate interviewer administered semi-structured interviews (SSI) with the frontline HWs and ANC clients, and partly field observations by a multidisciplinary team led by an economist. The SSI with the clients were conducted at the exit points when the clients concerned were leaving the clinics. There were fixed topics of interest, defined in light of the study objectives (Fitzpatrick and Boulton 1994).

HWs were investigated on their knowledge, views and experience on ANC services related to IPTp. Among other things, interest was on factors influencing the performance of frontline HWs in ANC services, availability of essential supplies for IPTp and costs incurred by the service clients attending ANC clinics, and the psychosocial and cultural factors influencing pregnant women's attendance and utilization of ANC services.

Exit interviews with ANC clients were aimed to eliciting the psychological and economic factors influencing the target service users' satisfaction and compliance with IPTp services, including the perceived and real cost of care, as in most health service research undertakings (Lilford and Harrison 1994). The respondents were investigated about their knowledge on

IPTp, reasons for their decision to contact the ANC clinic at which they were interviewed, and their perception of SP in terms of its safety and efficacy; and the direct and indirect cost related to ANC seeking.

Ethical Considerations

The study team adhered to the guidelines of the Council for International Organization of Medical Sciences (CIOMS 2002), and received national ethics clearances from the governments of Tanzania and Denmark. A copy of this clearance was presented to the district government authorities. Also this copy and an official letter from the office of the district councils were presented to all the HF administration and local (villages/ward) governments authorities in which the study HFs and were located. Before their enrolment, the study participants were asked for their consent to participate. Those who were willing but did not want to sign the consent forms were allowed. Among those who hesitated were the illiterate ones and those who feared that their names or finger prints would be used for security investigations if they could give sensitive information. The target study participants were also informed of the estimated time for each interview session, right to withdraw from the study without giving reasons or facing penalty, and anonymity of the information provided. Participants were also allowed to ask questions if they felt so. Debriefing about the study was given to the district and ward authorities during the implementation of the study. All the study participants were informed that the study findings would be submitted to the district and national authorities and for publications in international journals or other outlets.

Data Processing and Analysis: Two data bases were used for entering data from ANC clients and those from HWs. This paper mainly provides the quantitative information that was analyzed using STATA version 8.2 computer program (STATA Corp. Inc., Texas, USA). Specifically, focus is on the descriptive frequencies of the responses obtained to particular study questions/themes, supported some statistical tests aimed to establish the statistical similarities or differences or associations between some of the observations made or proportions of the responses per specific study questions. Logistic regression analysis was also undertaken, but the output obtained has been presented elsewhere. The responses obtained were mostly categorical in nature and varied between several questions, and as reflected in the study results section. Therefore, the percentages shown for various aspects of the findings were calculated based on the responses obtained per specific questions rather than necessarily on the overall study sample. Statistical tests were conducted using mainly Spearman's chi-square ($\chi 2$) tests for categorical data while a t-test technique was applied on the limited type of the continuous data related to age and income of the respondents. Statistical significance in the differences observed was considered when at a p-value ≤ 0.05.

Results

Designation Characteristics of the HWs Involved

In total, 35 and 43 HWs were involved in Mkuranga and Mufindi, respectively. Of the 78 HWs interviewed, 25 (32.1%) were medical attendants, 18 (23.1%) were clinical officers, 9 (11.5%) were public health nurses, 8 (10.3%) were nurse midwives, 8 (10.3%) were maternal MCH Aides, and the rest 7 (8.9%) included laboratory and assistant health officers. Of the 78 HWs, 50 (64.1%) were found at government HFs and the rest at private HFs. Furthermore, 16 (20.5%) and 11 (14.1%) of the respondents were found at health centre and hospital levels, respectively while 51 (65.4%) were found at dispensary levels. The mean number of years of working at the HF at which they were interviewed was 8.3 years and the range was 0.5 – 24 years.

Socio-Economic Related and Other Characteristics of the ANC Clients

►***ANC clients:*** Out of the 821 interviewed in both districts, 590 (71.9%) were found at government clinics, 143 (17.4%) at faith-based clinics, and 88 (10.7%) at commercial clinics.

Among the 417 respondents in Mkuranga, 344 (82.5%) were married, 44 (10.6%) were single and the rest include cohabiters, separated and widows. In Mufindi, 359 (88.4%) of the respondents were married, 34 (8.4%) were single and the rest include the cohabiters, separated and widows. In Mkuranga, age of the respondents ranged between 15 and 46 years while the mean age was 23.6 years. In Mufindi, age ranged between 15 and 47 years while the mean and median ages were 25 and 26 years, respectively. A student t-test indicated that the differences in the respondents mean age between the two districts was not statistically significant. Participation in farming as the main occupation was reported by 303 (72.84%) and 340 (84.2%) of the respondents in Mkuranga and Mufindi, respectively. In Mkuranga, engagement in retail business was reported by 52 (12.5%) of the respondents while this activity and casual labor in Mufindi employed 23 (5.7%) and 8 (1.99%) of the respondents, respectively. Only 57 (13.7%) and 8 (1.9%) of the respondents in Mkuranga and Mufindi, respectively were civil servants. The rest were either jobless or students/pupils or sick for a long time. More than 55% of the respondents per district were living in poor house conditions. Moreover, 264 (63.31%) and 253 (62.62%) of the respondents in Mkuranga and Mufindi, respectively had not earned cash money one month before this study. The mean income earned one month before this study in Mkuranga was 15,753.3 shillings (US$ 13.1) (ranging 0-45,000 shillings (US$0-37.5)) and the median income was 5,000 shillings (US$ 4.2; n=256). In Mufindi, the mean monthly income earned by 151 respondents one month before was 26,780.1 shillings (US$ 22.3) (ranging 0-300,000 shillings (US$0-250)) while the median income was 10,000 shillings (US$ 8.33; n=243). The mean monthly income in Mkuranga was significantly lower than of their counterparts in Mufindi ($t=-4.125$; $p<0.0001$). The overall mean family size of 807 respondents from both districts was 4. When the family size was categorized into large family size (> 4 people) and small family size (≤ 4 people), the median family size of the group of the respondents from large families was 6.6 (range: 5-23) and for those from average family sizes was 2.9 (range: 1-4).

Of the respondents in Mkuranga 238 (57.1%) had attained at least standard seven primary education while 179 (42.9%) never went to school. Of their counterparts in Mufindi, 356 (88.6%) had attained at least standard seven while 46 (11.4%) never went to school. Based on chi-square test, the literacy level was significantly higher in Mufindi than in Mkuranga ($p<0.001$).

Over 50% of the respondents had more than one deliveries and having attended ANC clinic several times while out of all the 417 respondents in Mkuranga, 329 (73.3%) had delivered at least once before while 88 (26.7%) were in their first pregnancies. In Mufindi, 327 (81.1%) out of 403 respondents had delivered at least once before their current pregnancies while 76 (18.9%) were in their first pregnancies.

Safety of IPTp with SP

►***Taking SP knowingly or Unknowingly:*** Among the ANC clients, awareness that pregnant women attending ANC clients were receiving anti-malarial drugs ranged from moderate in Mkuranga (about 59% of 416 respondents) to high in Mufindi (about 81% of 394 respondents). Considering the proportions of the responses indicating 'Yes' (they receive the anti-malarial drug) for IPTp versus 'No', the ANC clients found in Mufindi were significantly more informed about IPTp than their counterparts in Mkuranga ($\chi^2(1)=13.1$; $p<0.001$). Recognition that SP was the drug administered for IPTp also varied between the two districts, as in Mkuranga, 174 (67.9%) ANC clients and 176 (34.3%) of their counterparts in Mufindi, were able to identify SP as the drug recommended. Others, including 78 (30.5%) and 138 (42.6%), respectively were unaware that SP was the drug recommended while the rest of the respondents reported drugs other than SP. The alternative drugs mentioned including antipyretics such as panadol/paracetamol, and other antimalarial drugs such as amodiaquine and CQ. Several respondents among those who were unaware believed that SP was the name of a drug that was different from orodar and fansidar®.

Moreover, 123 (29.6%) out of 416 of the ANC clients met in Mkuranga stated to have been given SP for IPTp during the particular study days while 64 (15.4%) were unsure if they received drugs for IPTp. In Mufindi, 137 (34.8%) out of 394 ANC clients reported to have received SP while 78 (19.8%) were unsure. The rest of the respondents in each district denied to have received SP for IPTp. Statistically, it is seemed that acknowledgement for having received SP for IPTp was significantly higher in Mufindi than in Mkuranga ($p=0.001$).

Looking at the combined dataset for both districts, further analysis indicated that awareness about pregnant women attending ANC clinics receiving anti-malarial drug for IPTp was significantly higher among the ANC clients who had at least attained standard seven primary education than those who either never went to school at all (($\chi^2(1)=14.7$; $p<0.001$)). Also, 441 (78.6%) out of all the ANC clients approached in both districts were found at government clinics while only 120 (21.4%) were met at private clinics. Statistically, awareness that IPTp was administered, regardless of the type of the drug, was significantly higher among the government clinic ANC clients than those at private clinics ($\chi^2(1)=38.2$;

p<0.001)). Even by looking at each districts data separately, it was noted that the ANC clients found at government clinics were significantly more informed than those at private clinics (70.0% out of 247 respondents versus 42.0% out of 169 respondents, p<0.001), albeit for Mkuranga district only. In Mufindi, a similar trend in the responses was observed, although statistically the difference was not significant (data not shown).

Moreover, out of the 561 ANC clients who responded to the question related to their pregnancy experience, 97 (17.3%) and 464 (82.7%) were primigravidæ and multigravidæ, respectively. Among these, the multigravidæ women were significantly more awareness than the primigravidæ women ($\chi^2(1)=9.4$; p=0.002)).

As generally viewed by several HWs, unawareness that SP was the drug recommended for IPTp might be disadvantageous to pregnant women who might have end up either inappropriately using anti-malarial drugs through self-medication practices at community level or failing to comply with the instruction given by the HWs at clinic levels, wherefore, risking their pregnancies (data not shown).

►***Perceived and Real Treatment Outcomes of SP:*** In light of their experience with previous use of SP, perceptions were given about the benefits and risks of SP. Experience with adverse effects whether during pregnancy period or not was reported by 53 (24.3%) and 55 (20.9%) of the ANC clients who stated responded to the question on this issue in Mkuranga and Mufindi, respectively. However, the observed difference between the two districts was not statistically significant. Probed further about what they would do if they were allowed to choose the drug for use against malaria during pregnancy, 47 (13.7%) and 14 (4.8%) of the ANC clients who responded in Mkuranga and Mufindi, respectively were still in favor of SP. Some of the reasons given include the convenience of taking a full dose once, having minor side effects that were tolerable and common for most drugs, un-bitter taste unlike experience for CQ and other drugs, and because it was the drug recommended by the government for saving the lives of the mothers and their fetuses. The rest of the respondents would opt for drugs other than SP. This was due to reasons related to the perceived serious adverse treatment effects and lack of antipyretic effect of SP. The observed difference was statistically significant (p=0.001), indicating a higher support to SP in Mufindi than in Mkuranga.

Experience with ANC clients who feared to take SP during the current year (study period) was reported by 8 (22.9%) and 10 (23.3%) of the HWs in Mkuranga and Mufindi, respectively. These clients expressed feeling adverse treatment effects after taking SP. No statistically significant differences were noted between the two districts regarding these experiences. Several HWs added that if SP was delivered in several quantities and not only once for full dose completion, compliance would be lower as was the case with CQ.

Regarding the question about whether or not the need for receiving SP at the clinic for IPTp was one of the influencing factors for pregnant women's attendances, it was noted that 56% and 70% of the ANC clients in Mkuranga and Mufindi, respectively wanted to know the foetal progress and being examined about their general health conditions. Only <5% of the the ANC clients in each district revealed their interest in receiving IPTp doses. Moreover, 78 and 6 of the reporters among the ANC clients approached in Mufindi and Mkuranga, respectively reported the frontline HWs' failure to advise them about the utilization and timing of the IPTp doses and how to recognize danger signs during pregnancy. Concerning health education, 68 (93.2%) of the same type of respondents in Mufindi were reported not having been advised on malaria prevention on the study days, and this seemed one of the disappointments to the potential ANC clients to utilize IPTp services.

►***Compliance with DOT for IPTp:*** The factors contributing to the low adherence to DOT for IPTp, as reported by the frontline HWs in both districts

Most of the HWs in both districts were aware of the policy warning that SP and ferrous/folic acid tablets should not be administered concurrently (MOH 2004). Nonetheless, 5.2% out of 63 HWs who gave their experience admitted having been administering the two types of drugs concurrently, and lack of information about the policy warning was reported as a cause. In Mufindi, DOT was avoided after the frontline HWs have noted that some of the clients arrived at the clinic while they were alcoholic after taking local brews commonly locally known as *Ulanzi* and *Komoni*.

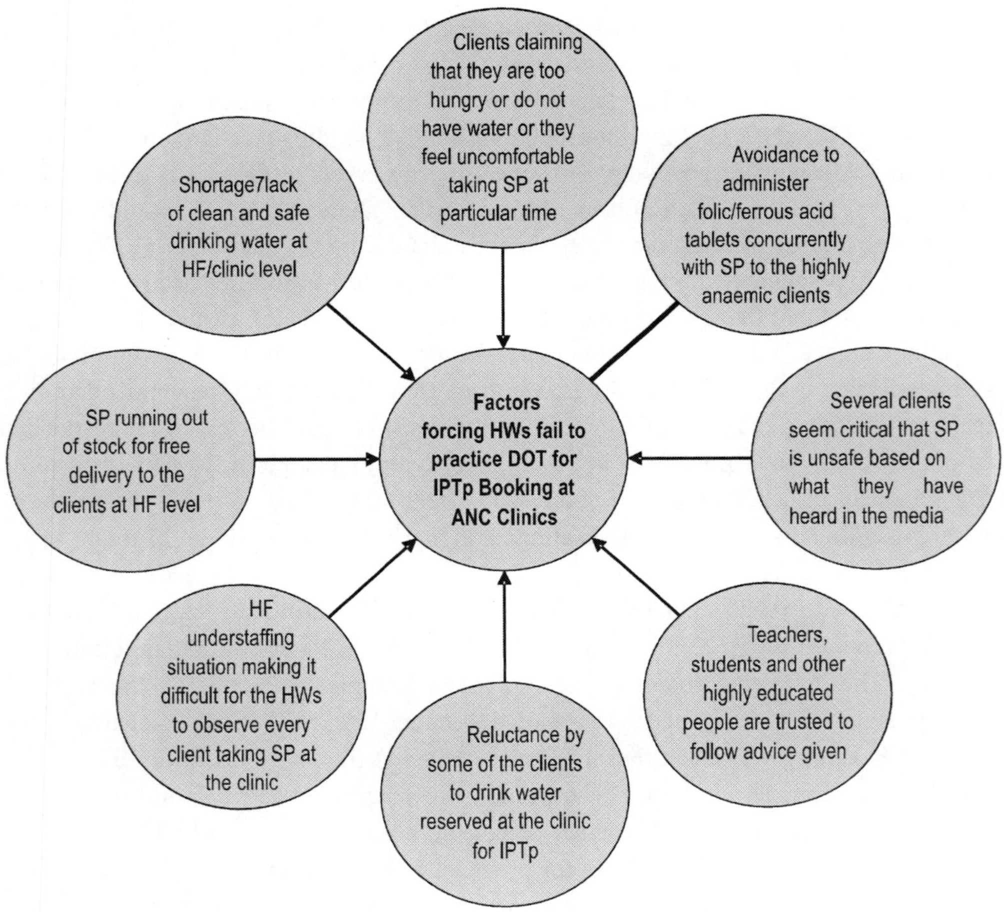

Figure 1. Key factors contributing to low compliance with DOT for IPTp by the frontline HWs and ANC clients, as reported by the frontline HWs in Mkuranga and Mufindi districts, Tanzania.

HF running out of water supply for IPTp under DOT was reported by 44% of all the HWs in Mkuranga and only 12.2% of their counterparts in Mufindi, the difference seeming statistically significant (p=0.002). Experience with ANC clients buying water for taking IPTp at the HFs was reported by >50% of the HWs in Mkuranga and only by about 19% in Mufindi, again the difference being statistically significant (p=0.001). Experience with ANC clients who were allowed to take SP at home for IPTp was shown by 33.3% and 37.5% of the HWs in these districts, respectively, the difference was not statistically significant. All these factors as summarized in figure 1 seemed to contribute to improper drug use, perceived low efficacy and safety of the drug in various social contexts.

The ANC clients who reported to have received IPTp on the particular study days were asked to show the types of the drug tablets they had received. This was aimed to confirm if DOT was effectively practiced and the possible risk/disadvantage of allowing the clients take SP for IPTp at home. A significantly higher proportion of the respondents in Mufindi than in Mkuranga (about 45% versus about 30%) believed to have received drugs for IPTp ($\chi^2(2)=34.3$; $p<0.001$), although they did not specify the type of the drug they had received.

Specifically, 123 ANC clients in Mkuranga and 179 of their counterparts in Mufindi acknowledged reception of SP at the clinic on the particular study days. Out of these respondents, 54 (43.9%) and 20 (11.2%) respectively showed the real tablets of SP to the interviewers. Others, including 8 (6.5%) and 4 (2.2%) in Mkuranga and Mufindi, respectively showed tablets other than SP, although they believed it was SP. Testimony that DOT has been practiced on the particular study days was shown by 59 (47.9%) and 152 (84.9%) clients confronted in the latter districts, respectively. Statistically, a significantly higher proportion of the respondents were allowed to take SP at home in Mkuranga district than in Mufindi ($\chi^2(2) = 49.5$; $p<0.001$). The drugs other than SP tablets that were shown include mebendazole, ferrous and vitamin tablets. These are among the services which are recommended for pregnant women attending ANC clinic (MOH 2004).

Costs of Accessing IPTp Services

In their view, 22 (62.9%) and 24 (55.8%) of the HWs in the Mkuranga and Mufindi, respectively expressed reservations about government policy of provision of essential ANC services free of charge (Mubyazi et al., 2006b; MOH 1993). As expressed by 9 (25.7%) and 8 (18.6%) of the interviewees in Mkuranga and Mufindi respectively, it was difficult to provide free service under shortage of essential supplies.

Less than 50% of the total HWs interviewed in both districts, particularly 17 (48.6%) and 21 (48.8%) in Mkuranga and Mufindi districts, respectively were aware that the government recommends delivery of the essential ANC services free of charge at all types of HFs.

It was generally noted that IPTp services are not absolutely delivered for free as the suggested in the national MCH policy implementation guidelines. The following sections reveal:

Official User Fees

Testimony was given by the HWs that officially user fees exist, especially at private HFs and these have an influence on ANC attendances by those who feel, or really, unable to pay.

Payment of user-fees on the study day was reported by a significantly higher proportion of the ANC clients in Mkuranga than in Mufindi (i.e. 36.7% versus 7.0%; $\chi^2(1)=103.89$; $p<0.001$)). User-fees on blood and urine screening was reported to have been paid by 112 (27.3%) out of 411 ANC clinic respondents from both districts.

Experiences with payment difficulties of user fees was more reported by the ANC clients from Mkuranga than from Mufindi, and the observed differences were statistically significant (Table 1 and Table 2). User-fee payment difficulties at the clinics other than those at which the clients concerned were found under this study was faced by a significantly higher proportion of the respondents in Mkuranga than those in Mufindi (Table 1). Nineteen (5.6%) of 338 clients found in Mufindi reported having not contacted clinics owned by the Mufindi Tea Company due to the existence of user fees for people who were neither employed by the Company nor relatives of the Company's employees.

Table 1. Reasons given by the ANC clients about reasons for their decision to avoid contacting ANC clinics other than the ones at which they were interviewed (*chi-square test for comparing the responses from the two districts, interest being on travel distance and user fees components*).

Type of clinic not contacted and why	Mkuranga (N=417)	Mufindi (N=406)	P-value
• *Why not contacted a government clinic*	(n=145)	(n=39)	-
Reasons related to long travel distance	103 (71.03%)	22 (56.41%)	
Reasons related to direct and official cost of ANC	0 (0%)	0 (0%)	
Reasons other than distance and official user fees	42 (28.97%)	17 (43.59%)	
• *Why not contacted a private-for-profit clinic*	(n=331)	(n=398)	<0.019
Reasons related to long travel distance	181 (54.68%)	138 (34.67%)	
Reasons related to direct and official cost of ANC	97 (29.31%)	60 (15.08%)	
Reasons other than distance and official user fees	53 (16.01%)	200 (50.25%)	
• *Why not contacted a Faith-based /Mission clinic*	(n=276)	(n=352)	<0.001
Reasons related to long travel distance	160 (57.97%)	145 (41.19%)	
Reasons related to direct and official cost of ANC	44 (15.94%)	43 (12.22%)	
Reasons other than distance and official user fees	72 (26.09%)	164 (46.59%)	
• *Why not contacted clinics owned by any other agencies*	(n=5)	(n=338)	-
Reasons related to long travel distance	0 (0%)	162 (47.93%)	
Reasons related to direct and official cost of ANC	0 (0%)	19 (5.62%)	
Reasons other than distance and official user fees	5 (100%)	157 (46.45%)	

(-) sign indicates that the chi-square test was not conducted for that case due to presence of 0 result.

The point indicated as '*reasons other than user fees and travel distance*' that influenced some respondents not contact clinics other than the ones at which they were interviewed were mainly related to the perceived quality of care, having faced no complication or serious condition that would prompt one to visit a particular HF, and lack of awareness.

►***Fees on Drugs:*** None of the ANC clients in both districts reported existence of user fees at government HFs as a dissuading factor for their decision to avoid visiting government clinics (Table 1). However, this did not mean that government HFs were not implementing user fees, rather the fees were affordable to the latter types of the respondents. For instance, existence of user fees at private HFs for ANC services was reported by several ANC clients, and confirmed by the private HWs who reported experience with occasional stock outs of ANC SP for free delivery, wherefore, being forced to advise their clients to buy SP elsewhere or at the same HF like other types of the patients. From the latter two categories of the respondents, that is HWs and ANC clients who reported payments for drugs, 1 dose of 3 tablets of SP was charged between 300 and 500 shillings (US$0.25-0.41).

Table 2. Experience with user-fee payment for ANC at several non-government HFs in Mkuranga and Mufindi districts (*chi-square tests for Yes and No responses*).

Questions Asked and Responses	Mkuranga	Mufindi	P-values
	N (%)	N (%)	
• *Have you paid for ANC at this clinic today?* (1 = Yes)	151 (36.74%)	28 (7.04%)	<0.001
• (If paid) *Do the user-fees as you have paid today have any influence on your attendance to ANC clinic in the future?* (1=Yes)	32 (20.0%)	5 (9.43%)	0.078
• *Have you ever faced user-fee payment difficulty (including either total inability to pay or paying, but with a feeling of too high cost) at this clinic?* (1= Yes)	28 (56.0%)	5 (23.8%)	0.013
• *Have you ever faced difficulty paying for ANC at other clinics?* (1=Yes)*	54 (12.98%)	16 (4.0%)	<0.001

*Indicates that the last question was posed even if the respondent said 'No' in the preceding one(s).

►***Fees on non-drug services:*** Screening for HIV was reported by a number of the ANC clients to cost 1200 shillings (about US$1) at Irene-Kilimahewa mission dispensary. At this dispensary, screening for venereal diseases (VDRL) including syphilis was charged 500 shillings (US$0.41), and this service was reported by the HWs as essential especially for the pregnant women visiting the clinic for the first time in their current pregnancies. Pregnancy Test (PT) was another type of the service occasionally delivered under payment at the private HFs. This service, however, was for those who personally volunteered to confirm either whether they were pregnant or the gestational age of their pregnancies, otherwise it was not necessary. According to the frontline HWs at several HFs, it was unfortunate that not all the clients understood this, as some took it for granted that this service was one of the essential services to be delivered for free according to government exemption policy for MCH services. PT was charged 2000 shillings (about US$1.7) at the Arafa-Kiparang'anda private-for-profit dispensary. At this dispensary, a dose of ferrous/folic acid tablets was charged at 100 shillings, also this being essential for all the pregnant women attending whether private or public clinics as per national focused ANC guidelines (MOH 2004). Although these prices seemed low from the HWs' viewpoint, episodes about the women who failed to pay and end asked for waiver/payment exemptions were reported by the HWs at Irene-Kilimahewa and Mwalusembe faith-based dispensaries, as well as Arafa-Kiparang'anda dispensary.

Paying for exercise books that were sometimes used at the clinic instead of ANC cards was also reported by the ANC clients, and confirmed by the HWs who reported experience with occasional stock outs of ANC cards for free delivery. As reported by a number of the clients and confirmed by the HWs, the price per exercise book ranged between shillings 200 and 300 (US$ 0.2 – 0.25). The mean monetary expenditure on food was shillings 146.7 (US$0.1), ranging between 20 shillings and 600 shillings ((US$0.02-0.5) in both districts. This amount was considered generally affordable and acceptable for those who actually paid.

In the shortage of ANC cards, particularly at private HFs, as reported by HWs at Usokami Mission Dispensary in Mufindi and Arafa-Kiparang'anda private-for-profit Dispensary in Mkuranga, the HF management concerned was sometimes forced to produce photocopies in the town. As viewed by 29.4% and 11.6% of the HWs in Mkuranga and Mufindi, respectively, the cost of these was unavoidably recovered from charging the ANC clients.

Furthermore, 6 (17.1%) and 4 (9.3%) of the HWs in Mkuranga and Mufindi, respectively were unhappy with the widespread confusion in the community about the services that should be accessed freely. This contributes to failure by some women to attend MCH clinics especially at private HF for basic services. Even at the government HFs pregnant women sometimes are charged for being treated like other kinds of patients after they had been diagnosed of malaria or other illness conditions, as it happens when the clients with complications are required to share the cost for emergency services such as paying for fuel used by the HF ambulance or hiring a car at their own cost. This has lowered some patients' trust in the HWs who are believed to charge the clients illegally (unofficially).

Unofficial Charges

Experience with unofficial payments to HWs was reported by only 4 (0.9%) out of 415 ANC respondents in Mkuranga and only 7 (1.7%) out of 403 respondents in Mufindi. In this regard, payment of 500-1000 (US$ 0.41-0.83) was associated with the respondents' need for immediate attention or special services such as access to drugs instead of being directed to buy drugs elsewhere. Moreover, 2 and 4 respondents in Mkuranga and Mufindi respectively stated to have decided on their own to provide an incentive to HWs in appreciation of HWs' provision of good services under stressed circumstances.

Transport Costs

►***Cost related to the distance traveled:*** As illustrated in Table 1 above, cost related to traveling to and from ANC clinics was an issue from the perspective of the ANC clients. The frontline HWs were concerned about travel distance, time and financial cost when participating in MCH services delivered at mobile/outreach clinic stations, as described later.

Regardless of the organization owning the HFs at which the ANC clients were interviewed, 292 (70.2%) and 270 (67.3%) of the respondents in Mkuranga and Mufindi, respectively reported to have been influenced by the short travel distance in their decision to contact the respective study clinics on the particular study days. Having postponed or delayed attending clinic during their current pregnancies due to inconvenience related to transport (including avoidance of the long travel distance and lack of money for transport) was reported a few ANC clients, particularly 32 (2.3%) and 9 (2.3%) in the latter districts, respectively.

For the clients who had walked from home to the clinics on the particular study days, 265 (64.5%) out of 411 ANC respondents in Mkuranga and 315 (79.3%) out of 397 in Mufindi did not incur financial cost on paying for bus fare, but reported time lost on travel as the main inconvenience. The amount paid for transport depended mainly on the means of transport used. Ninety (60.8%) out of 148 ANC clinic respondents in Mkuranga and 32 (38.6%) out of 99 of their counterparts in Mufindi reported to have paid for public cars (*a local minibus popular as 'daladala' or a lorry*). The mean fare paid for the car was 129 shillings (about US$ 0.1) in Mkuranga and shillings 936 (US$ 0.8) in Mufindi. The cost of a one-way travel by car ranged 200 – 2000 shillings (US$0.2 -1.7) in both districts. This amount was unaffordable to some women, it was reported. The mean payment for hiring a bicycle was 233.3 shillings (US$0.2), ranging between 300 and 2000 shillings (US$ 0.3-1.7). Therefore, those who avoided paying more for a bicycle were prompted to leave the clinic before receiving all the desired services. Episodes of delaying to attend ANC clinic until one had obtained money for direct transport cost were reported by 25 (6.0%) of 415 ANC clinic respondents in Mkuranga and 9 (2.3%) of 397 respondents in Mufindi.

► ***Financial expenditures other than bus/bicycle fares:*** These were categorized as direct costs and indirect costs. Direct costs involved the money spent on the way for buying soft drinks or foods, as testified by 44 (5.4%) of 812 ANC clinic respondents in both districts. Buying these materials was common among the clients who were accompanied by young children, including pregnant women who were either lactating or closely taking care young children. Indirect costs were explained in terms of the productive time lost while travelling to and from the clinic, and this was perceived to discourage some potential clients to attend ANC clinic for IPTp and other essential services.

In Mkuranga, 29 (82.9%) of the HWs reported to have occasionally been incurring expenses by paying out of their pockets for transport (bicycle hire or car fare) towards mobile clinic stations. Also, 21 (60.0%) HWs reported to have been buying food and drink at late hours, respectively. Concern about arriving at the clinic at late hours when he clients are already tired of waiting longer to receive health education related to safe motherhood including the prevention of malaria in pregnancy, was reported. Moreover, working beyond the ordinary official working hours without receiving financial compensated was reported to demoralize the frontline HWs and contributing to sub-standard implementation of the IPTp guidelines.

Cost Related to Time Lost while Waiting for ANC Services

►***Opportunity cost of the time lost*:** Views were obtained from the ANC clients who responded to the question concerning time lost while waiting for services at the clinic on the particular study days, excluding the time spent with the interviewer. Of the ANC clients interviewed in Mkuranga and Mufindi, 136 (32.6%) and 158 (39.2%), respectively were comfortable with the time they had spent at the clinic. In contrast, 202 (48.4%) and 170 (42.2%) of the ANC clients in these districts, respectively reported to have lost a longer time than expected, the observed difference was statistically significant (p=0.039). The rest of the respondents in these districts were somewhat indifferent about the length of the time lost. A common view among the respondents who complained about the time lost was that this was a dissuading factor to the potential clients to attend clinic for basic services.

Forty-two (10.4%) and 8 (1.6%) out of 405 and 384 ANC clients interviewed in Mkuranga and Mufindi respectively viewed that they would not be ready to revisit the same clinic or unless they decide to arrive earlier so that they could be among the first clients to be attended and leave home earlier. This was especially reported in account of those who were spending a considerable time on the way to and from the clinic. It was argued that working up earlier at home to begin traveling to the clinic could interrupt with the domestic duties usually attended by the women concerned, as some women have a responsibility of preparing food first for their families, prepare and even escort young children to school.

In both districts, long waiting time at the clinics was mainly faced on Mondays, Wednesdays and Fridays when the number of patients is often high at the under-staffed HFs where the HWs faced a heavy workload by having to serve many patients.

►***Financial expenditures:*** Buying foods or drinks while waiting for service for a long time at the clinic was pinpointed by the ANC clients in the same way as explained above about a similar practice on traveling. It was lamented that like the very young children, pregnant women normally need to eat something more frequently than normal, so waiting for service longer forces those with cash to buy some foods or drinks.

Discussion

Perceived Versus Real Safety of SP for IPTp Against Malaria

According to WHO, the programmatic effectiveness of an anti-parasitic drug is determined by not only the efficacy of the drug in question against the parasite, but also the drug's characteristics, including its affordability and acceptability to the target population within the existing ANC delivery systems, among other things (WHO 2001). Clients may perceive a drug anyhow depending on the information they may have about it rather than their real experience with the use of such a drug. Any drug is subject to stimulate public concerns/debate about its safety, whether it is recommended as a new treatment regimen or has been under use for many years. It is imperative for the target users and the frontline HWs to be properly informed of the real treatment benefits and possible albeit rare risks of the recommended drug. Sadly, this study found a considerable proportion of the ANC clients who were unaware that SP was recommended for IPTp and those unaware that pregnant women attending clinics were receiving IPTp doses. Although one study in Tanzania recently noted no statistically significant association between clients' knowledge about- and their utilization of IPTp (Nganda et al., 2004), the report about the HWs who for some reasons including the work-pressure failing inform their clients adequately about the drug administered to them testifies that some of the clients may use it as a loophole for avoiding SP. This is very likely considering the widespread and often amplified general public fear about possible adverse drug treatment outcomes, as noted of the reservations expressed about SP treatment outcomes prompting several clients in this study to show their preferences to drugs other than SP. Owing to an amplified public perception on SP adverse treatment effects in Tanzania (Hetzel et al., 2007; Nsimba 2006; Mubyazi et al., 2005a; Mubyazi and Gonzalez-Block 2005), as in other countries e.g. Uganda (Mbonye et al., 2006ab), Kenya and Malawi (Hill and Kazembe 2006), there is also possibility that even those who denied to prefer to drugs other than SP did so in a way of pleasing the interviewers who might have been considered part of the healthcare system whose interest were to hear positively from their respondents about their perception of SP.

Moreover, it is likely that pregnant women walking a number of kilometers to and from seeking ANC may either arrive at the clinic or at home when they are already too tired to consume SP comfortably. The consequence of taking the drug when one is too tired and hungry means a lot in terms of the treatment outcome of the drug such as SP that may be unnecessarily perceived negatively by its users.

Perceived Efficacy of SP versus Other Anti-Malarial Drugs

Apparently, the present study populations, including both the frontline HWs and ANC clients did not explicitly question on the ability of SP to clear the malaria parasites as compared to other anti-malarial drugs. This implies that they might have been confident that SP was an effective drug, despite the perceived/reported adverse treatment effects. However, a small proportion of the clients who reported to prefer drugs other than SP if they were allowed may include those who have low trust in both its efficacy and safety.

Consequences of DOT Failure

Allowing the ANC clients eligible for IPTp to take SP at home instead of being directly observed by the qualified HWs is likely to remain in the context where the HFs are not equipped with adequate supplies including SP, safe drinking water, and skilled and motivated frontline HWs. The resent study reveals that the existing environment for such supplies dos not allow everywhere and always in both study districts. This mirrors the possibility that some of the clients could avoid taking SP if they were not directly observed at the clinics or as reported by the HWs, some of the clients may end up incorrectly taking the drug and eventually complain about its efficacy and safety. Outcome quality of care, including the perceived benefit and risks of SP for IPTp is an important component in the analysis of demand for ANC services (Ribera et al., 2007).

Cost of Accessing IPTp Services

► ***User fees:*** Previous studies reported the practice of user fees for ANC services, other than IPTp, in Tanzania (Mubyazi et al., 2006; Boller et al., 2003; Quijada and Comfort 2002). This study verifies this for the general ANC services, and occasionally for IPTp when SP is paid for. The HWs reported about the general public over-generalizing that the government policy recommends free ANC without exclusion of particular services, and the chances such a perception contributes disappointing some of the clients who are occasionally charged. In social contexts where the private sector may be dominant over the public sector, it is obvious that charging a considerable proportion of the clients is common, and therefore, the consequences of this to IPTp delivery and coverage remains an empirical research question (Mubyazi et al., 2008; Mubyazi et al., 2005a). As reported about costs associated with living far away from ANC clinics, official user-fees remain a challenge to IPTp scaling up in Tanzania, unless there is a way of exempting the poorest ones as has traditionally been done by the compassionate HWs or HF management of the faith-based HFs (Mubyazi et al., 2006a; Mamdani and Bangser 2004).

It was noted that most of the study participants in both districts were living in poor conditions, almost around the poverty line of US$1 per day. Therefore, the reported user fees for some essential services e.g. screening for HIV, syphilis and other services, might be a constraint. That is, possibility of failure to attend clinics for ANC services including IPTp by the pregnant women who are constrained by poverty to affording the screening for HIV and other services that cost more than their daily income cannot be ruled out (Baiden et al., 2005).

It is argued that high direct payment and fear of unofficial costs are acute barriers to the use of maternal services (Kowalewski et al., 2002). As noted from the present study, unofficial charges for ANC services are uncommon in the two districts since they were experienced by < 2% of all the ANC clients interviewed. However, possible fear by the respondents to disclose the real fact if they considered that the researchers were government officials investigating among other things the illegal medical practice by the service providers among whom some are closely related or friends. Moreover, several respondents might not have been sure of which types of the services were supposed to be delivered for free in line with the government exemption policy.

► ***Travel Cost:*** The present study adds evidence on the value people place on travel distance and the consequent financial and opportunity cost influencing their decision to contact HFs for healthcare (Mrisho et al., 2007; Mamdani and Bangser 2004; Dor et al., 1987). One study in Ghana found that one-third of the women were disappointed by traveling more than 5km to reach a modern ANC clinic (Overbosch et al., 2004). Also in Kenya (van Eijk et al., 2006) and Nepal (Wagle et al., 2003), a walking distance of >1 hour significantly discouraged some pregnant women to attend ANC clinic, as was reported from Nigeria (Adam and Salihu 2002; Okonofua et al., 2002). Thus, despite the good intentions for recommending IPTp, the experiences and views expressed by the ANC clients gives an impression that this service remains inaccessible free of cost to pregnant women residing far away from the service delivery points, meanwhile facing difficulties in raising cash for their basic needs including healthcare services.

►***Waiting time:*** However efficacious and safe SP and any other drug recommended might be in various socio-economic contexts, the question remains about its deliverability. It is evident from this study that understaffing lowers the timing of the ANC services desired by the target clients. Interestingly, the policy authorities in Tanzania understand this challenge, albeit the solution remains unforeseen as the healthcare system is under-funded (Mubyazi et al., 2008). The present study also support anticipation by some of the authors of this paper (Mubyazi et al., 2005b) and other authors (Ribera et al., 2007) that free services could be possible if the target clients were not experiencing costs related to waiting time and financial expenditures on food or drinks while waiting for services or while traveling to and from ANC clinics.

Conclusion

When institutionalizing policies, national and international authorities often mention more than suggesting solutions related to the operational barriers against the recommended malaria- and healthcare interventions in local settings. Adding evidence that social perceptions on- and the real deficiencies of anti-malarial drug efficacy, safety and costs are a challenge for rolling back malaria in Tanzania, as elsewhere in Africa, this study suggests that possibilities be looked at such as instituting a cross the board subsidies for ANC services in favor, coupled by increased investments in HF supply conditions including supply of essential materials and staff recruitment and motivation of the HWs implementing the services.

Authors Contributions

The study was conceived by GMM for his PhD, who participated in every stage of the study from data collection through final report writing, conceiving the idea of and actually drafting this manuscript. The rest provided advice on the design of the research protocol, administrative support and commented on the research report and this manuscript. Dr. LEG Mboera tirelessly followed up the logistic issues, offered equipment for use in data collection, and advised on statistical consultation at NIMR. Prof. ICB and Dr. PB led the supervision/mentoring process for GMM's PhD study at the University of Copenhagen, Denmark, in collaboration with Drs. PM, JB, KSH and ØEO.

Acknowledgement

This study was funded by the Bill and Melinda Gates Foundation through the Gates Malaria Partnership (GMP) under coordination by the London School of Hygiene and Tropical Medicine, UK in collaboration with the DBL – Center for Health Research and Development, Denmark and National Institute for Medical Research (NIMR), Tanzania. Data collection was assisted by Fagason J. Mduma, Nyangoma-J Mubyazi, Elly Mashauri, Raymond J. Ole-Mungaya, Ruth Kamugwawa, Dorcas Mujwauzi-Mubyazi, Theresa E. Manumbu, Anna Rwegoshora, and Libent Bankobeza. Abdulatif Rashid and George Kambanga drove the project car safely throughout the study period. The study received support from regional and district health authorities and study populations. Data analysis was assisted by Bruno Mmbando and database preparation by Kesheni Senkoro, both working at NIMR, Tanzania. NIMR Director General (Dr Andrew Y. Kitua) on behalf of the Ministry of Health and Social Welfare of Tanzania approved a PhD study leave for GMM.

Conflict of Interest. The authors declare no conflict of interest related to this study.

References

Adam, Y. M. & Salihu, H. M. (2002). Barriers to antenatal and obstetric care services in rural Kano. *Journal of Obstetric Gynaecology*, 2002, *6(22)*, 600-603.

Anders, K., Marchant, T., Chambo, P., Mapunda, P. & Reyburn, H. (2008). Timing of intermittent preventive treatment during pregnancy and the implications for current policy on early uptake in north-eastern Tanzania. *Malaria Journal*, *7*, 79.

Baiden, F., Baiden, R., Williams, J., Akweongo, P., Clerk, C., Philips, D. J. & Hodgson, A. (2005). Review of antenatal-linked voluntary counselling and HIV testing in sub-Saharan Africa: Lessons and Options for Ghana. *Ghana Medical Journal*, *39(1)*, 8-13.

Boller, C., Wyss, K., Mtasiwa, D. & Tanner, M. (2003). Quality and comparison of antenatal care in private and public providers in Dar Es Salaam, United Republic of Tanzania. *Bull WHO*, *81(2)*, 116-1220.

Borghi, J., Ensor, T., Somanathan, A., Lissner, C. & Mills, A. (2006). Mobilizing financial resources for maternal health. *Lancet*, *368*, 1457-1465.

Brabin, B. J. (1983). An analysis of malaria in pregnancy in Africa. *Bulletin of WHO*, *61*, 1005-1016.

CIOMS (2002). International Ethical Guidelines for Biomedical Research Involving Human Subjects. *Council for International Organisations of Medical Sciences* (CIOMS), *ISBN 92 9036 0755*.

Dor, A., Gertler, P. & Der Gaag, J. (1987). Non-price rationing and the choice of medical care providers in rural Cote d'Ivoire. *Journal of Health Economics*, *6(4)*, 291-304

Drummond, M., Sculpher, M. J., Torrance, M. J., O'Brien, B. J. & Stoddart, G. L. (2005). Methods for economic evaluation of health care programmes. *Oxford University Press*.

East African Network on Malaria Treatment (EANMAT) (2001). Monitoring antimalarial drug resistance within national malaria control programmes: the EANMAT experience. *Trop. Med. Int. health, 6(10)*, 1-8.

Ensor, T. & Cooper, S. (2004). Overcoming barriers to health service access: influencing the demand side. *Health Policy and Planning, 19(2)*, 69-79.

Eriksen, J., Tomson, G., Mujinja, P. & Warsame, M. Y. (2007). Assessing health worker performance in malaria case management in a rural Tanzanian district. *Trop. Med. Int. Health, 12(1)*, 52-61.

Filler, S., Kazembe, P., Thigpen, M., Macheso, A., Parise, M. E., Newman, R. D., Steketee, R. W. & Hamel, M. (2006). Randomized Trial of 2-Dose versus Monthly Sulfadoxine-Pyrimethamine Intermittent Preventive Treatment for Malaria in HIV-Positive and HIV-Negative Pregnant Women in Malawi. *Journal of Infectious Diseases, 194(3)*, 286-93.

Fitzpatrick, R. & Boulton, M. (1994). Qualitative methods for assessing health care. *Quality in Health Care, 3*, 107-113.

Frederickx, I. (1998). Health in rural Tanzania: the determinants of health status, health care demand and health care choice: Discussion Paper Series DPS 98.03. *Katholieke Universiteit Leuven*, Centre for Economic Studies.

Gates Malaria Partnership (GMP), DBL - Institute for Health Research and Development (2005). Evaluation of the Intermittent Preventive Treatment component of the Accelerated Child Survival and Development Project in The Gambia. *Final report.*

Goodman, C., Abdulla, S., Coleman, P., Mubyazi, G., Kikumbih, N., Okorosobo, T. & Mills, A. (2006). Choosing the first-line drug for malaria treatment-how can cost-effectiveness analysis inform policy? *The Economics of Infections*. Edited by Jennifer A. Roberts. Oxford University Press, UK.

Goodman, C., Coleman, P., Hanson, K., Meek, S. & Mills, A. (2003). Economics of Malaria Control in sub-Saharan Africa. *Global Forum for Health Research*, WHO, Geneva.

Greenwood, B. (2004). The use of antimalarial drugs to prevent malaria in the populations of malaria endemic countries. *Am. J. Trop. Med. Hyg., 70(1)*, 1-7.

Greenwood, B. (2006). Review: Intermittent preventive treatment- a new approach to prevent malaria in children in areas with seasonal malaria transmission. *Trop Med Int. Health, 11(10)*, 983-991.

Greenwood, B., Alonso, P., ter Kuile, F., Hill, J. & Steketee, R. (2007). Malaria in Pregnancy: priorities for Research. *Lancet Infect Dis., 7(2)*, 169-74.

Hamel, J., Dufour, S. & Fortin, D. (1993). *Case study methods*. Newbury Park, CA: Sage Publications.

Hanson, K., Hanson, K., Goodman, C., Lines, J., Meek, S., Bradley, D. & Mills, A. (2004). *The economics of malaria control interventions*. Global Forum for Health Research, WHO, Geneva.

Hardon, A., Boonmongkon, P., Streefland, P., Tan, M., Hongvicatana, L., van de Geest, S., van Staa, A., Varkevisser, C., Acuin, C., Chowdhury, M., Bhuiya, A., Sringeryuang, L., van Dongen, E. & Gerrits, T. (2001). Applied Health Research: Anthropology of health and health care. A manual. Revised Edition. *Het Spinhuis*, Netherlands.

Hetzel, M. W., Iteba, N., Makemba, A., Mshana, C., Lengeler, C., Obrist, B., Schulze, A., Nathan, R., et al., (2007). Understanding and improving access to prompt and effective malaria treatment and care in rural Tanzania: the ACCESS Programme. *Malaria Journal, 6*, 83.

Hill, J. & Kazembe, P. (2006). Reaching Abuja Targets for intermittent preventive treatment of malaria in pregnancy in African women: a review of progress and operational challenges. *Tropical Medicine and International Health, 11(4)*, 409-418.

Holtz, T. H., Kachur, S. P., Roberts, J. M., Marum, L. H., Mkandala, C. & Macheso, A. (2004). Use of antenatal services and IPT for malaria among pregnant women in Blantyre, Malawi District. *Trop. Med. Int. Health, 9(1)*, 77-82.

http://www.bioline.org.br/request?th07036: Select clips for media coverage around the partners' forum on maternal, newborn and child health. Dar Es Salaam, Tanzania, 17-20 April, 2007.

Kirkwood, B. R. & Sterne, A. C. (2003). Essentials of medical statistics. 2nd Edition. *Blackwell Sci.*, UK.

Kone-Pefoyo and Rivard, M. (2006). Poverty and socio-cultural factors in the use of maternal health services. *Rev Epidemiol Sante Publique, 54(6)*, 485-95.

Kowaleski, M., Mujinja, P. & Jahn, A. (2002). Can mothers afford maternal health care costs? User costs of maternity services in rural Tanzania. *African Journal of Reproductive Health, 6(1)*, 65-73.

Langer, A., Villar, J., Romero, M., Nigenda, G., Piaggio, G., Kuchaisit, C., Rojas, G., Al-Osimi, M., Miguel, B. J., Al-Mazrou, Y., et al., (2002). Are women providers satisfied with antenatal care? Views on a standard and simplified, evidence-based model of care in four developing countries. *BMC Women's Health, 2*, 7.

Lilford, R. & Harrison, S. (1994). Health services research: what it is, how to do it, and why it matters? *Health Services Management Research, 7(4)*, 214-219.

Malaria Consortium: Tanzania Roll Back Malaria Consultative Mission Report. *Malaria Consortium*, London, UK, 17th February 2004.

Mamdani, M. & Bangser, M. (2004). People's experiences of health services in Tanzania: a literature review. *Women's Dignity Project*, Tanzania. www.womensdignity.org/peoples_experience.pdf

Mapping Malaria Risk in Africa (MARA) (2000). Tanzania Malaria Transmission Risk. *Ministry of Health in collaboration with Tanzania Health Interventions Project* (TEHIP) *and MARA*. http:www.malvacdecision.net/overview%20%Malaria%Control%20DMF (accessed on 18th July 2007).

Mbonye, A. K. (2006b). A new approach to deliver malaria prevention interventions to pregnant women at community level in Uganda. *PhD Thesis, University of Copenhagen*, Denmark.

Mbonye, A. K., Magnussen, P. & Bygbjerg, I. C. (2007), Intermittent preventive treatment of malaria in pregnancy: the effect of new delivery approaches on access and compliance rates in Uganda. *Tropical Medicine & International Health, 12, 4*, 519-531.

Mbonye, A. K., Neema, S. & Magnussen, P. (2006a). Perceptions on use of sulfadoxine-pyrimathamine in pregnancy and the policy implications for malaria control in Uganda. *Health Policy, 77(3)*, 279-89.

Menendez, C. (1995). Malaria during pregnancy: a priority area of malaria research and control. *Parasitology Today, 11(5)*, 178-83.

Ministry of Health - Tanzania (1993). Proposals for Health Sector Reform. *Ministry of Health (MoH), Dar Es Salaam.*

Ministry of Health - Tanzania (2004). Focused antenatal care malaria and syphilis in pregnancy: orientation package for service providers. *Dar Es Salaam, Ministry of Health- Reproductive and Child Health Unit & NMCP.*

Mrisho, M., Schellenberg, J., Mushi, A., Obstrist, B., Mshinda, H., Tanner, M. & Schellenberg, D. (2007). Factors affecting home deliveries in Tanzania. *Trop. Med. Int. Health, 12(7)*, 862-872.

Mubyazi, G., Bloch, P., Byskov, J., Hansen, K., Olsen, Ø. & Magnussen, P. (2005b). Economic and other contextual determinants of the acceptability and viability of intermittent preventive treatment of malaria during pregnancy in Tanzania. *Acta Tropica, MIM Conference Abstracts, 95S(2005b)*, S1-S506, 252.

Mubyazi, G., Bloch, P., Kamugisha, M., Kitua, A. & Ijumba, J. (2005a). Intermittent preventive treatment of malaria during pregnancy in Tanzania: a qualitative study of knowledge, attitudes and perceptions of district health managers, antenatal service staff and pregnant women in Korogwe district, northeastern Tanzania. *Malaria Journal, 4*, 31.

Mubyazi, G., Massaga, J., Kamugisha, M., Mubyazi, J. N., Magogo, G. C., Mdira, K. Y., Gesase, S. & Sukwa, T. (2006a). User charges in public health facilities in Tanzania: effect on revenues, quality of services and people's health seeking behaviour for malaria illnesses in Korogwe district. *Health Services Management Research, 19(1)*, 23-35.

Mubyazi GM and Gonzalez-Block MA (2005). Research influence on national antimalarial drug policy in Tanzania: case study of changing from chloroquine to sulfadoxine-pyrimethamine. *Malaria Journal, 4*, 51.

Mubyazi, G. M., Bygbjerg, I. C., Magnussen, P., Olsen, O., Byskov, J., Hansen, K. S. & Bloch, P. (2008). Prospects, achievements, challenges and opportunities for scaling up malaria chemoprevention in pregnancy in Tanzania: the perspective of national level officers. *Malaria Journal, 7*, 135.

Mubyazi, G. M., Kamugisha, M., Mushi, A. & Blas, E. (2004). Implications of decentralization for the control of tropical diseases in Tanzania: evidence from a case study of four districts. *International Journal of Health Planning and Management, 19*, S167-185.

Mubyazi, G. M., Mushi, A. K., Shayo, E., Mdira, K., Ikingura, J., Mutagwaba, D., Malecela, M. & Njunwa, K. J. (2007b). Local Primary Health Care Committees and Community-Based Health Workers in Mkuranga District, Tanzania: Does the Public Recognise and Appreciate Them? *Ethno-Medicine, 1(2)*, 27-35.

Mutabingwa, T. K. (1994). Malaria and pregnancy: epidemiology, pathophysiology, and control options. *Acta Tropica, 57*, 239-254.

Mutabingwa, TK (2002). Antimalarial Intermittent Treatment during Pregnancy in Africa. In *PREMA-EU Newsletter*, Issue 1, November.

National Bureau of Statistics, Tanzania (2002). National Population Census 2002: District Data. *National Bureau of Statistics, Dar Es Salaam, United Republic of Tanzania* 2002.

Nganda, R. Y., Drakeley, C., Reyburn, H. & Marchant, T. (2004). Knowledge of malaria influences the use of insecticide treated nets but not intermittent presumptive treatment by pregnant women in Tanzania. *Malaria Journal, 3*, 42.

Nsimba, E. D. (2006). How sulfadoxine-Pyrimethamine was perceived in some rural communities after phasing out chloroquine as a first-line drug for uncomplicated malaria in Tanzania: lessons to learn towards moving from monotherapy to fixed combination therapy. *Journal of Ethnobiology and Ethnomedicine*, *2*, 5.

Overbosch, G. B., Nsowah-Nuamah, N. N. N., van den Boom, G. J. M. & Damnyag, L. (2004). Determinants of antenatal care use in Ghana. *Journal of African Economies*, *13(2)*, 277-301.

Phillip-Howard, P. A., Behrens, R. H. & Dunlop, J. (1989). Steven-Johnson syndrome due to pyrimethamine/sulfadoxine during presumptive self therapy of malaria. *Lancet*, *2(8666)*, 803-4.

Priya, N. (2002). Gender Dimensions of User fees: Implications for Women's Utilisation of Health Care. *Reproductive Health Matters*, *10(20)*, 127-134.

Quijada, C. & Comfort, A. (2002). Maternal health financing profile in Tanzania. Working Paper No. 003. *Partnership for Health Reform* (*PHRplus*), Abt. Associates Inc., Bethesda MD, USA.

Ribera, M. J., Hausmann-Muela, S., D'Alessandro, U. & Grietens, P. K. (2007). Malaria in pregnancy: what can social sciences Contribute? *PLoS Medicine*, *4(4)*, e92, 0001-0005.

Rugemalila, J. B., Wanga, C. L. & Kilama, W. L. (2006). Sixth African Malaria day in 2006: how have we come after the Abuja Declaration? *Mal J.*, *5*, 102.

Schellenberg, D., Cisse, B. & Menendez, C. (2006). The IPTi Consortium: research for policy and action. *Trends in Parasitology*, www.malariaconsortium.org/data/files/pages/ipt_4.pdf (accessed 7th September 2006). Doi:10.1016/j.pt.2006.05.006.

Scholz, R. W. & Olaf, T. (2002). Embedded Case Study Methods: Integrating Qualitative and Quantitative Knowledge. *Thousand Oaks*: *Sage Publications*, 392.

Smith, P. G. & Morrow, R. H. (1996). *Field Trials of Health Interventions in Developing Countries: A tool Box*. 2nd Edition. Macmillan.

Snow, R. W. (2004). The invisible victims: A special supplement Issue. *Nature*, *430*, 934-935.

Somi, M., James, B. R. G., Farshid, V., Njau, J. D., Kachur, P. S. & Abdulla, S. (2007). Economic burden of malaria in rural Tanzania: variations by socioeconomic status and season. *Trop. Med. Int. Health*, *12(10)*, 1139-1147.

Steketee, R. W., Nahlen, B. L., Parise, M. E. & Menendez, C. (2001). The burden of malaria in pregnancy in malaria-endemic areas. *Am. J. Trop. Med. Hyg. 64 (Supple 1-2)*, 28-35.

Tarimo, D. S. & Malekela, D. A. (2006). Health workers perceptions on chloroquine and sulfadoxine/sulfalene-pyrimethamine monotherapies: implications for the change to combination therapy of artemether/lumefantrine in Tanzania. *East African Journal of Public Health*, *4(1)*, 43-46.

Tellis, W. (1997, July). Introduction to case study [68 paragraphs]. *The Qualitative Report* [On-line serial], *3(2)*. Available: http://www.nova.edu/ssss/QR/QR3-2/tellis1.html

ter Kuile, F. O. & Steketee, R. W. (2007). Intermittent Preventive Therapy with Sulfadoxine-Pyrimethamine during Pregnancy: Seeking Information on Optimal Dosing Frequency. *Journal of Infectious Diseases*, *196*, 1574-6.

United Republic of Tanzania (URT)-MKUKUTA (2005). Poverty at the District Level in Mainland Tanzania: Brief 2 Poverty and Human Development Report 2005. *Research*

Analysis Technical Working Group of the MKUKUTA Monitoring System, Ministry of Planning, Economy and Empowerment, Dar Es Salaam, United Republic of Tanzania.

Vallely, A., Vallely, L., Changalucha, J., Greenwood, B. & Chandramohan, D. (2007). Intermittent preventive treatment for malaria in pregnancy in Africa: what's new, what's needed? *Malaria Journal*, *6*, 16.

van Eijk, A. M., Ayisi, A. G., tel Kuile, F. O., Otieno, J. A., Odondi, M. J. O., Rose, D. H., Kager, P. A., Steketee, R. W. & Nahlen, B. L. (2004). Implementation of intermittent preventive treatment with sulfadoxine-pyrimethamine for control of malaria in pregnancy in Kisumu, western Kenya. *Trop Med Int. Health*, *9(5)*, 630-7.

Verhoeff, F. H., Brabin, B. J., Chimsuku, L., Kazembe, P., Russel, W. B. & Broadhead, R. L. (1998). An evaluation of effects of intermittent sulfadoxine-pyrimethamine treatment in pregnancy on parasite clearance and risk of low birth-weight in rural Malawi. *Ann. Trop. Med. Parasit*, *92(2)*, 141-50.

Wagle, R. R., Sabroe, S. & Nielsen, B. B. (2004). Socio-economic and physical distance to maternity hospital as predictors for place of delivery: an observation study from Nepal. *Pregnancy and Child Birth*, *4*, 8.

White, N. (2005). Intermittent Presumptive Treatment for Malaria. *PLoS Medicine*, *vol. 2*/Issue 1/e1/e3.

WHO and UNICEF (2003b). Antenatal Care in Developing Countries: Promises, Achievements and Missed Opportunities: Analysis of Trends, levels and differentials. *WHO*, Geneva.

WHO: Implementation research: bridging the gap between efficacy trials and application. *TDR Newsletter No. 71*, 9th February 2004b.

WHO: The Abuja Declaration and the Plan of Action: An extract from The African Summit on Roll Back Malaria, Abuja 25 April 2000. WHO/CDC/RBM/2000.17

WHO: The use of antimalarial drugs: chemoprophylaxis treatment of malaria in special groups. *WHO* 2001, www.rbm.who.int/cmc_upload/0/000/014/923/am_3.htm#p3.1.

Williams, H. A., Durrheim, H. A. & Shretta, D. (2004). The process of changing national malaria treatment policy: lessons from country-level studies. *Health Policy and Planning*, *19(6)*, 356-370.

Worrall, E., Morel, C., Shunmay, Y., Borghi, J., Hill, J., Wiseman, V. & Mills, A. (2007). The economics of malaria in pregnancy-a review of the evidence and research priorities. *Lancet Infectious Diseases*, *7*, 156-168.

www.repoa.or.tz/documents_storage/PHDR%200520Brief%202%20English.pdf

Yin, R. K. (1994). *Case Study Research: designs and methods*. 2nd Edition. Sage Publications.

Zach, L. (2006). Using a multiple case-study design to investigate the information-seeking behaviour of arts administrators. www.thefreelibrary.com: (accessed 2nd November 2007).

In: Antimalarial Drugs: Costs, Safety and Efficacy
Editors: Emanuel Csizmadia and Istvan Kalnoky
ISBN: 978-1-60741-432-2

Chapter II

A Potential Therapeutic Strategy for Malaria: Reversal of Quinoline Resistance

L. M. Elandaloussi and P. J. Smith
Department of Pharmacology, University of Cape Town,
Observatory 7925, South Africa

Abstract

The resistance to antimalarial drugs, especially chloroquine, of *Plasmodium falciparum* has contributed to an increase in morbidity and mortality due to malaria in recent years. It has been well established that chloroquine-sensitive parasites accumulate more drug within *P. falciparum* food vacuoles than their resistant counterparts. Mechanisms underlying drug resistance in malaria remains unclear but three proteins have been implicated in quinoline resistance: Pgh-1 (P-glycoprotein homologue 1); PfCRT (*Plasmodium falciparum* chloroquine resistance transporter) and PfMRP (*Plasmodium falciparum* multidrug resistance protein). Whether these proteins act as channels or transporters of quinoline is still to be determined. Quinoline-reversing agents, a class of compounds unrelated to quinoline, are believed to act on these proteins. Although they do not have any intrinsic anti-malaria activity, they have the property of being able to reverse drug resistance. Recent advances in target orientated synthesis and structure activity relationship should be beneficial for the understanding of the mode of action of these agents and design of improved drugs for the control of malaria. Polymorphisms in the corresponding genes of the quinoline transporters (*pfcrt*, *pfmdr1* and *pfmrp*) have been detected and identified as potential molecular markers for parasite resistance to quinoline antimalarials. The integration of these molecular markers in surveillance program would be crucial for the monitoring of drug resistance and the management of strategies for the reversal of resistance. Resistance of *P. falciparum* to all the major drugs used for the treatment of malaria has evolved quickly after their introduction. The use of chemosensitisers could represent a potential therapeutic strategy to overcome failure treatments due to the increasing problem of drug resistance. This chapter discusses currently known quinoline transporters implicated in drug resistance, reversing agents and their potential as therapeutic strategy.

Introduction

Drug resistance, especially multidrug resistance, and difficulties in eradicating the mosquito vector have been the basis of malaria resurgence over the past 30 years. In addition, massive problems with logistic, planning, allocation of resources and a lack of operational research have contributed greatly to the failure of malaria eradication. Chloroquine was the antimalarial treatment of choice as it was the most common, well-tolerated and cost-effective drug for prophylaxis and therapy of malaria. It was widely used before the first resistant parasites were detected in 1959 in South America and a year later in South Asia. Since this time, resistance has spread rapidly and it is now present in all regions where malaria is endemic. The emergence and spread of drug-resistant *Plasmodium falciparum* strains has severely compromised the effectiveness of these drugs and contributed to a huge increase in morbidity and mortality from malaria.

The biochemical basis of chloroquine action and resistance are not completely understood. Early clinical investigations of the antimalarial activities of chloroquine noted that drug action was limited to those stages of the parasite life cycle which were actively degrading hemoglobin [Fairley, 1947]. The parasite degrades the hemoglobin in the food vacuole, and uses the amino acids as a major nutrient source. When ferrous haem is released from globin it oxidizes into the ferriprotoporphyrine IX which is toxic to the parasite. The parasite has evolved a novel pathway for the detoxification of this by incorporating it into an insoluble crystalline form called haemozoin or malaria pigment. The current hypothesis for chloroquine action is that this drug interferes with haemozoin formation resulting in toxic haem accumulation in the parasite that leads to its death. However, chloroquine is concentrated in the acidic vacuole of the parasite and it is clear that resistant parasites accumulate less chloroquine than sensitive isolates. The mechanism by which chloroquine-resistant parasites minimize chloroquine accumulation is controversial. Early studies had shown that verapamil was capable of reversing chloroquine resistance by increasing chloroquine accumulation in parasitised erythrocytes (Martin et al., 1987; Krogstad et al., 1987a; Bray et al., 1994]. These, and other observations have led to a number of hypotheses implicating three proteins as potentially acting as drug transporters or channels. The three proteins are Pgh-1 (P-glycoprotein homologue 1); PfCRT (*Plasmodium falciparum* chloroquine resistance transporter) and PfMRP (*Plasmodium falciparum* multidrug resistance protein).

Due to increases in the incidence of infection of U.S. army troops in Vietnam with chloroquine-resistant *P. falciparum*, a large drug screening programme were initiated by the Walter Reed Army Institute of research, leading to the development of mefloquine and halofantrine [Ohnmacht et al., 1971; Colwell et al., 1972; Schmidt et al., 1978a and 1978b]. Mefloquine is most effective against multidrug resistant strains of *P. falciparum* although reports indicate that mefloquine resistance is now established in several endemic regions of the world [Hameed, 2003]. Mefloquine resistance was first observed in the 1980s in South-East Asia

[Boudreau et al., 1982] and since then in vitro and in vivo susceptibility to mefloquine has been shown to decrease [Vijaykadga et al., 2006; Na-Bangchang and Congpuong, 2007]. Other antimalarials that have been developed include the quinine-like compounds such as amodiaquine and proguanil and the antifolate antagonists (pyrimethamine and sulfadoxine). More recently, a new class of compounds, the sesquiterpene endoperoxide have emerged with the isolation of artemisinin from a traditional Chinese medicinal herb Qinghao (Artemisia annua) [Klayman, 1985]. So far, there has been no clinical evidence of resistance of *P. falciparum* to artemisinin derivatives. Nevertheless, the generation of artemisinin-resistant mutants of *P. falciparum* after mutagenic treatment with N-methyl-N'-nitronitrosoguanosine has demonstrated the possibility of the development of resistance to this new anti-malarial [Inselburg, 1985]. In addition, a recent study has provided evidence of an association between in vitro and in vivo artemisinin resistance in Central African Republic [Menard et al., 2005] indicating that artemisinin resistance could emerge. Resistance commonly develops within 10-15 years after the introduction of an antimalarial [Peters et al., 1987; Bjorkman and Phillips-Howard, 1990]. Currently, sulfadoxine/pyrimethamine combined with artesunate is the first line treatment in several African countries as recommended by the WHO [2006]. Following the spread of chloroquine resistance, the combination of amodiaquine and sulfadoxine/pyrimethamine became the treatment of choice. However, high prevalence of chloroquine-, amodiaquine- and Sulfadoxine-Pyrimethamine-resistance appeared shortly after its introduction [Abacassamo et al., 2004]. The increase in sulfadoxine/pyrimethamine resistance and chloroquine resistance transporter (pfcrt) resistant haplotype could also compromise the introduction of the artemisinin-based combination consisting of artesunate/ sulfadoxine/pyrimethamine and amodiaquine strategy [Enosse et al., 2008] and resistance to this therapy could appear in few years.

Resistance of *P. falciparum* to all the major drugs used for the treatment of malaria has emphasised the need to develop novel antimalarial or to find a mechanism that circumvents the phenomena of drug-resistance. As there is not yet a useful vaccine against this disease, the major forms of treatment and control still rely on the use of mosquito-control and chemotherapeutic agents. This chapter will review the current knowledge about the mechanism of quinoline resistance and the potential of resistance reversal as therapeutic agents.

Quinoline Resistance

Current hypotheses to explain chloroquine resistance include modification in drug transport [Sanchez et al., 2003], altered binding of chloroquine to the heme [Bray et al., 1998] and changes in digestive vacuole pH [Dzekunov et al.,2000; Ursos et al., 2000].

Most notably, chloroquine resistance has been associated in vitro and in vivo with point mutations in two genes, pfmdr 1 (multidrug resistance) and pfcrt (chloroquine resistance transporter), which encode the *P. falciparum* digestive-vacuole transmembrane proteins Pgh1 [Reed et al., 2000], and PfCRT [Fidock et al., 2000] respectively.

Pgh1

Observations of reduced chloroquine accumulation in chloroquine-resistant *P. falciparum* and the ability of verapamil and a number of other unrelated agents to reverse chloroquine resistance prompted mechanistic comparison of chloroquine resistance in the parasite with multidrug resistance in mammalian cancer cell lines [Martin et al., 1987]. The mechanism of multi-drug resistance in tumor cells has been identified to result from an increased drug efflux that is mediated by increased expression of a P-glycoprotein [Cornwell et al., 1986]. Multidrug resistant tumor cells are able to expel a large range of chemically distinct anti-tumor drugs [Skovsgaard, 1978]. The multidrug resistance phenotype is believed to result from the overexpression of an ATP-dependent drug exporter [Riordan et al., 1985] and can be inhibited by several drugs including the calcium channel blockers [Tsuruo et al., 1984]. A 170-kDa protein located on the plasma membrane has been identified as a likely candidate accounting for the phenomenon of multidrug resistance in tumor lines [Endicott and Ling, 1989]. This P-glycoprotein is an ATP-dependent pump encoded by the mdr gene which is amplified in tumor lines resistant to multiple drugs and can be photoaffinity labelled by both drugs [Safa, 1992; Cornwell et al., 1986] and ATP [Cornwell et al., 1987; Georges et al., 1991].

P. falciparum has been shown to possess at least two *mdr*-like genes (*pfmdr1* and *pfmdr2*), one of which has been suggested to confer the chloroquine resistant phenotype. *Pfmdr1* has been sequenced [Foote et al., 1989] and has been shown to encode a 160 kDa P-glycoprotein homologue (Pgh1). Mammalian *mdr* genes typically share 50% homology with *pfmdr1* [Foote et al., 1989]. The *P. falciparum* P-glycoprotein is of interest because its putative transport function is unknown and because it has been linked to the chloroquine resistance phenotype. Cowman et al. [1991] showed that Pgh1 is localised primarily to the membrane of the digestive vacuole of *P. falciparum* trophozoites and that a small fraction appears to be localised to the parasite membrane. Pgh1 has been shown to bind nucleotides by photoaffinity labelling [Karcz et al., 1993], which is consistent with a role in drug transport. However, photoaffinity studies using a photoreactive analogue of chloroquine failed to demonstrate an interaction of chloroquine with Pgh1 in *P. falciparum* [Foley et al., 1994]. Pgh1 is expected to share at least some of these features with other P-glycoproteins, although presently only ATP-binding has been demonstrated for Pgh1 [Karcz and Cowman, 1991]. Pgh1 belongs to the superfamily of ATP- binding cassette transporters (ABC). The typical ABC transporter, including Pgh1, is formed by two highly homologous halves (62% homology) connected by a hydrophilic linker region. Each half contains six predicted transmembrane domains, glycosylation consensus sequences, and one consensus site for ATP-binding [Walker et al., 1982]. P-type ATPases, such as Pgh1, are characterised by the presence of a phosphorylated intermediate and can be inhibited by vanadate, a transition state analogue of phosphate. Oligomycin, an inhibitor of the mitochondrial membrane ATPase by preventing phosphoryl group transfer has been shown to inhibit P-gp mediated drug transport [Hollo et al., 1994; Homolya et al., 1993].

Initially, Pgh1 present on the food vacuole membrane was thought to expel drugs from this organelle and therefore overexpression of Pgh1 was expected to increase the rate of removal of chloroquine from *P. falciparum* thereby rendering the parasite chloroquine resistant. It was also proposed that amino-acid substitution favouring expulsion might occur in the protein. However, the protein is orientated with its nucleotide-binding domain exposed to the parasite cytoplasm [Karz et al., 1993], which suggests pumping of substrate into the food vacuole rather than out. Nevertheless, mutation in *pfmdr1* may have changed the substrate specificity of the wild-type (chloroquine sensitive) protein in such a way that chloroquine became a poor substrate. The same mutation associated with chloroquine resistance may also have affected translocation of essential endogenous substrates of Pgh1 into or out of the digestive vacuole. It has been difficult to correlate any overexpression or mutation in this protein with chloroquine resistance. Foote et al. [1989] found that the *mdr* gene was amplified in some resistant isolates but not in any sensitive ones, while Wilson et al. [1989] correlated amplification of the same gene with increased mefloquine, but not chloroquine resistance. To determine if *pfmdr1* was linked to chloroquine resistance, Wellems et al. [1990] performed a genetic cross between chloroquine-resistant and chloroquine-sensitive clones of *P. falciparum*. Their result showed that the rapid efflux is controlled by a single gene or a closely related group of genes but there was no linkage between the rapid efflux, chloroquine-resistant phenotype and *pfmdr1*. Analysing the complete sequence of two chloroquine-resistant (CQR) and 5 chloroquine-sensitive (CQS), Foote et al. [1990] were able to predict the CQS/CQR status of a further 34 out of 36 isolates. They predicted that both a *pfmdr1* allele competent for chloroquine-resistance and a mutation in a second unknown gene is required for chloroquine-resistance. However, further studies showed that the level of chloroquine resistance in a number of field isolates of a *P. falciparum* did not correlate with the level of Pgh1 expression [Cowman et al., 1994] and there was no correlation between particular alleles of *pfmdr1* and chloroquine resistance [Wilson et al., 1993]. Despite compelling evidence for common resistance reversal mechanism in the 2 cell types, this model has been questioned by several investigators [Sanchez et al., 1997; Bray et al., 1999].

Further studies indicated that the level of chloroquine resistance in a number of field isolates did not correlate with the level of Pgh1 expression [Cowman et al., 1994]. It has then been suggested that several alleles of *pfmdr1* are closely linked to chloroquine resistance [Foote et al., 1989]. In contrast, another study demonstrated that chloroquine resistance segregated independently of the *pfmdr1* and *pfmdr2* genes in a genetic cross between a chloroquine-sensitive and a chloroquine-resistant strain [Wellems et al., 1990, 1991]. Using a heterologous expression system for *pfmdr1* gene to express Pgh1 in CHO cells, Van Es et al. [1994] found that wild-type Pgh1 could mediate chloroquine accumulation while chloroquine-resistant associated mutated forms could not. This finding demonstrates that there is more than one chloroquine-resistance mechanism which probably involves different sets of genes, depending on the *P. falciparum* isolate analysed. In view of these conflicting data, no consistent molecular explanation which could account for a role of Pgh1 in chloroquine-resistance has yet been found. Recently, nuclear-receptor mediated responses to drug exposure has been proposed as a mechanism of regulation in *P. falciparum* : This is based on the observation that pre-treatment with phenobarbitone resulted in an increased expression of Pgh1 associated with a decreased susceptibility to chloroquine and the presence of a putative nuclear receptor gene revealed by whole genome analysis [Johnson et al., 2008].

Even though it has been extensively investigated, the role of Pgh1 in the mechanism of chloroquine resistance has not yet been elucidated. Nevertheless, Pgh1 can modulate sensitivity of *Plasmodium* to several antimalarials including mefloquine, halofantrine and artemisinin [Reed et al., 2000; Sidhu et al., 2005; 2006]. Overexpression of pfmdr1 has been associated with cross-resistance to mefloquine, halofantrine and quinine [Duraisingh and Cowman, 2005]. In vitro selection for mefloquine resistance resulted in cross-resistance to halofantrine and increased sensitivity to chloroquine associated with amplification and over expression of pfmdr1 [Wilson et al., 1989; Cowman et al., 1994]. In addition, allelic-exchange studies demonstrated that point mutations in pfmdr1 were associated with an increase in quinine-resistance and a decrease in mefloquine and artemisinin resistance [Reed et al., 2000]. The parasite susceptibility to the intrinsic antiplasmodial activity of verapamil has also been shown to be influenced by mutations in pfmdr1 [Hayward et al., 2005a]. Since mutations in pfmdr1 have similar effect on the susceptibility to the lipophilic drugs verapamil, mefloquine and halofantrine, it was suggested that these drugs share a common mechanism of drug resistance. Altogether, overexpression and/or polymorphism in pfmdr1 appear to be involved in the modulation of susceptibility and resistance to several antimalarials of the quinoline and arylamino alcohol group.

PFCRT

A number of studies have designated the pfcrt gene as the major component of chloroquine resistance: chloroquine resistance has been strongly linked to a K76T mutation in PfCRT, althouth other mutations have been linked to the resistant chloroquine phenotype both in *in vitro* and *in vivo* studies; a genetic cross between a chloroquine resistant line and a chloroquine sensitive line revealed a clear association between inheritance of verapamil-reversible chloroquine resistance and polymorphism in PfCRT [Fidock et al., 2000]; mutations within pfcrt, particularly changes from a charged amino acid residue (lysine K76) to an uncharged residue such as threonine (76T) appears crucial both in the acquisition of quinoline resistance and the reversibility of resistance by chemosensitisers [Cooper et al., 2002; 2005; Fidock et al., 2000; Lakshmanan et al., 2005; Warhurst et al., 2003]; and finally multiple in vivo studies also describe a strong association between K76T and increased treatment failure [Wellems and Plowe, 2001; Basco, 2002; Ochong et al., 2003], particularly for very young children in whom acquired immunity is believed to have little influence on the treatment outcome [Djimde et al., 2001a].

The mechanism by which pfcrt confers resistance remains unclear. It has been postulated that pfcrt could play a role in transmembrane chloride movement inducing a change in vacuolar pH, act as a chloroquine efflux pump or a channel of chloroquine. Pfcrt point mutations had been associated with a decrease in vacuolar pH [Fidock et al., 2000]. The heme detoxification pathway necessary for parasite survival is highly pH dependent as is the binding of chloroquine to heme [Leed et al., 2002; De Dios et al., 2003]. A decrease in vacuolar pH will facilitate the formation of unsoluble heme and consequently reduce the quantity of free heme available for the formation of toxic complex with chloroquine. A direct association between vacuolar pH and pfcrt mutations has been demonstrated in laboratory strains [Bennett et al., 2004]. However, in most cases, it is difficult to assess whether phenotypic features are produced by specific mutations or results from other indirect effect and, most likely, the alteration in vacuolar pH is not directly due to pfcrt mutation but rather to the lysosomatrophic effect of chloroquine. Therefore two models prevail to explain its role in chloroquine resistance. Mutated PfCRT would act either as a channel that might enable chloroquine to flow out of the food vacuole down its electrochemical gradient or a transporter of chloroquine that might expel chloroquine out of the digestive vacuole. pfcrt encodes a 48.6kDa protein with 10 predicted transmembrane domains located in the food vacuole membrane [Fidock et al., 2000] which groups with the drug/metabolite transporter superfamily [Tran and saier, 2004]. Evidence that the chloroquine resistance mechanism requires energy [Bray et al., 1992a; Krogstad et al., 1992; Sanchez et al., 2003] also prompted to an active carrier. In contrast, other study pointed out that energy deprivation or uncoupling the vacuolar proton gradient had no effect on the rate of chloroquine efflux from resistant parasites suggesting that mutated pfcrt is a gated aqueous pore allowing passive leak of protonated form of the drug out of the food vacuole [Warhurst et al., 2002; Zhang et al., 2004; Bray et al., 2006]. Both the charged drug leak and the active carrier model are consistent with substrate specificity. Furthemore, the ability of verapamil to reverse chloroquine resistance appears tightly linked to pfcrt [Ferdig et al., 2004]. Nevertheless, pfcrt point mutation S163R was demonstrated to abrogate verapamil reversible chloroquine-resistance in laboratory strain [Johnson et al., 2004].

Transfection experiments also indicated that acquisition of *pfcrt* 76T induces mefloquine hypersensitivity [Sidhu et al., 2002]. pfcrt mutation, especially S163R selected by halofantrine pressure conferred resistance to halofantrine and mefloquine that were not associated with pfmdr1 amplification or polymorphisms [Johnson et al., 2004] indicating a possible role for PfCRT in resistance to other anti-malarial compounds. In addition, this halofantrine-resistance selected line showed an increased sensitivity to chloroquine and a loss of verapamil-reversible chloroquine resistance [Johnson et al., 2004]. The observation that the reversal of chloroquine by verapamil is not universal is consistent with the hypothesis that multiple genes modulate the resistance to chloroquine. Nevertheless, the involvement of pfcrt in drug resistance other that chloroquine would need to be corroborated by field studies.

It is believed that PfCRT perform a vital function for the parasite as disruption in this gene has been found deleterious for the parasite [Waller et al., 2003]. However, neither the endogenous function of PfCRT nor its substrates are currently known. The substitution at position 76 is crucial for conferring chloroquine resistance and other changes that vary with independent evolutionary origins of chloroquine resistance can be directly involved in the chloroquine resistance mechanism or related with compensating the loss or reduction of the biological function of the protein [Hayward et al., 2005b]. Strikingly, analysis of compensatory changes associated with pfcrt point mutation showed an increased expression of genes encoding proteins involved in transport and or regulation of pH [Jiang et al., 2008]. These changes could be hypothesised to compensate for alteration in the functionality of PFCRT. In addition, discontinuation of chloroquine treatment has lead to a re-emergence of chloroquine sensitivity in the field [Wang et al., 2005] indicating that mutation 76T might inflict a fitness loss for the parasite. In the absence of drug pressure, mutation would be a disadvantage and should be abrogated, suggesting an alteration of normal cellular function and possibly an effect in maintaining the vacuolar pH.

Genes Other than PFCRT and PFMDR

The availability of *P. falciparum* genes with the genome sequencing project has provided the opportunity to search for candidate genes involved in drug resistance [Gardner et al., 2002]. Nine new candidates potentially associated with either quinine or chloroquine responses were recently reported [Mu et al., 2003]. Of these, six were associated with quinine or chloroquine resistance in a Southeast Asian sample. However, a latter study could not find any correlation between chloroquine or quinine response in eight of the nine candidates [Anderson et al., 2005]. Nevertheless, one of these candidates was potentially associated with artesunate response.

Genes recently identified as potential players in quinoline resistance include pfnhe-1 (sodium hydrogene exchanger) and pfmrp1 (multidrug resistance protein). Pfnhe-1 has been associated in vitro to quinine resistance [Ferdig et al., 2004]. Pfnhe-1 encodes a 1920 amino acid putative Na+/H+ exchanger (NHE) with 12 predicted transmembrane segments and a signal peptide cleavage site [Gardner et al., 2002; Ferdig et al., 2004]. A NHE activity in *P. falciparum* has been postulated to remove the increased cytolic acid burden caused by anaerobic glycolysis [Bosia et al., 1993]. An elevated PfNHE activity was found for strains with high levels of quinine resistance but its association with changes in pH was somewhat ambiguous [Bennett et al., 2007]. Mutation and/or overexpression of one of the multidrug resistance protein homologues found in the malarial parasite, PfMRP1 may further modulate the degree of multidrug resistance [Klokousas et al., 2003; 2004]. This gene has been annotated as a 1822 amino acid full-length ABC transporter (CAB63558). However, considerable controversy surrounds the precise contribution of PfMRP1, in part because no direct biochemical studies of PfMRP1 have yet been possible. In addition, immunomicroscopy techniques located this protein on the plasma membrane and not on the food vacuole [Klokousas et al., 2004], the site of chloroquine accumulation in the parasite. A recent field study in Iran detected the pfnhe allele associated with quinine resistance in vitro and the 191H and 437S pfmrp alleles [Ursing et al., 2006]. Nevertheless, data on their contribution to quinoline resistance lacks and would be needed in order to link polymorphisms and/or overexpression of these genes and resistance phenotype.

Molecular Markers for Quinoline Resistance

Monitoring of parasite resistance is essential for a rational use of antimalarial drugs. The susceptibility of *P. falciparum* can be assessed either by therapeutic responses (*in vivo* tests) or by measuring parasite growth (*in vitro* tests). Standardised tests have been developed initially for assessing the parasitological responses of *P. falciparum* to chloroquine in non-immune patients [WHO, 1973]. *In vivo* test permit to determine the threshold of treatment failure thus providing crucial information for adjusting antimalarial policy despite the constraints of their application in the field [WHO, 2003]. On the other hand, in vitro tests measuring the intrinsic susceptibility of the parasite to antimalarial drugs [WHO, 2001] do not take into account factors such as host immunity or pharmacokinetics, which also contribute to treatment failure. Similarly, the use of molecular markers presents the same inconvenient. Nevertheless, determination of in vitro susceptibility to drugs is useful for evaluating the frequency of resistant phenotype in a given population, the cross-resistance between drugs and the efficacy of new drugs [Warsame et al., 2001]. It is also essential for investigating the mechanisms underlying drug action and resistance [Foote and Cowman, 1994]. A better understanding of the molecular basis of drug resistance has led to the search of molecular markers for a less laborious follow-up of drug resistance. The level of resistance is likely to be regulated by multiple genes. Reverse genetics and candidate gene approaches have permitted the identification of several potential genetic markers of resistance.

Major single pfmdr1nucleotide polymorphism find to contribute to chloroquine resistance are N86Y and D1246Y [Basco et al., 1998; Duraisingh et al., 1997]. Molecular marker pfmdr1 N86Y plays an important role in predicting chloroquine and amodiaquine treatment failure in Papua New guinea [Marfurt et al., 2008] and this marker in combination with pfcrt 76T was predictive for treatment failure in Nigeria [Happi et al., 2006] and Kenya [Holmgren et al., 2006]. pfmdr1 level of amplification is also believed to confer mefloquine resistance and modulate chloroquine resistance [Duraisingh and Cowman, 2005; Reed et al., 2000]. However, difficulties in evaluating the number of copies of this gene have impeded large-scale field studies and most of the investigation has focused on determining relationship between single nucleotide polymorphisms and resistance [Basco et al., 1998; Povoa et al., 1998]. Involvement of pfmdr1 in chloroquine resistance remains unresolved whereas laboratories and field data support its implication in mefloquine resistance and others arylaminoalcohols. To date, point mutation in pfcrt K76T has been clearly associated with chloroquine resistance and can be used as a marker in surveillance for chloroquine -resistant *P. falciparum* malaria while other pfcrt polymorphisms linked to chloroquine resistance in vitro has to be confirmed in the field. In several studies, pfcrt mutant allele alone led to significant changes in chloroquine, amodiaquine and quinine sensitivity of the parasite in Mali [Djimde et al., 2001a] and Central African Republic [Menard et al., 2006]. Using DNA microarray-based technology, the usefulness of 24 markers including pfmdr1 and pfcrt in predicting treatment outcome with combination therapy of amodiaquine plus sulfadoxine-pyrimethamine was evaluated [Marfurt et al., 2008] and showed that the risk of treatment failure was associated with the total number of mutation in the analysed genes. In addition to these genes, recent findings have suggested that others loci may be involved in modulating *P. falciparum* quinoline response. Amongst these are pfmrp (multidrug resistance protein) [Klokouzas et al., 2004; Mu et al., 2003] and pfnhe-1 (sodium hydrogen exchanger) [Ferdig et al., 2004]; the latter specifically related to low levels of quinine resistance. Interestingly, a field survey in Iran reported a linkage of the 191H and 437S *pfmrp* alleles associated with decreased quinoline response [Ursing et al., 2006]. However, no co-variation and no association with quinolines were detected in a recent study on *P. falciparum* from Thailand [Anderson et al., 2005]. Therefore, the role of *pfmrp* is yet to be determined and differences between regions might also be expected.

Epidemiological differences in resistance exist in populations from different geographic origins [Menard et al; 2006; Duraisingh et al., 2005]. Therefore, the validity of molecular markers is likely to be dependent on the history of drug use in a given area [Djimde et al., 2001a]. Genotypic indices integrating molecular and clinical measures have been proposed by Djimde et al., [2001b]. These indices include the genetic resistance index and the phenotype failure index: the genetic resistance index is obtained by dividing the prevalence of a molecular marker by the prevalence of parasitological resistance; the phenotype failure index is obtained by dividing the prevalence of the marker by clinical failure rate. When combined with the local frequency of mutation these indices allow prediction of the local parasitological and clinical failure rate [Hastings, 2007]. These indices have been advocated as monitoring tools in WHO technical documentation [WHO, 2005] and several studies have confirmed their potential [Djimde et al., 2004; Tinto et al., 2005]. To date, application of molecular markers as a predicting tool for treatment outcome and drug policy in the field have been scarce. However, in Malawi where chloroquine was replaced by sulphadoxine-pyrimethamine as early as 1993 [Bloland et al., 1993], this approach has shown its potential in following drug resistance. Molecular markers had clearly demonstrated the decline of chloroquine resistant associated mutation pfcrt T76 confirmed by an increase efficacy in chloroquine treatment in clinical studies [Laufer et al., 2006]. Establishing the usefulness of molecular markers is a lengthy process requiring field survey and efficacy trials and has probably also been impeded by other factors influencing treatment outcome, mainly acquired immunity. Models that take into accounts these factors and the availability of data from in vitro and in vivo studies from diverse sites around the world would improve the predictability of these tools. The creation of a database of molecular markers has been proposed by Plowe et al. [2007] as a guide for the selection of first line drug to use and a tool that could accelerate the identification and validation of molecular markers.

Reversal of Drug Resistance

Verapamil was the first agent demonstrated to sensitise chloroquine –resistant strains of *P. falciparum* to chloroquine [Martin et al., 1987]. This resistance reversal agent has little intrinsic anti-malarial activity [Martin et al., 1987]. Since then, several other compounds belonging to different pharmacological classes such as the calcium channel blockers, antidepressants, calmodulin antagonists and anti-histamines, have shown promising capabilities as chemosensitisers (Figure 1). These are not only functionally diverse but also structurally. Verapamil was the first and remains the most studied reversal agent however the basis for chemosensitisation remains unresolved. This compound is a known calcium channel blocker [Fleckenstein et al., 1967]; however, its action on malaria as a reversal agent has been demonstrated to be independent of calcium channels [Ye and Van Dyke, 1988]. Verapamil can only partially reverse chloroquine resistance and was shown to enhance chloroquine sensitivity in chloroquine-resistant parasites but had no effect on the chloroquine sensitivity of chloroquine-sensitive strains [Martin et al., 1987]. Early studies have suggested that two phenotypically distinct mechanisms for chloroquine-resistance exist, one that is verapamil reversible, and one that is not. The observation that the reversal of chloroquine resistance can be either fully or partially sensitive to verapamil [Ward et al., 1995] is consistent with the hypothesis that multiple gene products modulate the response to chloroquine.

Since chemosensitisers which reverse multidrug resistance of tumour cells are also capable of modulating chloroquine resistance, these agents were proposed to function in a similar manner, and therefore expected to stimulate a P-glycoprotein activity. Mutations in pfmdrl associated with resistance to mefloquine are also associated with decreased sensitivity to verapamil, suggesting a possible interaction between VP and Pgh1 [Hayward et al., 2005a]. In addition, allelic-exchange studies conclusively showed that *pfmdr1* sequence polymorphisms were associated with changes in susceptibility to mefloquine, halofantrine, quinine and the weakly antimalarial verapamil [Hayward et al., 2005a]. Although pfmdrl was originally considered the candidate gene responsible for chloroquine resistance, it was subsequently shown that mutations in the gene pfcrt were both necessary and sufficient for chloroquine resistance in the laboratory and in the field [Fidock et al., 2000; Mayengue et al., 2005; Tinto et al., 2005]. Nevertheless, it does not exclude that polymorphism in pfmdrl further modulate the level of chloroquine resistance and possibly interact with verapamil. Other agents such as cyclosporin A, an immunosuppressive used in organ transplantation [Borel et al., 1996] could possibly interact with Pgh1. This compound displays an anti-malarial activity [Bell et al., 1996] and it has been demonstrated to reverse multidrug resistance in mammalian cancer cells [Rosenberg et al., 2005]. Sequence polymorphisms in pfmdrl altered the susceptibility of parasites to cyclosporin A and synergistic antimalarial interactions between cyclosporin A and quinine, mefloquine or halofantrine and antagonism between cyclosporin A and chloroquine occured [Gavigan et al., 2007]. The amino acid sequence and copy number of Pgh1 was suggested to influence cyclosporin susceptibility as a result of a direct interaction between the drug and the protein, or via indirect effects on the physiology of the digestive vacuole.

The ability of verapamil to increase steady-state chloroquine accumulation was found to be totally insufficient to explain the increase in chloroquine activity by the drug. In contrast, when chloroquine accumulation was increased by raising the medium pH, the corresponding shift in sensitivity to chloroquine could be accurately predicted [Bray et al., 1994]. In addition, verapamil increase the vacuolar pH for chloroquine-resistant parasites to a value close to that measured for chloroquine-sensitive parasites, without an effect on vacuolar pH in chloroquine-sensitive *P. falciparum* [Ursos et al., 2000]. The role of pH in chloroquine resistance and its reversibility is highly controversial [Wissing et al., 2002; Sanchez et al., 2003; Hayward et al, 2006] and to which extend pH could contribute to these mechanisms remains subject to debate. pfcrt is believed to play a key role in chloroquine resistance and also in its reversibility by verapamil [Cooper et al., 2002; 2005; Lakshmanan et al., 2005; Warhust et al., 2003]. Chloroquine resistance and its reversibility are clearly linked to the presence of specific sequences in the pfcrt gene. Parasites transformed with mutant pfcrt were found to exhibit an increased sensitivity to verapamil [Fidock et al., 2000]. PfCRT K76T is clearly associated in determining chloroquine sensitivity in *P. falciparum* strains from the new and old world and to modulate the degree of verapamil reversibility in chloroquine-resistant lines [Lakshmanan et al., 2005]. Verapamil reversibility was found more pronounced in clones expressing recombinant pfcrt from the old world than in parasites isolates from the new world [Mehlotra et al., 2001]. Polymorphisms found in pfcrt include the CVIET haplotype found mainly in parasites from the Old world and the SVMNT found in *P. falciparum* strains from the New world (Figure 2). Parasites carrying the SVMNT haplotype were less responsive to verapamil chemosensitisation when compared to those carrying the CVIET haplotype [Mehlotra et al., 2001]. Interestingly, only the CVIET haplotype acquired increased vacuolar pH after verapamil treatment [Mehlotra et al., 2001] and it was therefore suggested that chemosensitisation resulted from the observed change in the vacuolar pH. Other studies have challenged the pH model since no differences could be found in the vacuolar pH from chloroquine-sensitive or chloroquine-resistant parasites [Hayward et al., 2006]. Verapamil also modulates the parasite sensitivity to quinine and quinidine [Cooper et al., 2002] but has no effect on mefloquine sensitivity [Oduola et al., 1993]. Similarly to chloroquine reversal, verapamil has been demonstrated to decrease the IC50 of quinine in strains carrying the K76T, K76N or K76I [Cooper et al., 2002].

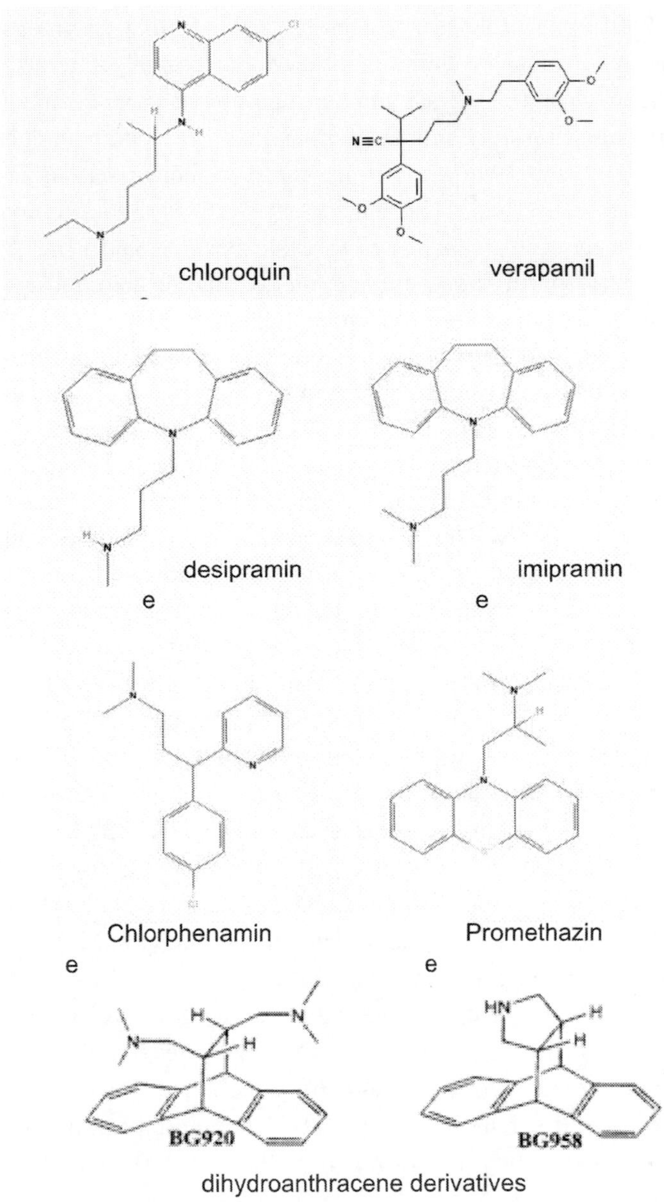

Figure 1. Chemical struture of chloroquine and some chloroquine resistance reversers.

Chloroquine susceptibility	pfcrt codons					Location
	72	73	74	75	76	
Sensitive	C	V	M	N	K	All region (Wild type)
Resistant	C	V	M	N	T	South America, Papua New Guinea
Resistant	C	V	I	E	T	Southeast Asia, Africa
Resistant	S	V	M	N	T	South America, Papua New Guinea

Figure 2. Geographic distribution of the major pfcrt haplotypes associated with chloroquine susceptibility.

Structure-activity profiling and three-dimensional quantitative structure-activity relationship (QSAR) studies revealed a common pharmacophore with critical features for potent chloroquine -chemosensitizing activity which could also account for the activity of a number of unrelated chloroquine resistance-reversers [Bhattacharjee et al., 2002]. A model based on structure-activity relationships study in dihydroanthracene derivatives was consistent with a binding site for pfcrt mutants carrying the CVIET haplotype [Alibert et al., 2002]. Similarly to verapamil, dihydroethanoanthracenic (DEA) derivatives reversal of resistance in *P. falciparum* is specific for resistant parasites and fully or partially reverses resistance in chloroquine-resistant parasites from different origins [Millet et al., 2004; Pradines et al., 2002]. Advantage of some of these DEA would be the low cost of synthesis and the absence of recognised psychotropic effect such as those observed with desipramine, imipramine and chlorpheniramine use in human [Sangalli, 1997; Stahl, 1984]. Altogether, these data would suggest that most chloroquine resistance reversers bind to the same site on pfcrt as chloroquine and subsequently blocking chloroquine by competition. However, this model does not accommodate other agents known to reverse chloroquine resistance such as NP30 which does not display the same structural features and has been demonstrated to reverse both chloroquine and mefloquine [Ciach et al., 2003]. Nonylphenolethoxylates, such as NP30, a surfactant, appeared phenotypically and genotypically distinct from verapamil [Ciach et al., 2003]. NP30 did reverse mefloquine resistance whereas no effect of verapamil could be detected. In contrast, only verapamil could reverse chloroquine resistance in another isolate. Interestingly, verapamil or NP30 dramatically decreased the resistance to quinine and quinidine. Combination of verapamil and NP30 was not additive for its chloroquine reversibility. NP 30 was found to reverse mefloquine, quinine and quinidine resistance. This agent does not have known toxic pharmacological effect and its reduced cost makes it an appealing therapeutic alternative.

Target-orientated and diversity-orientated organic synthesis has been proposed as a novel approach to study mechanisms of drug resistance in *P. falciparum* parasites and its reversal by chemosensitisers [Chibale, 2002]. Generating random mutation of resistance proteins and screening for a specific phenotype followed by a search for mutations and/or chemosensitisers that affect a specific drug resistance pathway could be a viable strategy and also shed light on the resistance pathway. Diversity-orientated synthesis approach [Schreiber, 2000] could be applied to identify the mutant target for the chemosensitisers and/or the molecular sequence of the mutant gene [Chibale, 2002]. This approach could offer the means to simultaneously identify resistance proteins that could serve as target for therapeutic intervention and chemosensitisers modulating the function of these proteins [Komarov et al., 1999; Mayer et al., 1999].

Despite the potential chemotherapeutic advantage of this strategy, few clinical studies have been conducted. Resistance-reversal agents which have been further tested in human trials include the tricyclic anti-depressants desipramine [Basco et al., 1990] and imipramine, and the antihistamines chlorphenamine and promethazine. Apart from their toxicity in humans, binding of some resistance reversers (e.g. desipramine) and pharmacokinetic interactions of the combination have limited their efficacy in human trials [Warsame et al., 1992; Basco et al., 1991]. Unlike desipramine, chlorpheniramine [Sowunmi and Oduola, 1997], imipramine [Adam et al., 2004] and promethazine [Oduola et al., 1998] were more successful in reversing chloroquine resistance in human trials. Plasma proteins inhibit desipramine chloroquine resistance reversing effect, and this effect is more pronounced with desipramine than other chemosensitisers [Suzuki et al., 1985]. Thus, the discrepancy observed between desipramine and imipramine in reversing chloroquine resistance in malaria patients could be attributed to variation in plasma protein binding properties of these agents. Clinical applications have been partly impeded by toxicity problems encountered with antidepressant and antihistamines. Antidepressants mediate the inhibition of neurotransmitter uptake by the biogeneic amine transporters [Stahl, 1984] and antihistamines compete with histamine for receptor sites on effector cells [Sangalli, 1997]. However, SAR studies might prove useful in designing safe, efficient and cost-effective resistance reversers. The development of such a therapy to restore chloroquine sensitivity would represent a challenge in future years.

Conclusion

The gene pfcrt appears to be the major determinant of chloroquine resistance whereas pfmdr1 modulates the level of resistance and is probably responsible for the resistance to other drugs such as mefloquine. Combination therapy with combinations such as Sulfadoxine/Pyrimethamine/Amodiaquine has shown the limit of this strategy with the rapid emergence of resistant haplotypes to each of the individual drug used. Discovery of novel anti-malarials is essential; however, the emergence and spread of resistance is likely to appear following intensive use of any particular drug. Chloroquine remains the least expensive and the safest anti-malarial drug to use in pregnant women and children. Combining this drug with resistant reversal agents is therefore an attractive strategy at the condition that the additional drug does not significantly increase the cost burden and that the combination therapy remains safe and efficient. It might be a more viable strategy for developing countries than introducing a novel anti-malarial drug. The coast of mefloquine, halofantrine or artesunate therapy is prohibitively high for those living in malaria-endemic countries and a combination of chloroquine with a resistance reversal agent might be a more economically viable alternative.

References

Abacassamo, F; Enosse, S; Aponte, JJ; Gómez-Olivé, FX; Quintó, L; Mabunda, S; Barreto, A; Magnussen, P; Rønn, AM; Thompson, R; Alonso, PL. Efficacy of chloroquine, amodiaquine, sulphadoxine-pyrimethamine and combination therapy with artesunate in Mozambican children with non-complicated malaria. *Trop Med Int Healt* 2004, 9, 200-8.

Adam, ME; A/Karim, ELI; Elkadaru, AY; Ibrahim, KEE; Berger, BJ; Wiese M; Babiker, HA. Imipramine induced complete reversal of chloroquine in Plasmodium falciparum infection in Sudan. *Saudi Pharmaceutical Journal*, 2004, 12, 130-5.

Alibert, S; Santelli-Rouvier, C; Pradines, B; Houdoin, C; Parzy, D; Karolak-Wojciechowska, J; Barbe, J. Synthesis and effects on chloroquine susceptibility in Plasmodium falciparum of a series of new dihydroanthracene derivatives. *J Med Chem*., 2002, 45, 3195-209.

Anderson, TJ; Nair, S; Qin, H; Singlam, S; Brockman, A; Paiphun, L; Nosten, F. Are transporter genes other than the chloroquine resistance locus (pfcrt) and multidrug resistance gene (pfmdr) associated with antimalarial drug resistance? *Antimicrob Agents Chemother*, 2005, 49, 2180-8.

Basco, LK; Le Bras, J. Reversal of chloroquine resistance with desipramine in isolates of Plasmodium falciparum from Central and West Africa. *Trans R Soc Trop Med Hyg*., 1990, 84, 479-81.

Basco, LK; Ringwald, P; Le Bras, J. In vivo-in vitro test for chloroquine potentiation by cyproheptadine against Plasmodium falciparum.*Trans R Soc Trop Med Hyg*., 1991, 85, 206-7.

Basco, LK; Ringwald, P. Molecular epidemiology of malaria in Yaounde, Cameroon. III. Analysis of chloroquine resistance and point mutations in the multidrug resistance 1 (pfmdr 1) gene of Plasmodium falciparum. *Am J Trop Med Hyg*., 1998, 59, 577-81.

Basco, LK. Molecular epidemiology of malaria in Cameroon. XII. In vitro drug assays and molecular surveillance of chloroquine and proguanil resistance. *Am J Trop Med Hyg*., 2002, 67, 383-7.

Bell, A; Roberts, HC; Chappell, LH. The antiparasite effects of cyclosporin A: possible drug targets and clinical applications. *Gen Pharmacol*., 1996, 27, 963-71.

Bennett, TN; Kosar, AD; Ursos, LMB; Dzekunov, S; Sidhu, ABS; Fidock, DA; Roepe, PD. Drug resistance-associated pfCRT mutations confer decreased Plasmodium falciparum digestive vacuolar pH. *Mol Biochem Parasitol*, 2004, 133, 99-114.

Bennett, TN; Patel, J; Ferdig, MT; Roepe, PD. Plasmodium falciparum Na+/H+ exchanger activity and quinine resistance.*Mol Biochem Parasitol*, 2007, 153, 48-58.

Bhattacharjee, AK; Kyle, DE; Vennerstrom, JL; Milhous, WK. A 3D QSAR pharmacophore model and quantum chemical structureactivity analysis of chloroquine(CQ)-resistance reversal. *J Chem Inf Comput Sci*., 2002, 42, 1212-20.

Bjorkman, A; Phillips-Howard, PA. Drug-resistant malaria: mechanisms of development and interferences for malaria control. *Trans R Soc Trop Med Hyg*., 1990, 84, 323-324.

Bloland, PB; Lackritz, EM; Kazembe, PN; Were, JB; Steketee, R; Campbell, CC. Beyond chloroquine: implications of drug resistance for evaluating malaria therapy efficacy and treatment policy in Africa. *J Infect Dis*., 1993, 4, 932-7.

Borel, JF; Baumann, G; Chapman, I; Donatsch, P; Fahr, A; Mueller, EA; Vigouret, JM. In vivo pharmacological effects of cyclosporin and some analogues. *Adv Pharmacol*, 1996, 35, 115-246.

Bosia, A; Ghigo, D; Turrini, F; Nissani, E; Pescarmona, GP; Ginsburg, H. Kinetic characterisation of the Na+/H+ antiport of Plasmodium falciparum. *J Cell Physiol*, 1993, 154, 527-534.

Boudreau, EF; Webster, HK; Pavanand, K; Thosingha, L. Type II mefloquine resistance in Thailand. *Lancet*, 1982, 2, 1335.

Bray, PG; Howells, RE; Ritchie, GY; Ward, SA. Rapid chloroquine efflux phenotype in both chloroquine-sensitive and chloroquine-resistant Plasmodium falciparum. *Biochem Pharmacol*, 1992[a], 44, 1317-24.

Bray, PG; Howells, RE; Ward, SA. Vacuolar acidification and chloroquine sensitivity in Plasmodium falciparum. *Biochem Pharmacol*, 1992b, 43, 1219-27.

Bray, PG; Boulter, MK; Ritchie, GY; Howells, RE; Ward, SA. Relationship of global chloroquine transport and reversal of resistance in Plasmodium falciparum. *Mol Biochem Parasitol*, 1994, 63, 87-94.

Bray, PG; Mungthin, M; Ridley, RG; Ward, SA. Access to hematin: the basis of chloroquine resistance. *Mol Pharmacol*, 1998, 54, 170-9.

Bray, PG; Janneh, O; Raynes, KJ; Mungthin, M; Ginsburg, H; Ward, SA. Cellular uptake of chloroquine is dependent on binding to ferriprotoporphyrin IX and is dependent of NHE activity in Plasmodium falciparum. *J Cell Biol.*, 1999, 145, 363-76.

Bray, PG; Mungthin, M; Hastings, IM; Biagini, GA; Saidu, DK; Lakshmanan, V; Johnson, DJ; Hughes, RH; Stocks, PA; O'Neill, PM; Fidock, DA; Warhurst, DC; Ward, SA. PfCRT and the transvacuolar proton electrochemical gradient: regulating the access of chloroquine to ferriprotoporphyrin IX. *Mol Microbiol.*, 2006, 62, 238-51.

Chibale, KA. Chemical approach towards understanding the mechanism and reversal of drug resistance in Plasmodium falciparum: is it viable? *IUBMB Life*, 2002, 53, 249-52.

Ciach, M; Zong, K; Kain, KC; Crandall, I. Reversal of mefloquine and quinine resistance in Plasmodium falciparum with NP30. *Antimicrob Agents Chemother*, 2003, 47, 2393-6.

Colwell, WT; Brown, V; Christie, P; Lange, J; Yamamoto, K; Henery, DW. Antimalarial arylaminopropanols. *J Med Chem.*, 1972, 15, 771-4.

Cooper, RA; Ferdig, MT; Su, XZ; Ursos, LM; Mu, J; Nomura, T; Fujioka, H; Fidock, DA; Roepe, PD; Wellems, TE. Alternative mutations at position 76 of the vacuolar transmembrane protein PfCRT are associated with chloroquine resistance and unique stereospecific quinine and quinidine responses in Plasmodium falciparum. *Mol. Pharmacol*, 2002, 61, 35-42.

Cooper, RA; Hartwig, CL; Ferdig, MT. pfcrt is more than the Plasmodium falciparum chloroquine resistance gene: a functional and evolutionary perspective. *Acta Trop.*, 2005, 94, 170-80.

Cornwell, MM; Safa, AR; Felsted, RI; Gottesman, MM; Pastan, I. Membranes vesicles from multidrug-resistant human cancer cells contain a specific 150 to 170 kDa protein detected by photoaffinity labeling. *Proc Natl Acad Sci.*, U. S. A., 1986, 83, 3847-50.

Cornwell, MM; Tsurno, T; Gottesman, MM; Pastan, I. ATP-binding properties of P-glycoprotein from multidrug-resistant KB cells. *FASEB J.*, 1987, 1, 51-4.

Cowman, AF; Karcz, S; Galatis, D; Culvenor, JG. A P-glycoprotein homologue of Plasmodium falciparum is localized on the digestive vacuole. *J cell biol.*, 1991, 113, 1033-42.

Cowman, AF; Galatis, D; Thompson, JK. Selection for mefloquine-resistance is linked to amplification of the pfmdr1 gene and cross-resistance to haslofantrine and quinine. *Proc Natl Acad Sci.*, U. S. A., 1994, 91, 1143-7.

de Dios, AC; Tycko, R; Ursos, LMB; Roepe, PD. NMR studies of chloroquine - ferriprotoporphyrin IX complex. *J Phys Chem A.*, 2003, 107, 5821-5.

Djimde, A; Doumbo, MD; Cortese, JF; Kayentao, K; Doumbo, S; Diourte, Y; Coulibaly, D; Dicko, A; Su, XZ; Nomura, T; Fidock, DA; Wellems, TE; Plowe, CV. A molecular marker for chloroquine resistant falciparum malaria. *N Engl J Med.*, 2001[a], 344, 257-63.

Djimde, A; Doumbo, OK; Steketee, RW; Plowe, CV. Application of a molecular marker for surveillance of chloroquine-resistant falciparum malaria. *Lancet*, 2001b, 358, 890-1.

Djimdé, AA; Dolo, A; Ouattara, A; Diakité, S; Plowe, CV; Doumbo, OK. Molecular diagnosis of resistance to antimalarial drugs during epidemics and in war zones. *J Infect Dis.*, 2004, 190, 853-5.

Duraisingh, MT; Cowman, AF. Contribution of the pfmdr1 gene to antimalarial drug-resistance. *Acta Trop.*, 2005, 94, 181-90.

Duraisingh, MT; Drakeley, CJ; Muller, O; Bailey, R; Snounou, G; Targett, GA; Greenwood, BM; Warhurst, DC. Evidence for selection for the tyrosine-86 allele of the pfmdr 1 gene of Plasmodium falciparum by chloroquine and amodiaquine. *Parasitology*, 1997, 114, 205-11.

Dzekunov, SM; Ursos, LM; Roepe, PD. Digestive vacuoles pH of intact intraerythrocytic Plasmodium falciparum either sensitive or resistant to chloroquine. *Mol Biochem Parasitol*, 2000, 110, 107-24.

Endicott, JA; Ling, V. The biochemistry of P-glycoprotein-mediated multidrug resistance. *Annu Rev Biochem.*, 1989, 58, 137-71.

Enosse, S; Magnussen, P; Abacassamo, F; Gómez-Olivé, X; Rønn, AM; Thompson, R; Alifrangis, M. Rapid increase of Plasmodium falciparum dhfr/dhps resistant haplotypes, after the adoption of sulphadoxine-pyrimethamine as first line treatment in 2002, in southern Mozambique. *Malar J.*, 2008, 7, 115.

Fairley, NH. Sidelights on malaria in man obtained by subinoculation experiments. *Trans Soc Trop Med Hyg.*, 1947, 40, 621-76.

Ferdig, MT; Cooper, RA; Mu, J; Deng, B; Joy, D; Su, XZ; Wellems, TE. Dissecting the loci of low level quinine resistance in malaria parasites. *Mol Microbiol.*, 2004, 52, 985-97.

Fidock, DA; Nomura, T; Talley, AK; Cooper, RA; Dzekunov, SM; Ferdig, SM; Ursos, LM; Sidhu, AB; Naude, B; Deitsh, KW; Su, XZ; Wootton, JC; Roepe, PD; Wellems, TE. Mutations in the Plasmodium falciparum digestive vacuole transmembrane protein PfCRT and evidence for their role in chloroquine resistance. *Mol Cell*, 2000, 6, 861-71.

Fleckenstein, A; Kammermeier, H; Doring, HJ; Freund, HJ. On the method of action of new types of coronary dilatators with simultaneous oxygen-saving myocardial effects, prenylamine and iproveratril. *2. Z. Kreislauf*, 1967, 56, 839-58.

Foley, M; Deady, LW; Ng, K; Cowman, AF; Tilley, L. Photoaffinity labelling of chloroquine-binding proteins in Plasmodium falciparum. *J Biol Chem,* 1994, 269, 6955, 61.

Foote SJ; Thompson JK; Cowman AF; Kemp DJ. Amplification of the multidrug resistance gene in some chloroquine-resistant isolates of P. falciparum, *Cell*, 1989, 57, 921-30.

Foote, SJ; Kyle, DE; Martin, RK; Oduola, AM; Forsyth, K; Kemp, DJ; Cowman, AF. Several alleles of the multidrug-resistance gene are closely linked to chloroquine resistance in Plasmodium falciparum. *Nature*, 1990, 345, 255-8.

Foote, SJ; Cowman, AF. The mode of action and the mechanism of resistance to antimalarial drugs.*Acta Trop*., 1994, 56, 157-71

Gardner, MJ; Hall, N; Fung, E; White, O; Berriman, M; Hyman, RW; Carlton, JM; Pain, A; Nelson, KE; Bowman, S; Paulsen, IT; James, K; Eisen, JA; Rutherford, K; Salzberg, SL; Craig, A; Kyes, S; Chan, MS; Nene, V; Shallom, SJ; Suh, B; Peterson, J; Angiuoli, S; Pertea, M; Allen, J; Selengut, J; Haft, D; Mather, MW; Vaidya, AB; Martin, DM; Fairlamb, AH; Fraunholz, MJ; Roos, DS; Ralph, SA; McFadden, GI; Cummings, LM; Subramanian, GM; Mungall, C; Venter, JC; Carucci, DJ; Hoffman, SL; Newbold, C; Davis, RW; Fraser, CM; Barrell, B. Genome sequence of the human malaria parasite Plasmodium falciparum. *Nature*, 2002, 419, 498-511.

Gavigan, CS; Shen, M; Machado, SG; Bell, A. Influence of the Plasmodium falciparum P-glycoprotein homologue 1 (pfmdr1 gene product) on the antimalarial action of cyclosporin. *J Antimicrob Chemother*, 2007, 59, 197-203.

Georges, E; Zhang, JT; Ling, V. Modulation of ATP and drug binding by monoclonal antibodies against P-glycoprotein. *J Cell Physiol*., 1991, 148, 479-84.

Hameed, A. Antimalarial drug resistance in the Eastern Mediterranean Region. *East Mediterr Health J*., 2003, 9, 492-508.

Happi, CT; Gbotosho, GO; Folarin, OA; Bolaji, OM; Sowunmi, A; Kyle, DE; Milhous, W; Wirth, DF; Oduola, AM: Association between mutations in Plasmodium falciparum chloroquine resistance transporter and P. falciparum multidrug resistance 1 genes. and in vivo amodiaquine resistance in P. falciparum malariainfected children in Nigeria. *Am J Trop Med Hyg*., 2006, 75, 155-61.

Hastings, IM. Molecular markers as indicators of antimalarial drug failure rates. *Tropical Medicine and International Health*, 2007, vol 12 no 11, 1298-1301.

Hayward, R; Saliba, KJ; Kirk, K. Mutations in pfmdr1 modulate the sensitivity of Plasmodium falciparum to the intrinsic antiplasmodial activity of verapamil. *Antimicrob Agents Chemother*, 2005a, 49, 840-2.

Hayward, R; Saliba, KJ; Kirk, K. pfmdr1 mutations associated with chloroquine resistance incur a fitness cost in Plasmodium falciparum. *Mol Microbiol*., 2005b, 55, 1285-95.

Hayward, R; Saliba, KJ; Kirk, K. The pH of the digestive vacuole of Plasmodium falciparum is not associated with chloroquine resistance. *J Cell Sci*., 2006, 119, 1016-25.

Hollo, Z; Homolya, L; Davis, CW; Sarkadi, B. Calcein accumulation as a fluorometric functional assay of the multidrug transporter. *Biochem Biophys Acta*, 1994, 1191, 384-8.

Holmgren, G; Gil, JP; Ferreira, PM; Veiga, MI; Obonyo, CO; Bjorkman, A. Amodiaquine resistant Plasmodium falciparum malaria in vivo is associated with selection of pfcrt 76T and pfmdr1 86Y. *Infect Genet Evol*., 2006, 6, 309-14.

Homolya, L; Hollo, Z; Germann, UA; Pastan, I; Gottesman, MM; Sarkadi, B. Fluorescent cellular indicators are extruded by the multidrug resistance protein. *J Biol Chem*., 1993, 268, 21493-6.

Inselburg, J. Induction and isolation of artemisinin-resistant mutants of Plasmodium falciparum. *Am J Trop Med Hyg*., 1985, 34, 417-8.

Jiang, H; Patel, JJ; Yi, M; Mu, J; Ding, J; Stephens, R; Cooper, RA; Ferdig, MT; Su, XZ. Genome-wide compensatory changes accompany drug- selected mutations in the Plasmodium falciparum crt gene. *PLoS ONE*, 2008, 3, e2484.

Johnson, DJ; Fidock, DA; Mungthin, M; Lakshmanan, V; Sidhu, AB; Bray, PG; Ward, SA. Evidence for a central role for PfCRT in conferring Plasmodium falciparum resistance to diverse antimalarial agents. *Mol Cell*, 2004, 15, 867-77.

Johnson, DJ; Owen, A; Plant, N; Bray, PG; Ward, SA. Drug-regulated expression of Plasmodium falciparum P-glycoprotein homologue 1: a putative role for nuclear receptors. *Antimicrob Agents Chemother*, 2008, 52, 1438-45.

Karcz, S; Cowman, AF. Similarities and differences between the multidrug resistance phenotype of mammalian tumor cells and chloroquine resistance in P. falciparum. *Exp Parasitol*, 1991, 73, 233-40.

Karcz, SR; Galatis, D; Cowman, AF. Nucleotide binding properties of a P-glycoprotein homologue from Plasmodium falciparum. *Mol Biochem Parasitol*, 1993, 58, 269-76.

Klayman, DL. Qinghaosu (artemisinin): an antimalarial drug from China. *Science*, 1985, 228, 1049-55.

Klokouzas, A; Shahi, S; Hladky, SB; Barrand, MA; van Veen, HW. ABC transporters and drug resistance in parasitic protozoa. *Int J Antimicrob Agents*, 2003, 22, 301-17.

Klokouzas, A; Tiffert, T; van Schalkwyk, D; Wu, CP; van Veen, HW; Barrand, MA; Hladky, SB. Plasmodium falciparum expresses a multidrug resistance-associated protein. *Biochem Biophys Res Commun*., 2004, 321, 197-201.

Komarov, PG; Komarova, EA; Kondratov, RV; Christov-Tselkov, K; Coon, JS; Chernov, MV; Gudkov, AV. A chemical inhibitor of p53 that protects mice from the side effects of cancer therapy. *Science*, 1999, 285, 1733-7.

Krogstad, DJ; Gluzman, IY; Kyle, DE; Oduola, AMJ; Martin, SK; Milhous, W; Schlesinger, PH. Efflux of chloroquine from Plasmodium falciparum: mechanism of resistance, *Science*, 1987, 238, 1283-5.

Krogstad, DJ; Gluzman, IJ; Herwaldt, BL; Schlesinger, PH; Wellems, TE. Energy dependence of chloroquine accumulation and chloroquine efflux in Plasmodium falciparum, *Biochem Pharmacol*., 1992, 43, 57-62.

Lakshmanan, V; Bray, PG; Verdier-Pinard, D; Johnson, DJ; Horrocks, P; Muhle, RA; Alakpa, GE; Hughes, RH; Ward, SA; Krogstad, DJ; Sidhu, AB; Fidock, DA. A critical role for PfCRT K76T in Plasmodium falciparum verapamil-reversible chloroquine resistance. *EMBO J*., 2005, 24, 2294-305.

Laufer, MK; Thesing, PC; Eddington, ND; Masonga, R; Dzinjalamala, FK; Takala, SL; Taylor, TE; Plowe, CV. Return of chloroquine antimalarial efficacy in Malawi. *N Engl J Med*., 2006, 355, 1959-66.

Leed, A; DuBay, K; Ursos, LM; Sears, D; De Dios, AC; Roepe, PD. Solution structures of antimalarial drug-heme complexes. *Biochemistry*, 2002, 41, 10245-55.

Marfurt, J; Müller, I; Sie, A; Oa, O; Reeder, JC; Smith, TA; Beck, HP; Genton, B. The usefulness of twenty-four molecular markers in predicting treatment outcome with combination therapy of amodiaquine plus sulphadoxine-pyrimethamine against falciparum malaria in Papua New Guinea. *Malar J.*, 2008, 7, 61.

Martin, SK; Oduola, AM; Milhous, WK. Reversal of chloroquine resistance in Plasmodium falciparum by verapamil. *Science*, 1987, 235, 899-901.

Mayengue, PI; Ndounga, M; Davy, MM; Tandou, N; Ntoumi, F. In vivo chloroquine resistance and prevalence of the pfcrt codon 76 mutation in Plasmodium falciparum isolates from the Republic of Congo. *Acta Trop.*, 2005, 95, 219-25.

Mayer, TU; Kapoor, TM; Haggarty, SJ; King, RW; Schreiber, SL; Mitchison, TJ. Small molecule inhibitor of mitotic spindle bipolarity identified in a phenotype-based screen. *Science*, 1999, 286, 971-4.

Mehlotra, RK; Fujioka, H; Roepe, PD; Janeeh, O; Ursos, LMB; Jacobs-Lorena, V; McNamara, DT; Bockarie, MJ; Kazura, JW; Kyle, DE; Fidock, DA; Zimmerman, PA. Evolution of a unique Plasmodium falciparum chloroquine-resistance phenotype in association with pfcrt polymorphism in Papua New Guinea and South America. *Proc Natl Acad Sci.*, 2001, 98, 12689-94.

Menard, D; Matsika-Claquin, MD; Djalle, D; Yapou, F; Manirakiza, A; Dolmazon, V; Sarda, J; Talarmin, A. Association of failures of seven-day courses of artesunate in a non-immune population in Bangui, Central African Republic with decreased sensitivity of Plasmodium falciparum. *Am J Trop Med Hyg.*, 2005, 73, 616-21.

Menard, D; Yapou, F; Manirakiza, A; Djalle, D; Matsika-Claquin, MD; Talarmin, A. Polymorphisms in pfcrt, pfmdr1, dhfr genes and in vitro responses to antimalarials in Plasmodium falciparum isolates from Bangui, Central African Republic. *Am J Trop Med Hyg.*, 2006, 75, 381-7.

Millet, J; Torrentino-Madamet, M; Alibert, S; Rogier, C; Santelli-Rouvier, C; Mosnier, J; Baret, E; Barbe, J; Parzy, D; Pradines, B. Dihydroethanoanthracene derivatives as in vitro malarial chloroquine resistance reversal agents. *Antimicrob Agents Chemother*, 2004, 48, 2753-6.

Mu, J; Ferdig, MT; Feng, X; Joy, DA; Duan, J; Furuya, T; Subramanian, G; Aravind, L; Cooper, RA; Wootton, JC; Xiong, M; Su, XZ. Multiple transporters associated with malaria parasite responses to chloroquine and quinine.*Mol Microbiol.*, 2003, 49, 977-89.

Na-Bangchang, K; Congpuong, K. Current malaria status and distribution of drug resistance in East and Southeast Asia with special focus to Thailand. *Tohoku J Exp Med.*, 2007, 211, 99-113.

Ochong, EO; van den Broek, IV; Keus, K; Nzila, A. Short report: association between chloroquine and amodiaquine resistance and allelic variation in the Plasmodium falciparum multiple drug resistance 1 gene and the chloroquine resistance transporter gene in isolates from the upper Nile in southern Sudan. *Am J Trop Med Hyg.*, 2003, 69, 184-7.

Oduola, AM; Omitowoju, GO; Gerena, L; Kyle, DE; Milhous, WK; Sowunmi, A; Salako, LA. Reversal of mefloquine resistance with penfluridol in isolates of Plasmodium falciparum from south-west Nigeria. *Trans R Soc Trop Med Hyg.*, 1993, 87, 81-83.

Oduola, AM; Sowunmi, A; Milhous, WK; Brewer, TG; Kyle, DE; Gerena, L; Rossan, RN; Salako, LA; Schuster, BG. In vitro and in vivo reversal of chloroquine resistance in Plasmodium falciparum with promethazine. *Am J Trop Med Hyg.*, 1998, 58, 625-629.

Ohnmacht, CJ; Patel, AR; Lutz, RE. Antimalarials 7. Bis (trifluoromethyl)-(2-piperidyl)-4-quinolinemethanols. *J Med Chem*., 1971, 14, 926-8.

Peters, W. *Chemotherapy and Drug Resistance in Malaria*. London, Academic Press, 1987. p659-786.

Plowe, CV; Roper, C; Barnwell, JW; Happi, CT; Joshi, HH; Mbacham, W; Meshnick, SR; Mugittu, K; Naidoo, I; Price, RN; Shafer, RW; Sibley, CH; Sutherland, CJ; Zimmerman, PA; Rosenthal, PJ. World Antimalarial Resistance Network (WARN) III: Molecular markers for drug resistant malaria. *Malaria J*., 2007, 6, 121.

Povoa, MM; Adagu, IS; Oliveira, SG; Machado, RLD; Miles, MA; Warhurst, DC. Pfmdr 1 Asn1042Asp and Asp1246Tyr polymorphisms, thought to be associated with chloroquine resistance, are present in chloroquine-resistant and -sensitive Brazilian field isolates of Plasmodium falciparum. *Exp Parasitol*, 1998, 88, 64-8.

Pradines, B; Alibert-Franco, S; Houdoin, C; Mosnier, J; Santelli-Rouvier, C; Papa, V; Rogier, C; Fusai, T; Barbe, J; Parzy, D. In vitro reversal of chloroquine resistance in Plasmodium falciparum with dihydroethanoanthracene derivatives. *Am J Trop Med Hyg*., 2002, 66, 661-6.

Reed, MB; Saliba, KJ; Caruana, SR; Kirk, K; Cowman, AF. Pgh1 modulates sensitivity and resistance to multiple antimalarials in Plasmodium falciparum. *Nature*, 2000, 403, 906-9.

Riordan, JR; Deuchars, K; Kartner, N; Alon, N; Trent, J; Ling, V. Amplification of P-glycoprotein genes in multidrug-resistant mammalian cell lines. *Nature*, 1985, 316, 817-9.

Rosenberg, MF; Callaghan, R; Modok, S; Higgins, CF; Ford, RC. Three-dimensional structure of P-glycoprotein: the transmembrane regions adopt an asymmetric configuration in the nucleotide-bound state. *J Biol Chem*., 2005, 280, 2857-62.

Safa, AR. Photoaffinitylabeling of P-glycoprotein in multidrug-resistant cells. *Cancer Investig*., 1992, 10, 295-305.

Sanchez, CP; Wunsch, S; Lanzer, M. Identification of a chloroquine importer in Plasmodium falciparum: differences in import kinetics are genetically linked with the chloroquine-resistant phenotype. *J Biol Chem*., 1997, 272, 2652-8.

Sanchez, CP; Stein, W; Lanzer, M. Trans stimulation provides evidence for a drug efflux carrier as the mechanism of chloroquine resistance in Plasmodium falciparum. *Biochemistry*, 2003, 42, 9383-94.

Sangalli, BC. Role of the central histaminergic neuronal system in the CNS toxicity of the first generation H1-antagonists. *Prog Neurobiol*, 1997, 52, 145-57.

Schreiber, SL. Target-oriented and diversity-oriented organic synthesis in drug discovery. *Science*, 2000, 287, 1964-8.

Schmidt, LH; Crosby, R; Rasco, J; Vaughan, D. Antimalarial activities of various 4-quinolinemethanols with special attention to WR-142,490 (mefloquine). *Antimicrob Agents Chemother*, 1978[a], 13, 1011-30.

Schmidt, LH; Crosby, R; Rasco, J; Vaughan, D. Antimalarial activities of various 9-phenanthrenemethanols with special attention to WR-122,455 and WR-171,669 (mefloquine). *Antimicrob Agents Chemother*, 1978b, 14, 292-314.

Sidhu, AB; Verdier-Pinard, D; Fidock, DA. Chloroquine resistance in Plasmodium falciparum malaria parasites conferred by pfcrt mutations. *Science*, 2002, 298, 210-13.

Sidhu, AB; Valderramos, SG; Fidock, DA. pfmdr1 mutations contribute to quinine resistance and enhance mefloquine and artemisinin sensitivity in Plasmodium falciparum. *Mol Microbiol.*, 2005, 57, 913-26.

Sidhu, AB; Uhlemann, AC; Valderramos, SG; Valderramos, JC; Krishna, S; Fidock, DA. Decreasing pfmdr1 copy number in plasmodium falciparum malaria heightens susceptibility to mefloquine, lumefantrine, halofantrine, quinine, and artemisinin. *J Infect Dis.*, 2006, 194, 528-35.

Skovsgaard, T. Carrier-mediated transport of daunorubicin, adriamycin, and rubidazone in Ehrlich ascites tumour cells. *Biochem Pharmacol*, 1978, 27, 1221-7.

Suzuki, Y; Sugiyama, Y; Sawada, Y; Iga, T; Hanano, M. Assessment of contribution of alpha 1-acid glycoprotein to serum binding of basic drugs using serum treated with sulphosalicylic acid and DEAE-cellulose. *J Pharm Pharmacol*, 1985, 37, 712-7.

Sowunmi, A; Oduola, AM. Comparative efficacy of chloroquine/chlorpheniramine combination and mefloquine for the treatment of chloroquine- resistant Plasmodium falciparum malaria in Nigerian children. *Trans R Soc Trop Med Hyg.*, 1997, 91, 689-93.

Stahl, SM. Regulation of neurotransmitter receptors by desipramine and other antidepressant drugs: the neurotransmitter receptor hypothesis of antidepressant action. *J Clin Psychiatry*, 1984, 45, 37-45.

Tran, CV; Saier, MH Jr. The principal chloroquine resistance protein of Plasmodium falciparum is a member of the drug/metabolite transporter superfamily. *Microbiology*, 2004, 150, 1-3.

Tsuruo, T; Iida, H; Kitatani, Y; Yokota, K; Tsukagoshi, S; Sakurai, Y. Effects of quinidine and related compounds on cytotoxicity and cellular accumulation of vincristine and adriamycin in drug-resistant tumor cells. *Cancer Res.*, 1984, 44(10), 4303-4307.

Ursing, J; Zakeri, S; Gil, JP; Bjorkman, A. Quinoline resistance associated polymorphisms in the pfcrt, pfmdr1 and pfmrp genes of Plasmodium falciparum in Iran. *Acta Trop.*, 2006, 97, 352-6.

Ursos, LM; Dzekunov, SM; Roepe, PD. The effects of chloroquine and verapamil on digestive vacuolar pH of P. falciparum either sensitive or resistant to chloroquine. *Mol Biochem Parasitol*, 2000, 110, 125-34.

van Es, HH; Renkema, H; Aerts, H; Schurr, E. Enhanced lysosomal acidification leads to increased chloroquine accumulation in CHO cells expressing the pfmdr1 gene. *Mol Biochem Parasitol*, 1994, 68, 209-19.

Vijaykadga, S; Rojanawatsirivej, C; Cholpol, S; Phoungmanee, D; Nakavej, A; Wongsrichanalai, C. In vivo sensitivity monitoring of mefloquine monotherapy and artesunate-mefloquine combinations for the treatment of uncomplicated falciparum malaria in Thailand in 2003. *Trop Med Int Health*, 2006, 11, 211-9.

Tinto, H; Sanou, B; Dujardin, JC; Ouédraogo, JB; VAN Overmeir, C; Erhart, A; VAN Marck, E; Guiguemdé, TR; D'Alessandro, U. Usefulness of the Plasmodium falciparum chloroquine resistance transporter T76 genotype failure index for the estimation of in vivo chloroquine resistance in Burkina Faso. *Am J Trop Med Hyg.*, 2005, 73, 171-3.

Walker, JE; Saraste, M; Runswick, MJ; Gay, NJ. Distantly related sequences in the alpha- and beta-subunits of ATP synthase, myosin, kinases and other ATP-requiring enzymes and a common nucleotide binding fold. *EMBO J.*, 1982, 1, 945-51.

Waller, KL; Muhle, RA; Ursos, LM; Horrocks, P; Verdier-Pinard, D; Sidhu, AB; Fujioka, H; Roepe, PD; Fidock, DA. Chloroquine resistance modulated in vitro by expression levels of the Plasmodium falciparum chloroquine resistance transporter. *J Biol Chem.*, 2003, 278, 33593-601.

Wang, X; Mu, J; Li, G; Chen, P; Guo, X; Fu, L; Chen, L; Su, X; Wellems, TE. Decreased prevalence of the Plasmodium falciparum chloroquine resistance transporter 76T marker associated with cessation of chloroquine use against P. falciparum malaria in Hainan, People's Republic of China. *Am J Trop Med Hyg.*, 2005, 72, 410-4.

Ward, SA; Bray, PG; Mungthin, M; Hawley, SR. Current views on the mechanisms of resistance to quinoline-containing drugs in Plasmodium falciparum. *Ann Trop Med Parasitol*, 1995, 89, 121-4.

Warhurst, DC; Craig, JC; Adagu, IS. Lysosomes and drug resistance in malaria. *Lancet*, 2002, 360, 1527-9.

Warhurst, DC. Polymorphism in the Plasmodium falciparum chloroquine- resistance transporter protein links verapamil enhancement of chloroquine sensitivity with the clinical efficacy of amodiaquine. *Malar J.*, 2003, 2, 31.

Warsame, M; Wernsdorfer, WH; Bjorkman, A. Lack of effect of desipramine on the response to chloroquine of patients with chloroquineresistant falciparum malaria. *Trans R Soc Trop Med Hyg.*, 1992, 86, 235-6.

Warsame, M; Wernsdorfer, WH; Payne, D; Bjorkman, A. Susceptibility of Plasmodium falciparum in vitro to chloroquine, mefloquine, quinine and sulfadoxine/pyrimethamine in Somalia: relationships between the responses to the different drugs. *Trans R Soc Trop Med Hyg.*, 2001, 85, 565-9.

Wellems, TE; Panton, LJ; Gluzman, IY; Rosario, VE; Gwadz, RW; Walker-Jonah, A; Krogstad, DJ. Chloroquine resistance not linked to mdr-like genes in a Plasmodium falciparum cross. *Nature*, 1990, 345, 253-255.

Wellems, TE; Walker-Jonah, A; Panton, LJ. Genetic mapping of the chloroquine-resistance locus on Plasmodium falciparum chromosome 7. *Proc Natl Acad Sci.*, U. S. A., 1991, 88, 3382-6.

Wellems, TE; Plowe, CV. Chloroquine-resistant malaria. *J Infect Dis.*, 2001, 184, 770-6.

Chemotherapy of malaria and resistance to antimalarials. Geneva, World Health Organisation, 1973 (WHO Rechnical Report Series, N° 529).

In vitro micro-test (Mark III) for the assessment of the response of Plasmodium falciparum to chloroquine, mefloquine, quinine, amodiaquine, sulfadoxine/pyrimethamine and artemisinin. Instructions for use of the in vitro micro test kit (Mark III). Geneva, World Health Organization, 2001 (CTD/MAL/97.20 Rev.2).

World Health Organisation (WHO): Assessment and Monitoring of Antimalarial Drug Efficacy for the Treatment of Uncomplicated Falciparum Malaria. Geneva, Switzerland, World Health Organization (WHO) 2003, WHO/HTM/RBM/2003.50.

World Health Organization (2005) Susceptibility of Plasmodium falciparum to Antimalarial Drugs: Report on Global Monitoring 1996-2004. WHO, Geneva.

World Health Organization (WHO) 2006. Guidelines for the treatment of malaria, WHO Press, Geneva, 266 pp.

Wilson, CM; Serrano, AE; Wasley, A; Bogenschutz, MP; Shankar, AH; Wirth, DH. Amplification of a gene related to mammalian mdr genes in drug-resistant Plasmodium falciparum. *Science*, 1989, 244, 1184-6.

Wilson, CM; Volkman, SK; Thaithong, S; Martin, RK; Kyle, DE; Milhous, WK; Wirth, DF. Amplification of pfmdrl associated with mefloquine and halofantrine resistance in P. falciparum from Thailand. *Mol Biochem Parasitol*, 1993, 57, 151-60.

Wissing, F; Sanchez, CP; Rohrbach, P; Ricken, S; Lanzer, M. Illumination of the malaria parasite Plasmodium falciparum alters intracellular pH. Implications for live cell imaging. *J Biol Chem*., 2002, 277, 37747-55.

Ye, ZG; Van Dyke, K; Reversal of chloroquine resistance in falciparum malaria independent of calcium channels. *Biochem Biophys Res Commun*., 1988, 155, 476-81.

Zhang, H; Paguio, M; Roepe, PD. The antimalarial drug resistance protein Plasmodium falciparum chloroquine resistance transporter binds chloroquine. *Biochemistry*, 2004, 43, 8290-6.

Reviewed by Martin Friede, World Health Organization, Initiative for Vaccine Research, Switzerland.

In: Antimalarial Drugs: Costs, Safety and Efficacy
Editors: Emanuel Csizmadia and Istvan Kalnoky
ISBN: 978-1-60741-432-2

Chapter III

Acceptability of Intermittent Preventive Treatment (IPT) for Malaria in Infants (IPTi) in Tanzania: Lessons to Learn from IPT in Pregnancy (IPTp) in Mkuranga and Mufindi Districts

Godfrey M. Mubyazi**[1,2]*, *[3]**Paul Bloch**, [3]**Pascal Magnussen**, [4]**Ib C. Bygbjerg**, [3]**Jens Byskov**, [3]**Øystein Olsen**, [1]**Leonard E.G. Mboera** and [5]**Kristian S. Hansen

[1]National Institute for Medical Research (NIMR), P.O. Box 9653 Dar Es Salaam, Tanzania; [2]Amani Medical Research Centre, P.O Box 81 Muheza, Tanzania; [3]University of Copenhagen, DBL-Centre for Health Research and Development, Institute of Veterinary Pathobiology, Faculty of Life Sciences, [4]Copenhagen, Denmark; University of Copenhagen, Faculty of Health Sciences, Department of International Health, Immunology and Microbiology, Copenhagen, Denmark; [5]University of Aarhus, Institute of Public Health, Department of Health Services Research, DK-8000 Aarhus C, Denmark.

Abstract

Although clinical trials on intermittent-preventive-treatment (IPT) for malaria in infants (IPTi) are underway in Africa following the notable benefit of IPT during pregnancy (IPTp) using sulfadoxine-pyrimethamine (SP), evidence on the socio-economic determinants of the acceptability and viability of IPTi within infant clinic settings is inadequate. This paper reports a study on the acceptability of IPTi in two Tanzanian districts implementing IPTp using SP. Data were collected from 24 focus-group-discussions (FGDs) with pregnant-women and infants' mothers; interviews with

* Correspondence author: email: gmmubyazi@yahoo.co.uk;gmubyazi@hotmail.com

823 antenatal clients, 78 antenatal workers and 14 district health-managers among whom some also participated in FGDs. Qualitative findings indicated IPTi being appreciated among all the study population groups, considering the malaria situation. However, reservations were expressed about IPTi if SP is officially recommended. Skeptics pinpointed the side-effects, lack of antipyretic-effect and the general treatment failures of the SP drug. Another concern was that IPTi may face operational challenges such as those currently facing IPTp implementation, including the shortage of essential supplies, poor health facility infrastructural conditions, and low numbers, skills and motivation of human-resources. Based on a hypothetical question eliciting the pregnant women's willingness to allow (WTA) their babies to receive SP for IPTi if officially SP was the drug of choice, logistic regression analysis of the data obtained indicated variations among the respondents within and between the districts about in the WTA their babies to receive IPTi-SP. In conclusion, IPTi has limited potential acceptability in the healthcare system if SP is recommended, and despite some of the respondents having expressed speculative concerns, there is need for strong public sensitization before and during IPTi implementation towards enhancement of community and frontline health-workers' compliance.

Keywords: Intermittent-treatment, infants, pregnancy, acceptability, practicability, malaria.

Background

Malaria is the leading parasitic infectious disease in sub-Saharan Africa (SSA) in terms of morbidity, hospitalisation and mortality [1]. Pregnant women and children under the age of five years, especially the infants, are the most vulnerable [2-3]. In SSA where 90% of the global burden of malaria is concentrated, at least one child dies of malaria every 40 seconds [4].

Intermittent preventive treatment (IPT) describes the administration of a full course of an antimalarial drug to the population at risk at specified time intervals, irrespective of the whether or not one is infected [5-15]. Previous policies emphasised malaria chemoprophylaxis in pregnancy and children under-five through the weekly use of chloroquine [3, 6, 15]. Increased evidence on parasite resistance to this drug in SSA prompted the World Health Organization (WHO) to recommend alternative antimalarials to be considered by SSA governments [16]. Sulfadoxine-pyrimethamine (SP) was recommended and is currently used for IPT during pregnancy (IPTp) [12]. Randomised-controlled trials in Tanzania and several other SSA countries have demonstrated the safety of SP for IPT in infants (IPTi) if properly administered through routine EPI (Expanded Programme for Immunization) services [13-14]. Other studies have also demonstrated that Amodiaquine (AQ) is another potentially useful drug for IPTi [9, 17-18]. Guidelines for the administration of both IPTp and IPTi emphasise the practice of direct observation therapy (DOT) protocol [16, 18].

The results from the completed and ongoing IPTi-SP trials may prompt policy-makers to officially approve the scaling-up of this novel intervention strategy in the national healthcare delivery systems [18-19]. However, the urgency of information on the possible operational challenges including its acceptability to the mothers or infants' caretakers is noted [6, 9, 11-12]. This is because not all interventions recommended based on clinical trials would be operationally feasible in real life contexts [20]. In other words, there is no guarantee that a new strategy like IPTi will be operationally effective without challenges. This includes the unknown long-term sustainability and target users' adherence, considering among other things, the questions about their socio-cultural acceptability [21].

Using two districts as a case, the present study investigated the perceived acceptability of IPTi from the viewpoints of the members of district council health management teams (CHMT), frontline health workers (HWs) at health facility (HF) level, pregnant women currently using antenatal care (ANC) services who were the expected mothers of infant children (infants), and the mothers of infant children whose children were eligible for child health services usually delivered at children's clinics in Tanzania.

Methods

Study design: This is a sub-study of the overall cross-sectional case study focusing on potential acceptability of IPTi based on data collected from multiple sources of information [22] in two districts- *Mkuranga* and *Mufindi*. But this study was not part of any clinical trial and therefore does not present findings from such kind of trials. Rather it was designed to explore the possible feasibility in terms of acceptability and practicability of the IPTi strategy in the local socio-cultural and healthcare system settings if such a strategy comes to be officially recommended in Tanzania. The data for this sub-study was collected between November 2005 and January 2007. Despite focus being on IPTi with SP, the experience of the study populations with the implementation of IPTp with SP in districts in areas with different malaria transmission intensities and socio-cultural and economic characteristics, was solicited.

Research Team. The overall study involved a multidisciplinary team from the following fields: health economics, sociology, medicine, pharmacology, public health, and health policy, planning and management.

Study areas: Two districts were covered, namely (i) *Mkuranga*, located on the Coast Region near Dar es Salaam along the Indian Ocean on the eastern part of Tanzania, and (ii) *Mufindi*, in the southern highlands of Tanzania, particularly located about ≥470km away from Dar es Salaam. Mkuranga has a stable and perennial transmission of malaria [23]. Most of the residents are small-scale farmers and earn less than US$1 per day [24]. Mufindi has two main climatic zones: the highland zone which is colder with temperatures ranging between 15°C and 20°C (November-February) with the minimum of 13.2 °C in July (District Council Comprehensive Health Plan, 2006-7, unpublished). It is one of the districts with unstable malaria transmission in Tanzania [23].

Study Participants

The district CHMT (previously called *District Health Management Team*) members who involved the district medical officer (DMO), district hospital medical officer in-charge, district reproductive and child health coordinator (DRCHC), district health officer (DHO), district health secretary (DHS), district nursing officer (DNO), and other CHMT members performing other roles [25-26]. These were involved as the officers responsible for health planning, health service supervision, monitoring and evaluation as well as district health service management in general.

The frontline HWs include those directly involved in ANC services (nursing and laboratory personnel) and their immediate superiors at HF level who are mainly the clinical officers (COs) or nursing officers (NOs). As HWs who confront ANC clients, they were expected to share their experience about women's perceptions of SP for malaria treatment as well as their own views.

Current ANC clients include pregnant women who were traced at HF level as they were attending ANC clinics on particular days. Follow up was made of other pregnant women in the villages falling within the catchment areas of either public or private HFs. This was done in an attempt to search for information from the women who by being interviewed far from HFs might be more open to express themselves than their counterparts who were traced at HFs, as it was experienced during the pilot phase of the present study. Infants' mothers (recent ANC users) were included based on the assumption that as the mothers of small children, they might have recently faced malaria episodes and possibly treated their children with anti-malarial drugs including SP and/or other antimalarial drugs. Such mothers were also expected to (a) have personally used SP for IPTp during the pregnancy period of their current babies or sometimes when they were not pregnant, (a) express themselves more confidently than pregnant women, as it was experienced by the research team during the pilot phase of this study.

Sampling

CHMT members at district level: District CHMT members and HWs were *purposefully.* Depending on who were available for the study within the planned period, 8 and 7 CHMT members in Mufindi and Mkuranga districts respectively were eventually involved.

HF-based study participants: In both districts, 28 HFs with ANC clinics were covered, targeting the frontline HWs and the ANC clients. Using a multistage sampling method, HFs were selected from different divisions and wards. In total, 10 dispensaries were randomly selected using a list of all the dispensaries in the district with ANC clinics. Of the selected dispensaries in Mkuranga 5 were private (non-governmental), among which 2 were owned by the religious/faith-based organization and 3 were private-for-profit/commercial). The rest 5 were owned by the government. Also, the only 1 district government hospital and only 2 government health centres (HC) in Mkuranga were directly selected without randomization as was done for the only 2 hospitals (1 government, 1 private) in Mufindi. In the later district, 3 government dispensaries were selected randomly (including 2 government, and 1 faith-based) while of the 10 dispensaries selected, only 2 were faith-based and the rest were government. Noting that most of the HFs were understaffed, the number of the different cadres of the HWs approached at each HF depended on the presence of the targeted staff cadres. Therefore, selection was done using a convenient sampling method to arrive at 78 HWs in total (35 in Mkuranga and 43 in Mufindi). Also, 417 and 406 ANC clients in

Mkuranga and Mufindi, respectively were selected as they were coming out of the HF after receiving the ANC services. Since on most of the study days, the ANC attendance rates were as low as ≤10 pregnant women, a simple random sampling method was applied only on days when the ANC attendance rates were relatively higher.

Village-based participants: Six villages were selected in each district based on a multistage random sampling strategy. From the villages, pregnant women and mothers of infants were purposefully selected to participate in group discussions. Two groups, each having 6-12 women were confronted per village, one group including pregnant women and another one the infants' mothers. Twelve groups were confronted per district.

Data Collection Methods

The research instruments including guides for focus group discussion (FGDs), in-depth-interview (IDI), and semi-structured interviews (SSI) were used and written in Swahili language. The tools were pre-tested and tried again in the pilot survey undertaken in Temeke and Ilala districts of Dar es Salaam and some rural settings of Mkuranga district. These tools contained the questions that were similar to those adopted in previous surveys in Korogwe district [26] and Muheza districts in Tanzania (Mubyazi GM 2006, unpublished data: *Annual Joint Scientific Conference Abstract of NIMR*), targeting district health managers, pregnant women and mothers' of infants.

Focus Group Discussion (FGDs): These involved (i) the district CHMT members in Mufindi only and (ii) pregnant women and infants' mothers at village levels. Conduction of a FGD with CHMT members in Mkuranga was not possible as the key members could not be gathered for a group meeting due to the work-pressure they were facing. Instead, such members participated in the IDI. As suggested by all the CHMT member participants in the FGD, the DMO, Pharmacists, DRCHC and DHS were followed later individually after the FGD to provide additional information. FGD with the pregnant women and infants' mothers were conducted separately since during the pilot survey it was noted that it was mostly the infants' mothers who were more open and dominant during the discussion than the pregnant women when the two were mixed in the same group. Field notes were taken by hand and validated later by transcription of the audio tapes.

Study themes

Although interest was in the perceived acceptability of IPTi using SP, the study broadly explored aspects related to the participants' experiences with and views on use of SP for IPTp, preferences to SP in the existence of alternative drugs, safety of SP, and logistics in the deliverability and utilization of SP for malaria chemoprevention in pregnancy and infants. The district CHMT members and some of the HWs were selected to comment on how they perceived about the feasibility of IPTi in local clinic settings in light of their experience with the implementation of IPTp and other health services at HFs.

Data Handling and Processing

Data were checked for quality each day immediately after collection. Debriefing sessions among the research team members were conducted to discuss strategies for improving the data collection. Dropping any misleading data during the data entry process was done. The responses to open-ended questions from the SSI were double entered along with the pre-coded ones in the database prepared in EPI-info version 6.1 (CDC Atlanta). Notes from IDI and FGDs were expanded immediately after collection by each fieldworker and discussed by the research team during debriefing. The handwritten notes and transcripts of the discussions taped on the particular day were compiled after being collated and expanded as the data collection process was going on. The overall transcription of taped discussions was done verbatim simultaneously with the handwritten notes at the end of data collection [22, 27].

Data Analysis

Quantitative data

Data from SSI were analyzed using STATA version 8.2 programme. Beginning with descriptive statistics indicating the frequencies of the responses obtained on specific questions, the next step was to undertake bivariate and multivariate logistic regression analyses of the data from the exit interviews with the ANC clients. The hypothetical question used to define the dependent variable stated as follows: "*Suppose when you breast-feed your child and want to protect her from malaria, and were asked by a health worker if you your baby could be given SP for malaria preventive treatment, would you allow your baby have SP*?". This question had three coded answer options: *yes*, *no* and *it depends* (this including the *maybe and Don't know* sorts of responses). This made it possible to obtain each of the individual respondent's perceived or stated *willingness to allow her baby to be given SP for IPTi* (WTA-IPTi), should the IPTi strategy be officially recommended in real health service situation. The dummy variables for the dependent question were 1=Yes and 0=Else (with 'No', 'Don't know', and missing values). The codes for the responses were defined in advance based on the experience obtained from the pilot survey phase. The design dummy variables for the predictor (explanatory) variables were defined accordingly, based on either the responses given to the study question or the characteristics of the study individuals (Table 3-6). Bivariate regression analysis was used as a basis for identifying the useful predictor variables for inclusion in the multivariate regression model (Table 1). This was in light of the study assumptions (Box 1), the aim being to get the first impression on the association between the dependent variable and each of the predefined predictor variables/covariates [28].

Despite recognition that intuitive model building runs a risk of ignoring (or improperly using) important relationships [29-30], analysis for the present study includes only the variables that seemed relevant to the study assumptions and objectives. Assessment was done on whether or not there were statistically significant differences in the stated WTA-IPTi between the ANC clients with different demographic characteristics, experiences and opinions in relation to the use of SP during or before the respondent's current pregnancy, SP treatment outcomes, and advantages of SP over other anti-malarial drugs (Tables 5-6). Spearman's chi-square tests were also conducted to indicate some relationships that were not directly reflected by the bivariate logistic regression models, for example, in comparing the statistical differences in the proportions of particular responses or characteristics. The difference in the result on a particular test was considered to be statistically significant when $p \leq 0.05$. Although in the regression analyses the odds ratios (OR) and their corresponding confidence intervals (CI) are often reported, the corresponding p-values were also reported on several occasions in attempt to inform the readers who may be interested knowing the significance status of the compared statistical differences in the observations. During the pilot survey phase and actual implementation of the present study it was noted that some women had visited ANC several times than the records shown on their ANC cards. But, in the regression analyzes carried out and presented in the present paper, the covariate that was fitted in the regression model was the number visits actually recorded on each of the respondents' ANC card.

Box 1. Theoretical assumptions concerning the predictor variables fitted in the logistic regression models

Gravidity: - women of high gravidity were expected to be more supportive to IPTi with SP than the primigravidæ who might have been less experienced with malaria in pregnancy and malaria attack to infants

Awareness of SP as a drug recommended for IPTp – Those aware were expected to know why IPTp was recommended and therefore understanding the possible benefits a similar intervention for the infants

Experience with adverse treatment outcome with SP – Those with such an experience were expected to be less supportive to SP for IPTi than those who had not (due to the perceived risks)

Previous use of SP – Those who previously used SP during current pregnancy or at other times were expected to have appreciated the benefit/advantage of SP for malaria treatment more than those who had not, assuming that the former had not experienced serious adverse effects

Preference to antimalarial drug other than SP – from the economic demand viewpoint, consumers may substitute goods available in the market, subject to their preferences. Therefore, those who expressed their preferences to drugs alternative to SP were expected to be less supportive to SP for IPTi than those who did not

Education – It was envisioned that health education helps people to accept an intervention. People with relatively higher education were expected to understand health education messages better than those with low levels of education.

Frequencies of ANC visits – The more a pregnant woman visited a clinic the more chances she was expected to have attended health education sessions including messages related to IPT. So, the more such clients were expected to be supportive to malaria preventive strategies through IPTp and IPTi than those with less visits

Place of interview – Government HFs were expected to comply with national guidelines by sensitizing their clients on SP because they have no profit motive unlike some (if not most) of HFs run NGOs. Among the latter HFs, HWs might be promote and prescribe other antimalarial drugs in stock due to easy accessibility or those preferred by the clients (*demand-driven prescription*).

Table 1. Description of the dummy variables developed from the explanatory variables and used in the bivariate and multivariate logistic regression models.

(a)	Education: This was a design variable categorised into three levels and each level having dichotomised as (1=having attained that level and 0 =not attained that level/else) School_1 (1 = attended at primary school at whatever level; 0 = not gone to school at all/else) School_2 (1 = completed form four secondary or higher; 0 = not reached that level/else)
(b)	Age of the respondent: (1 = less than 20 years; 0 = else (≥20 years/else)
(c)	Gravidity of the respondent: (1 = Multigravid; 0 = Primigravid/else)
(d)	ANC visits made as recorded on the ANC card: (1 = at least twice; 0 = 1st visit/else)
(e)	Awareness of the pregnancy trimester not recommended for using SP: (1 = aware; 0 = Not aware/else)
(f)	Whether previously used SP in the current pregnancy: (1 = Yes; 0 = No/else)
(g)	Whether previously used SP when not pregnant (1 = Yes; 0 =No/else)
(h)	Whether experienced SP adverse treatment outcomes: (1 = Yes; 0 = No/else)
(i)	Whether would opt for non-SP drug if given the opportunity: (1 = Yes; 0 = No/else)
(j)	Whether interviewed at a government health facility/clinic (1=Yes; 0=No/else)

***Qualitative data*:** These were analyzed manually, looking at the study themes, pattern and contents of the information obtained. Data analysis began during the data collection process [31-33]. Since each of the study team members listened to the audio-recorded interviews while noting down the key points from the study participants without interpreting them, the debriefing meetings allowed a shared discussion and comments after each one's notes were cross-checked with those taken by other research team members. A comprehensive interpretation of the general transcription was done thereafter, taking into account the common experiences and views versus the contrasting ones, as noted from the study populations in both districts.

Ethical issues: The study that received national ethical approval from the Ministry of Health and Social Welfare through the Medical Research Coordinating Committee. It adhered to the International Ethical Guidelines for Biomedical Research Involving Human Subjects [34], in seeking informed consent from all the authorities and target respondents/participants from the district level through the village and HF levels. This includes assurance given to the participants regarding anonymity of any confidential information provided, and asking for their approval to disseminate the un-confidential information obtained for official use and a wider and public audience, and asking the respondents to sign a consent form or give their thumbprint for those who were illiterate.

Results

Characteristics of the Study Population Groups

CHMT members: The study involved district: medical officers; nursing officers; pharmacists and assistant/acting pharmacists; health officers; laboratory technologists; TB and Leprosy coordinator (Mkuranga only); dental officer (Mufindi only); reproductive and child health coordinators (RCHC); and public health nurses who were co-opted members to the CHMT.

ANC workers: Of the 78 ANC workers interviewed, 25 (32.1%) were medical attendants (previously known as nurse auxiliaries), 18 (23.1%) were COs, 9 (11.5%) were public health nurse grade 'B' (PHNB), 8 (10.3%) were nurse midwives (NMD), 8 (10.3%) were maternal and child aides (MCHA) and the rest 7 (8.9%) included laboratory and assistant health officers. Moreover, of the 78 interviewees 50 (64.1%) were found working at government (public) HFs and the rest at private HFs (13 found at faith-based HFs, 9 at the Unilever Tea Company HF; 6 at other private-for-profit HFs). In terms of HF levels where the interviewees were found, 16 (20.5%) and 11 (14.1%) of the respondents were found at HC and hospital levels, respectively and the rest majority 51 (65.4%) were met at dispensary levels. Females HWs totalled 62 (79.5%) of all interviewees. On average, the respondents had worked for 8.3 years (range: 0.5–24 years) at the HF they were found.

Pregnant women traced at ANC clinics: The median age of the pregnant women was 25 years (range: 15-47 years (only for 810 respondents from both districts). Among the 823 interviewees, 165 (20.0%) stated to have never delivered any child before, as was confirmed by observation made on their ANC cards. In terms of formal education attained, literacy rate in Mufindi was significantly higher than in Mkuranga (Table 2).

Table 2. Level of education attained by the ANC clients interviewed in Mkuranga and Mufindi districts.

Level of schooling attained	Mkuranga (N=417)	Mufindi (N=402)
Not gone to school at all	179 (42.9%)	46 (11.4%)
Primary school but less than standard 7	49 (11.8%)	32 (7.9%)
Standard 7 primary school	180 (43.2%)	308 (76.2%)
Secondary school but less than form four	0	11 (2.7%)
Ordinary level secondary school (form four)	2 (0.5%)	4 0.9%)
High school	0	1 (0.5%)
Higher than high school (University or other)	7 (1.7%)	0

Attitudes towards SP and IPTi among the Frontline HWs

CHMT members: All the eight CHMT members in Mkuranga and only three of their counterparts in Mufindi doubted about wider acceptability of SP for IPTi. The reasons for their doubts are detailed later along with other respondents' expressions noted under the qualitative findings section.

Frontline HWs: Among the 78 interviewees, 42 (53.9%) had reservations on IPTi-SP. Thirteen (16.7%) of the HWs reported to have dealt with the ANC clients who claimed to have experienced adverse effects of the SP administered to them before. Moreover, 18 (23.1%) respondents reported to have dealt with the clients who were hesitant to take SP for IPTp in fear of SP treatment outcomes.

ANC clients: Asked if they would be willing to allow their infants to be given SP for IPTi, 27.8% out of 349 respondents to this question in Mkuranga stated to be willing; 24.6% were unwilling and the rest (47.6%) were uncertain (as they said 'It depends'). In Mufindi, 44.9% out of the 296 respondents stated to be willing; 23.9% were unwilling while the rest (32.2%) were uncertain. Considering those who said 'Yes' to the question - indicating their willingness to allow (WTA) their babies to receive IPTi with SP and those who said 'No' indicating their unwillingness (Figure 1), the WTA-IPTi was significantly higher in among the Mufindi respondents than their counterparts in Mkuranga ($\chi^2(1)=5.4$; $p=0.019$).

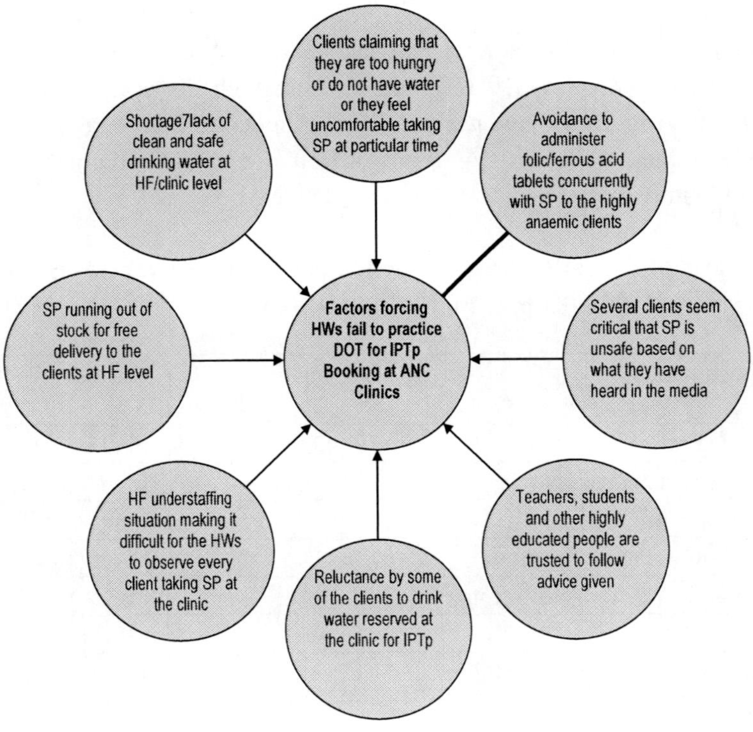

Figure 1. Key factors contributing to low compliance with DOT for IPTp by the frontline HWs and ANC clients, as reported by the frontline HWs in Mkuranga and Mufindi districts, Tanzania

SP was perceived as being too strong to infants. This was explained in terms of its causes on physical exhaustion (in the arm and leg joints) and dizziness to adult people, a situation that is less tolerable to infants. SP was also perceived to have no antipyretic effect (slowness in lowering fever and even raising body temperature) and causing nausea, and requiring its users to take much water or other soft drinks when taking it in order to avoid physical exhaustion and dizziness conditions while it is difficult to make an infant child to be forced to take adequate water /juices (Table 3). Some respondents reported to have heard that SP may cause stillbirth.

Table 3. Responses regarding experience with use of SP and reasons for not being willing to agree/allow SP for IPTi among the antenatal clients interviewed in Mkuranga and Mufindi district cases, Tanzania.

Particulars/Observations from Descriptive Analysis	Results for each District	
	Mkuranga	Mufindi
Why wouldn't you allow SP for IPTi? (*≥1 answer allowed*)	(n=74)	(n=68)
If too strong to adults then what about infants	64 (86.5%)	45 (66.2%)
Can kill my baby	1 (1.4%)	4 (5.9%)
My baby can get blindness	0 (0.0%)	9 (13.2%)
Other perceived effects (e.g. skin reaction)	4 (5.4%)	6 (8.8%)
Already the baby was prevented in the womb through EPI/IPTp services given to the mother	1 (1.4%)	2 (2.9%)
Never used it myself so can't give my baby/child	3 (4.1%)	2 (2.9%)
Silent/No reason given	1 (1.4%)	0 (0.0%)

Table 4 indicates the proportions of the respondents on specific questions based on which the explanatory variables used in the logistic regression models were defined. By comparing data for both districts combined, it was observed that WTA-IPTi in general terms was significantly higher among the clients: (i) interviewed at government HFs than those at private HFs (ii) who reported to have used SP previously during pregnancy than those who had not (iii) those who would opt for an anti-malarial drug other than SP if they were allowed to choose against SP than those who would not. Gravidity and age of the client had not shown any significant influence on WTA-IPTi. In both districts most of the respondents were found at government HFs (Table 4), albeit statistically the respondents interviewed at government HFs in Mufindi were significantly more than their counterparts in Mkuranga ($p<0.001$). This was expected because more private HFs were involved in Mkuranga than in Mufindi. Previous use of SP during the current pregnancy was reported by 55.2% of the clients in Mkuranga, significantly less than 73.2% of their counterparts with the same experience in Mufindi ($p<0.001$). Also, previous use of SP during the current pregnancy period was reported by 32.5% of the respondents in Mufindi as compared to a significantly less proportion of their counterparts with the same experience in Mkuranga ($p=0.001$). Preference to drugs other than SP was expressed by 13.7% of the respondents in Mkuranga, significantly less than 31.4% of their counterparts in Mufindi ($p=0.019$). In Mkuranga, 42.9% of the respondents had not acquired any formal education, this being significantly higher than 11.2% of their counterparts in Mufindi ($p<0.001$).

Table 4. Descriptive results on ANC clients' personal characteristics and experiences with pregnancy, use of SP, and attitudes towards SP for IPTi if recommended in Tanzania.

Explanatory variables defined based on the study questions and their design dummy variables (*missing responses were excluded in the statistical tests using chi-square*)	Mkuranga District		Mufindi District		P-Values
	No. of respondents (n)	*Frequenc of responses (%)*	*No. of respondents (n)*	*Frequency of responses (%)*	
Place of interview (1=Government clinic; 0=NGO clinic)					
Government	248	59.5	342	84.7	<0.001
Previous use of SP for malaria treatment during current pregnancy (1=Yes; 0=No)					
1=Yes	196	55.2	224	73.2	<0.001
Previous use of SP at times other than current pregnancy (1=Yes; 0=No)					
Yes	85	24.1	99	32.5	0.019
Previous experience with adverse effect of treatment with SP (1=Yes; 0=No)					
Yes	53	24.2	55	20.9	0.113
Awareness that SP is not recommended for IPTp at particular trimester of pregnancy (1=Yes, 0=No/Don't know)					
Yes	48	13.3	57	18.5	>0.05
Preferences to drugs other than SP if choice were allowed (1=Yes; 0=No)					
Yes	47	13.7	14	4.8	0.001
Number of deliveries (including abortions if any) ever had so far (1=None; 0=one or more)					
None	88	26.7	76	18.9	>0.05
Highest level of formal education attained so far (1=Never gone to school; 0=primary or more)					
Never gone to school	179	42.9	46	11.4	<0.001
Age in years based on confirmed on the ANC card (1=less than 20 years; 0=more than 20)					
Place of interview (1=Government clinic; 0=NGO clinic)					
Less than 20 years	69	16.5	45	11.2	>0.05
Number of visits to the clinic during the current pregnancy as reported (verbally) by the respondent (1=first visit; 0=two or more)					
First visit	147	35.7	168	41.6	>0.05
Number of the visits made to ANC clinic as shown on the respondents' ANC card (1=one visit; 0= two or more visits)					
1=One visit	161	38.8	176	44.4	>0.05

Note: As usual in logistic regression analyses, missing variables were coded and accounted for in developing the design dummy variables (Table 7 and Table 8). The chi-square tests indicated here are meant for comparing the statistical differences between the two districts per each of the variables listed.

Empirical Findings

The stated WTA-IPTi based on bivariate regression Analyses

Results from bivariate regression analyses using the data for each district are shown separately but in the same table. Notably, there were some common results across both districts as well as mixed results in terms of the association between the respondents' stated WTA-IPTi and the individual predictor variables (Table 5). The stated WTA-IPTi by the respondents who had previously used SP during their current pregnancy or sometimes when they were not pregnant was significantly higher than their counterparts who had not used SP any time previously, as expected *a priori* (Box 2). Only in Mufindi, the WTA-IPTi of the respondents aged 20 years or above (≥20) was significantly higher than of their counterparts who were younger (p=0.05). WTA-IPTi was significantly higher among the respondents who had visited clinics many times more than those who had fewer visits only in Mkuranga (p=0.030) while there was no any difference noted among their counterparts from Mufindi. The respondents found at government HFs expressed a higher WTA-IPTi than those found at the private HFs in both districts, but the association was statistically significant in Mkuranga only (p=0.009).

The stated WTA-IPTi based on a multivariate logistic regression analysis.

Table 6 shows the results from a multivariate regression analysis. The statistically significant predictor variables included in the model include those that had indicated either a higher odds ratio (OR) or a p≤0.05 in the previous bivariate regression model illustrated in Table 5. Through the elimination processes, several variables were dropped from the original multivariate regression model in attempt to find out the most parsimonious model. In comparison with the reference groups, the results on the data for each district treated separately indicated that the perceived/stated WTA-IPTi was:

- higher among the respondents who had previously used SP, both during their current pregnancy and sometimes when they were not pregnant than those who had not. However, the observed difference in the WTA-IPTi was statistically significant when comparing those who had had used or not used SP in their current pregnancies (p<0.001), in both study districts. On the other hand, the those who reported to have used SP previously were more likely to be willing to allow IPTi with SP than those who had not, but at the time they were not pregnant. However, the difference in the stated WTA-IPTi was statistically significant among the respondents found in Mufindi only (p=0.011).
- Knowledge of the gestational age of pregnancy in which SP is not recommended for IPTp was associated with a higher likelihood of the WTA-IPTi than not in the Mkuranga case, the difference was statistically significant (p=0.001). In the Mufindi case, the respondents who were knowledgeable about this recommendation were also more likely to be willing to allow IPTi-SP than those who were un-knowledgeable, but the difference was not statistically significant.
- Also, the age of the respondent consistently indicated to be a significant predictor of their WTA-IPTi (as noted in the bivariate analysis) in Mufindi case only where the

respondents aged ≥20 years were more likely to allow IPTi-SP than the younger ones (p=0.005). Other results have been interpreted accordingly in the discussion section.

FGDs and interviews

Among the different study participants, there was a mixture of perceptions regarding the advantages and practicability of IPTi with SP as categorised below.

Table 5. Results from bivariate logistic regression analyses of the association between the ANC clients' stated WTA-IPTi with SP and several explanatory variables: case study of Mkuranga and Mufindi districts, Tanzania (*the details shown in italics clarify explanatory variable concerned which was used for comparison against their reference variables* i.e. the comparison groups).

WTA-IPTi Predictor Variable (*Reference Group*)	MKURANGA district			MUFINDI district		
	OR	95% Confidence Interval		OR	95% Confidence Interval	
• Place of interview (1=*Government clinic*)	2.34	1.24	4.41	1.24	0.68	2.24
• Gravidity (1=*Multigravidæ*)	.56	0.30	1.05	1.21	0.72	2.03
• Age of the respondent (*≥20 years*)	.67	0.40	1.16	1.71	1.00	2.92
• Formal education (1=*attained at least some primary education i.e. ≤ std. 7*)	1.29	0.81	2.06	.65	0.35	1.21
• Attended secondary education or higher (1=*Yes*)	.41	0.05	3.29	2.10	0.77	5.74
• Number of ANC visits recorded on the ANC card (1=*≥ 2 visits*)	1.28	1.02	1.59	1.09	0.89	1.35
• Awareness that SP is not recommended for IPTp at some stage/age of pregnancy (1=*Yes*)	4.48	2.41	8.35	1.12	0.62	2.02
• Previous use of SP in current pregnancy (1=*Yes*)	6.50	3.78	11.18	7.57	4.48	12.79
• Previous use of SP when not pregnant (1=*Yes*)	3.05	1.83	5.09	2.44	1.53	3.89
• Experience with SP adverse treatment effects (1=*Yes*)	3.62	1.99	6.58	1.43	0.79	2.56
• Preference to drugs other than SP if allowed (1=*Yes*)	1.65	0.85	3.19	1.55	0.53	4.58

Note: The two explanatory variables related to the respondent's schooling were treated separately as design variables aimed at assessing whether or not the different levels of formal education had any different association with the dependent variable

Table 6. Results of fitting data to the multivariate logistic regression models in eliciting the ANC clients' perceived WTA-IPTi in Mkuranga and Mufindi districts, Tanzania if SP was the drug recommended *(the variables included are only those who were statistically associated with the dependent variable in the bivariate analyses).*

WTA-IPTi Predictor Variable (*Reference Group*)	MKURANGA district			MUFINDI district		
	OR	95% Confidence Interval		OR	95% Confidence Interval	
• Place of interview (1=*Government clinic*)	1.91	0.95	3.81	.79	0.39	1.62
• Gravidity (1=*Multigravidœ*)	.51	0.23	1.15	.93	0.45	1.94
• Age of the respondent (*≥20 years*)	1.09	0.55	2.16	3.11	1.41	6.83
• Awareness that SP is not recommended for IPTp at some pregnancy trimester (1=*Yes*)	3.24	1.57	6.66	.74	0.39	1.43
• Number of ANC visits recorded on the ANC card (1=*≥ 2 visits*)	1.04	0.79	1.35	.88	0.68	1.12
• Previous use of SP during current pregnancy (1=*Yes*)	4.83	2.71	8.62	9.66	5.32	17.54
• Previous use of SP when not pregnant (1=*Yes*)	1.31	0.71	2.45	2.06	1.18	3.58
• Experience with SP adverse treatment effects (1=*Yes*)	1.81	0.91	3.57	0.63	0.32	1.25

CHMT members: In Mkuranga district, the DMO was of the following view regarding people's perception of the efficacy of SP: "Imagine everyone would expect that by any means these kind of babies (newborn infants) would be protected through their parents who were given SP at clinics and whose mothers are advised to sleep under- and sometimes given ITNs free of charge. But why are they found symptomatic or parasitemic for malaria?". All of the CHMT members in Mkuranga anticipated the possibility of the general public to lose trust in SP after the new first-line drug combination therapy- 'artemether-lumefantrine' (ALu) (or coartem) has been officially introduced in January 2007.

In Mufindi district, similar views on the possibility of low target users' trust in SP for preventive and actual treatment of malaria were presented by two CHMT members. Contrary to the confidence expressed by the rest of the discussants in her group regarding community perception of SP after the introduction of ALu, the DRCHC for Mufindi expressed her speculated doubt: "*Unless there is systematic research undertaken to ascertain the feasibility of IPTi there is likely to be some non-compliance as it happened to IPTp when it was noted later that most of the pregnant women who initially were allowed to take SP at home were throwing the drug away*". Furthermore, the DRCHC viewed that children would be exposed to the use of drugs without confirmatory diagnosis that may perpetuate the growth of parasite resistance. This view was partly shared by her DMO who showed some reservation with the current practice of the Integrated Management of Childhood Illnesses (IMCI) in some districts through which children under the age of five years are given anti-malarial drugs on presumptive basis - without laboratory confirmation.

Box 2. Summary and description of the results obtained from the bivariate regression analyses to determine the association between the pregnant women's perceived WTA-IPTi (dependent variable) and the predictor (explanatory) variables listed in Table 4.

Common Findings in both Districts Either in Full or in Part

- *Place of interview*: In both districts, higher likelihood was noted among the respondents found at government HFs than those at private HFs, although the difference in the association was statistically significant in Mkuranga district only
- *Frequency of visits to clinics*: In both districts, higher likelihood was noted among those who had previously attended clinic more times than those attended less times, but the difference was not statistically significant in either the district case
- *Awareness that SP is not recommended for IPTp at some stage of pregnancy*: In both districts, there was a higher likelihood between those who were aware than those who were unaware, but the association was statistically significant only in the Mkuranga district case
- *Previous use of SP*: Notably and counter-intuitively, a higher likelihood was noted among the respondents who had experienced side-effects than those who had never. The association in each case was statistically significant
- *Preference to drugs other than SP*: In both districts, there was a higher likelihood that the respondents who expressed that they would opt for drugs other than SP if they were allowed than those who said that they would still prefer SP. However, the association was not statistically significant in any of the two district cases.

Completely Different Results between the Two Districts

- *Gravidity|Parity*: A lower association between the stated WTA-IPTi was noted among the multigravidæ than the primigravidæ in Mkuranga, and the association was marginally significant (p=0.069). In Mufindi, there was a higher likelihood that the multigravidæ were willing than the primigravidæ, but the difference was not statistically significant.
- *Age of the expected mother*: In Mkuranga, the respondents who were aged <20 years were more likely to be willing than the older ones (those aged ≥20 years). The converse was true in the Mufindi case. Nevertheless, there was no statistically significant difference in the stated WTA between the different groups of the respondents in either of the two districts.

Five out of the seven CHMT members in Mkuranga viewed that it would not be surprising to experience low or irregular number of infants living far from HFs not turning up for IPTi. This point was based on experience from IPTp implementation as some pregnant women living far from HFs fail to attend ANC clinic in time and/or regularly due to inconvenience of transport, hence failing to access IPTp doses. Climatic changes such as the long heavy rain seasons when most of the river streams are overflowing were also pointed out in Mkuranga as another possible hindering factor for the people living far from HFs where there are no reliable access-roads. Barriers related to travel distance did not feature as an issue in Mufindi as it was reported that most of the roads connecting HFs and villages were accessible throughout the year. On the other hand, the positive results of children brought for

EPI services at formal MCH clinics was generally viewed in both target districts as an encouraging prospect for high IPTi service coverage. Several CHMT members in Mkuranga and Mufindi viewed that it would probably be better if the infants' mothers/caretakers are not informed that the drug administered for IPTi is SP in order to reduce the number of parents/caretakers who would reject bringing their children for EPI services in fear of SP. Such a concern was not shared by the Mufindi district DMO who viewed that most of the parents appreciate EPI services, a situation likely to prevail if the public is adequately sensitised on IPTi-SP beforehand and regularly.

Frontline HWs: Nine respondents lamented that some of the adverse treatment effects of SP occasionally reported by people may seem minor or tolerable from the service providers' viewpoint, but may be important to discourage a considerable proportion of the population to use SP. Concern on the possible effect of ALu's introduction on the uptake of IPTp with SP was not raised by the respondents in Mufindi contrary to their counterparts in Mkuranga. In Mufindi, the HWs who were concerned about IPTi-SP claimed that often there was no malaria in the cold zone that would make most of the people who do not associate malaria with cold climates not to value IPTi as a necessary intervention. In Mkuranga, recognition about malaria being a big public health problem was noted, but more arguments reflected the worry that compliance would be low due to the target parents/caretakers of the infants perceiving SP negatively.

One HW in Mkuranga suggested the need for the health authorities concerned to ensure adequate supply of SP and antipyretics essential (especially) for the infants if IPTi is recommended in the healthcare system. Such an opinion was based on the view that SP has no antipyretic effect and many users complain that it even raises the body temperature (called *Homa* in Swahili). Based on their experience from private HFs in relation to IPTp implementation, shortage of SP was identified as a potential drawback to IPTi coverage at private HFs in Mkuranga. This point was related to the situation where sometimes ANC clients at private HFs only receive prescriptions for them to buy SP from drug shops, particularly when the HWs/providers claim not to have received supply of SP from the DMO's office for free delivery according to the government's health care financing policy [26, 50]. Similar problems were reported by the informants from Mufindi about the private HFs not receiving supplies of SP from the district health authorities.

Target ANC clients: Most of the pregnant women and infants' mothers questioned about the effects of SP during pregnancy and infancy stages. Some village FGD participants suggested the need for an anti-malarial drug alternative to SP which should be in syrup form if IPTi is to receive high community acceptability. SP was noted of having poor curative results to most of its users. As noted from one mother in Mkuranga, the following statement illustrates the common perceptions in the community about SP's treatment outcomes: "*Even adult people are advised to take much water with SP and find this as being difficult for them to tolerate, how about the infants who cannot be forced to take much water*". Statements similar to the latter were notes from a considerable number of individual interviewees and FGD participants in both districts. In Mufindi, it was revealed that during several FGDs that even drinking water is a less common habit especially during cold weather seasons (June-

August). Another concern raised in both districts, but mostly in Mkuranga was that if pregnant women were advised to eat adequately before and after taking SP, how possible will that be for the infants whose eating ability is usually low, leave alone the poor feeding capacity of many families in the district who mainly depend on cassava and take only one meal in the day?

IPTi with SP was positively appreciated by several pregnant women and infants' mothers in all of the 6 villages visited in Mkuranga. This was based on their experience with the frequent attacks of malaria to young children and the reported benefits of IPT implementation for the pregnant women who are also exposed to malaria. Such participants extended their acknowledgement to the government for recommending such a strategy. In contrast, FGD participants in Mkerezange village (in Mkuranga) expressed their doubts about SP despite their appreciation of the IPTi strategy. Their doubt was noted after one woman aged between 25–30 years had commented: "*IPTi would be a useful strategy, as long as a drug other than SP is recommended*". This point was supported by other participants in the same FGD. At Kitomondo village (Mkuranga), FGD participants argued that sometimes poor drug administration by HWs contribute to the observed poor treatment outcomes of SP, otherwise SP is a good drug if properly prescribed and used.

Optimizing effective implementation of IPTi from the CHMT and health workers' perspectives: Viewed as the most important factor to be considered by the malaria control authorities in their consideration to formally introduce IPTi-SP in Tanzania was the *need for enhancing the target service users' knowledge about the reason for IPTi and the usefulness of SP*. This could help changing users' perceptions of SP and foster compliance. Suggested actions to be taken include:

- strengthening and sustaining support to community sensitization on the benefits of SP-SP for infants over speculated risks
- Promoting HF-based deliveries: High proportion of women delivering at home and shying away from child health clinics where their children could receive immunization and other services was viewed as a potential conundrum to IPTi coverage. Therefore, strategies to encourage HF-based deliveries and registration of the newborns were suggested through a multi-sectoral action supported by community sensitization.
- Improving the human-resource-management situation: This was anticipated to increase the number and skills of HWs through: (a) training the existing ones, and (b) giving more attention to the needs of peripheral dispensaries often suffering from low quality services and understaffing.

Discussion

This study demonstrates the application of qualitative and quantitative data collection methods in eliciting people's perceptions and attitudes towards a proposed malaria treatment intervention in infants, based on their perceptions of a similar intervention currently implemented for pregnant women. It reveals that different actors in the healthcare system share some common experiences and opinions but also differ on some issues. Generally, the findings based on both the qualitative and quantitative methods demonstrate that IPTi is acceptable in the study districts subject to the type of the anti-malarial drug recommended. The reservations expressed by IPTi are related to the study participants' low trust in SP mainly on safety grounds from the users' perspective while the frontline HWs and district health managers were mainly concerned about the efficacy of SP and its delivery mechanism in the already human-resource and essential supply constrained healthcare system. For example, evidence from other districts in Tanzania indicates that IPTp implementation has faced constraints to the implementation of DOT due to drawbacks such as HF understaffing which occasionally contributes to the few frontline HWs' failure to observe the clients taking the drug; shortage of clean and safe water drinking along with SP tablets mainly at government HFs; and drug stock-outs for free delivery to the clients at private HFs in line with the government guidelines [26]. Similar findings have been reported from Malawi and Uganda [35], (also in Mubyazi GM and others, unpublished data from Muheza district, Tanzania). This is a challenge to the health system before the strategy is officially recommended and taken to national scale. A number of previous studies in Tanzania and elsewhere support the IPTi strategy, but the authors have proposed more studies on the operational challenges before the strategy is taken to national scale. This involves analysis of acceptability of IPTi with the recommended drug, efficacy and feasibility of drugs alternative to SP [6, 9, 12, 14, 19-20, 37]. Moreover, it is suggested that more research be conducted about the feasibility of IPTi service delivery mechanisms and on the more cost-effective anti-malarial drug that would be an alternative to SP that is increasingly facing trends in parasite resistance [9, 14, 21]. Thus, as Tenbensel [38] asserts "*The most important clues for best practice could be from an analysis of existing practice*". This study contributes to such a discussion and alerts the malaria control authorities, pharmaceutical companies and the research community at large regarding the perceived acceptability of IPTi in different socio-cultural and malaria transmission settings of Tanzania.

White [9] warns about possible low acceptability of SP for IPTi due to the negative attitudes people may have towards administering SP to asymptomatic children. This is supported by *Health Belief Theories* asserting that the likelihood of a person to adopt a recommended preventive health action depends on the feeling they have about their susceptibility to a disease and the consequences that may be experienced if they opt for taking action or not [39-41]. In the present study, district CHMT members and frontline HWs also questioned about the acceptability of IPTi with SP to the public which is informed about ALu's replacement of SP as the first-line drug against uncomplicated malaria following the trend in SP's treatment failures. This implies that health managers and frontline HWs may share the same negative perceptions as their target communities about the proposed drug/intervention, hence they may not have an incentive to promote IPTi unless they are also adequately sensitised and even supervised to ensure they comply with the guidelines. Previous studies in Tanzania found health professionals associating SP with adverse treatment outcomes [26, 42-43] and some of them questioning about the rationale for replacing chloroquine with SP as the first-line drug for uncomplicated malaria [42]. This suggests that it is not good to underscore the views of the frontline HWs regarding the possibility that infants' parents/caretakers may not bring their children for EPI and other basic child health services (including IPTi) if they are informed that their children would be given SP, this being due to the prevailing negative public association of SP with side effects. Alternatively, the children may be brought for immunization and other services but their parents/caretakers may pretend that such children are allergic to SP or use other means to ensure that the child is not given SP under DOT.

The Mkuranga DMO viewed that IMCI contributes to perpetuate parasite resistance to SP which is a challenge to IPTi implementation. This view is somehow shared by other authors' [44]. On one hand, we add that the community may be confused by the messages warning them to use drugs without appropriate medical check-up including laboratory confirmation meanwhile receiving messages which promote drug use on a presumptive basis as anticipated for IPTi and currently practiced under IMCI strategy. So far, it is yet unknown which anti-malarial drug will be recommended for IPTi in Tanzania since currently there are two arms of trials looking at the clinical potential of different antimalarial drugs. One arm is looking at amodiaquine (AQ) in northern Tanzania while the other one is looking at SP in southern Tanzania [17]. Here there are two important challenges: the first one is that the policy decision may be difficult to pass if the two randomized trial arms come up with different recommendations e.g. AQ versus SP i.e. each arm recommending the drug that has been tested. In this regard, it may call for more evaluations to be undertaken to assess the acceptability challenges since in different socio-cultural and economic settings communities may have different attitudes towards particular drugs. Secondly, in areas near the borders of countries where other anti-malarial drugs e.g. Mozambique where AQ is tried out apparently recommended, people may share the same preferences to anti-malarial drugs recommended in a neighbouring country. Such drugs may be crossing the border, filling the local commercial outlets and probably more accessible than the drug recommended in their mother country. This is another potential systemic challenge to the acceptability of and community compliance with the drug recommended for IPTi. For instance, from the present study, it was noted that a high degree of uncertainty about acceptability of IPTi with SP from the target clients' viewpoint was greatly attributed to the perceived intolerable strength of SP to infants. That is probably why 48% of the pregnant women in Mkuranga and 31% of their counterparts in Mufindi were undecided about their actual WTA-IPTi. This category of respondents might have shied away to express their position to the researchers who might have been considered to be part of the healthcare service system with main interest in hearing positive remarks about SP and IPTi. In the presence of an alternatively widely acceptable (positively perceived) drug in the open market (e.g. retail shops, drug stores in the streets), one would expect low target users' compliance. Need for considering how these challenges may be confronted is urgent before official launching of IPTi with whatever anti-malarial drug.

Findings from the bivariate logistic regression analyses indicate the importance of the clients' experience in the use of SP during or before their current pregnancy as the most important and reliable positive predictors of infants' caretakers' WTA-IPTi with SP. This suggests that people's experience with SP may demystify its perceived adverse effects and dilute anecdotal information about widely spread people's negative attitudes to SP. That is, people's preferences to particular malaria preventive or curative products may be enhanced by promoting people to use such products especially in situations whereby people have a range of products to choose (e.g. anti-malarials) and negative perceptions towards particular products (e.g. SP). This makes sense that pharmaceutical get more involved in promotion of the recommended drugs to enhance their target of the consumers.

Moreover, the empirical findings from regression models demonstrated that pregnant women found at government HFs were more likely to express their WTA-IPTi than their counterparts who were found at private HFs. However, statistically the association was significant in the Mkuranga study case only. This kind of likelihood in WTA-IPTi in the two study districts may be attributed to different approaches or intensities in health education and community/target SP uses' sensitisation messages undertaken at MCH clinics. The finding supports the study assumptions that government healthcare providers may have more less incentive to (i.e. motive behind) promoting anti-malarial drugs other than those recommended by he government than the private providers (Box 1).

Some of the odds for some of predictor variables changed more or less in a multivariate logistic regression model, depending on the number and types of the covariates fitted in the model. This is normally the case as a design issue of the model since the likelihood and significance of a particular covariate in the model may depend on the presence or absence of other covariates in the same model. Often multivariate models are used to control for the potential confounders [28-29, 45]. However, the consistent statistical significance of several variables e.g. previous use of the drug implies that some covariates are real predictors of the dependent variables regardless of the types of the covariates with which they are fitted in the same model. This implies that, the habit of using a particular product (including a medicine) may be positive determinant of the acceptability of the product concerned since the utility value of the consumer product be more realised though using it rather than reliance on what other people talk about the product. Therefore, promotion on the use of the product may be an entry point to marketing the product for its large-scale use (demand).

Literature indicates that education of women is an important determinant of their healthcare seeking behaviour and use of the MCH- and other reproductive health- services [46], including those related to malaria [47]. Therefore, it would be expected that the relatively higher WTA-IPTi in Mufindi than in Mkuranga may be attributed to the relatively higher literacy level in the former district, albeit this is weakly supported by empirical evidence from the present study. Nonetheless, the bivariate regression model case (Table 5) indicates that the stated WTA-IPTi was consistently lower among the women who had at least reached form four secondary education than those who had not in the Mkuranga case while the opposite was true for the Mufindi case. Therefore in the former district case, it may be explained that that there may be a positive association between the target drug consumers' intellectual ability to interpret the health messages provided and their critical sense. That is, the more people are formally educated the more they may be critical to health messages including those related to drug use, hence challenging the notion that higher levels of education necessarily have positive implications on people's adoption of the recommended intervention. This is controversy is very likely to be experienced in a situation whereby some people may question about using the drug while if people are already informed about the decreasing efficacy of the drug concerned and or its potential side-effects. Therefore, it would be inferred that unacceptability of an intervention like IPTi depends in some-ways on the experience people have with related interventions such as IPTp if the service delivery models including the type of treatment is the same. The latter argument/explanation may not apply in the case of Mufindi where the odds of WTA-IPTi were higher among the more educated people than the less educated ones (Table 5).

In Mufindi the results from bivariate and multivariate regression analyses were mixed (i.e. seemed controversial) on the issue of the association between the respondents' gravidity status and their WTA-IPTi. In the bivariate regression case, the likelihood of WTA-IPTi was higher among the multigravidæ than the primigravidæ, although the difference was not statistically significant. In the Mkuranga case, the likelihood was relatively lower among the multigravidæ than their counterparts, also the difference being statistically insignificant. A similar pattern of controversial likelihood in the WTA-IPTi was noted for several other variables, with some variations between the two study districts. Again, this could be a model design issue rather than the real situation since there was no statistically significant differences in most of the observations. The age of the respondent seemed consistently a significant predictor of WTA-IPTi in the Mufindi case. This may be due to the possibility of a greater confidence among the Mufindi respondents to express their position about the health intervention concerned than the young ones (especially if the primigravidæ). This situation was different in Mkuranga where older women expressed a less WTA-IPTi, possibly due various factors: for instance, the types of the respondents from each of the study districts might have had different experiences with SP. The socio-cultural and demographic variations in the two districts, some of which have not been covered under the present study, might contribute to the different in the study findings. Another reason may the specifications of the model [30, 48], which does not capture the un-measurable observation (*random/stochastic variable*). Model specification may provide results that may be misleading or ambiguous making it difficult to interpret them and come up with a plausible inference, as in socio-behavioural studies accounting psychosocial dimensions [45].

Moreover, a large part of the data was collected between November 2005 and December 2006 after the government has announced its plan for introducing ALu as the first-line drug for uncomplicated malaria treatment. Mkuranga was one of the few districts in the country where ALu was introduced on a pilot basis around mid 2006 at several government and non-government HFs. This included orientation of the frontline HWs. ALu was not piloted in Mufindi before its official introduction in 2007. Depending on the extent to which the target populations are sensitised, we view that IPTi-SP and IPTp-SP strategies are facing a great acceptability challenge in Tanzania and other countries where ACTs have been recommended for the treatment of uncomplicated malaria. Moreover, the present study is subject to other methodological limitations related, for instance, to the adoption of convenient sampling methods, interviewing fewer CHMT members in Mufindi district than in Mkuranga, and conducting FGDs only in the former district. Also, the study focused on IPTi-SP while promising research on the efficacy of IPTi-AQ is also currently conducted [17]. Most of the data were collected before the government had officially replaced SP with ALu for the treatment of uncomplicated malaria, a situation that may have an impact on the acceptability of SP for IPTi and even IPTp at present and in the future.

Conclusion

In light of the findings from this study, anecdotal and empirical evidence published elsewhere, we argue in support of other authors [5-6, 13-14, 51] that IPTi is a prospectively beneficial strategy for rolling back malaria in infants. Nonetheless, based on the low confidence the public may have in SP and the growing of SP treatment failure rates [9, 21], we suggest a number of measures before officially launching and scaling up the IPTi strategy in Tanzania: Firstly, studies aimed at finding a drug alternative to SP which can be delivered with the highest possible compliance rate. Secondly, studies conducted on socio-cultural factors acting as potential barriers to the acceptability of IPTi and how barriers can be addressed. This involves assessment of health-seeking behaviour for malaria both in pregnancy and infancy in the context of the newly introduced ACT. Thirdly, it is crucial to integrate social science research within the national and district malaria control operational research programmes. This would help to create a local evidence base for malaria-control decisions including the conduction of more systematic baseline survey with adequately analysed data. This may contribute to the evidence base for malaria-control decisions at local and national levels. Fourthly, the need for human resources in terms of numbers, skills and management (including motivation) since the delivery of health services is basically and mostly labour intensive process. Fifthly, supply of the recommended drug, whether SP, AQ or any other at all HF levels has to be ensured regardless of the type of and ownership of the HF. Sixthly, community sensitisation programmes about the existing and the proposed malaria-control interventions. Seventhly, as well as regular monitoring/supervision strategies need concerted efforts including a reliable financial resource base to support transport of the health personnel and CHMT involved in the service programme. Taking all these into account both in theory and practice may result in the IPTi strategy demonstrating high coverage and effectiveness. Strong health systems are essential to ensure that the planned (donor-driven) vertical initiatives (e.g. IPTi and IPTp) succeed [49].

Authors' Contributions

GMM conceived the study, worked fully on the project as part of his doctor of philosophy degree training, analysed the data, wrote the manuscript drafts and finalised them with co-authors' comments. The rest of the authors contributed their ideas from the conception of the study through technical advice to GMM during the progression of the study and data analysis, and commented substantially on the draft manuscripts. Dr. KSH spent more time working with GMM on the logistic regression analyses with comments from Dr. PB. PhD supervision was coordinated by Prof. ICB and Dr. PB.

Acknowledgement

This was part of a PhD study funded by the Bill and Melinda Gates Foundation through the Gates Malaria Partnership (GMP) coordinated by the London School of Hygiene and

Tropical Medicine in collaboration with the DBL Center for Health Research and Development, University of Copenhagen (Denmark) and National Institute for Medical Research (NIMR), Dar Es Salaam, Tanzania. Data collection assistants (F-Mduma, P-Kiluwa, R-J-Ole- Mungaya, D-Mubyazi, A-Rwegoshora; N-J-Mubyazi; E-Mashauri, L-Bankobeza, T-Manumbu, R-Kamugwawa, G-Kambanga, A-Rashid, A-Abdul and W-Lazarus); Kesheni Senkoro of NIMR-Tanzania assisted in preparing the database. Ministry of Health (MOH) granted national ethics clearance; Regional and District Health Authorities (special thanks to Drs. Ayubu Shekimweri-Mkuranga and Dr. D. Subi-Mufindi) for their tireless support and courtesy; study populations; NIMR Director General (Dr. Andrew Y. Kitua) approved the study for publishing and study leave permission for GMM. Neither GMP nor the Government of Tanzania is responsible for any personal views expressed by the authors of this study.

References

[1] Rosen, J. B. & Breman, J. G. (2004). Malaria intermittent preventive treatment in infants, chemoprophylaxis, and childhood vaccinations. *Lancet*, 2004, *363*, 1386-1388.

[2] Snow, R. W. (2004). The invisible victims: A special supplement Issue. *Nature*, *430*, 934-935, August 2004.

[3] Steketee, R. W., Nahlen, B. L., Parise, M. E. & Menendez, C. (2001). The burden of malaria in pregnancy in malaria-endemic areas. *Am. J. Trop. Med. Hyg.*, *64 (Supple 1-2)*, 28-35.

[4] Rugemalila, J. B., Wanga, C. L. & Kilama, W. L. (2006). Sixth African Malaria day in 2006: how have we come after the Abuja Declaration? *Mal J*, *5*, 102.

[5] Greenwood, B. (2007). Intermittent preventive treatment of malaria in infants. *Clinical Infectious Diseases*, *45(1)*, 26-28.

[6] Greenwood, B. (2006). Review: Intermittent preventive treatment- a new approach to the prevention of malaria in children in areas seasonal with malaria transmission. *Trop. Med. International Health*, *11(7)*, 983-991.

[7] Greenwood, B. (2004). The use of antimalarial drugs to prevent malaria in the population of malaria endemic countries. *American Journal of Tropical Medicine and Hygiene*, *70(1)*, 1-7.

[8] Macete, E., Aide, P., Apponte, J. J. et al., (2006). Intermittent treatment for malaria control administered at the time of routine vaccination in Mozambican infants: a randomized, placebo-controlled trial. *J. Infect Diseases*, 2006, *194(3)*, 276-85.

[9] Massaga, J., Kitua, A., Lemnge, M., Akida, J. A., Malle, L. N., Rønn, A., Theander, T. & Bygbjerg, I. C. (2003). Effect of intermittent treatment with amodiaquine and malarial fevers in infants in Tanzania: a randomised placebo-controlled trial. *Lancet*, *vol. 361*, 1853-1860.

[10] O'Meara, W. P., Breman, J. & McKenzie, E. (2005). The promise and potential challenges of intermittent preventive treatment for malaria in infants (IPTi): Review. *Mal Journal*, *4*, 33.

[11] Pool, R., Munguambe, K., Macete, E., Aide, P., Juma, G., Alonso, P. & Menendez, C. (2006). Community response to intermittent preventive treatment to infants (IPTi)

through the EPI system in Manhica, Mozambique. *Trop. Med. Int. Health, 11(11)*, 1670-1678.

[12] Vallely, A., Vallely, L., Changalucha, J., Greenwood, B. & Chandramohan, D. (2007). Intermittent preventive treatment for malaria in pregnancy in Africa: what's new, what's needed? *Malaria Journal*, *6*, 16.

[13] Schellenberg, D., Menendez, C., Kahigwa, E., Tanner, M., Mshinda, H. & Alonso, P. (2005). Intermittent treatment for malaria and anaemia control at time of routine vaccinations in Tanzanian infants: a randomized placebo-controlled trial. *Lancet*, 2005, *357(9267)*, 1471-7.

[14] Schellenberg, D., Cisse, B. & Menendez, C. (2006). The IPTi Consortium: research for policy and action. *Trends in Parasitology*, www.malariaconsortium.org/data/files/pages/ipt_4.pdf (accessed 7th September 2006). Doi:10.1016/j.pt.2006.05.006.

[15] Lobel, H. O. & Campbell, C. C. (1986). Malaria chemoprophylaxis and distribution of drug resistance. *Clinical Tropical Medicine Commun.*, *80*, 452-458.

[16] WHO and UNICEF: Antenatal Care in Developing Countries: Promises, Achievements and Missed Opportunities: Analysis of Trends, levels and differentials. *World Health Organization* (WHO), *Geneva* 2003.

[17] Chandramohan, D., Owusu-Agyei, S., Carneiro, I., Awine, T., Amposa-Achiano, K., Mensah, N., Jaffar, S., Baiden, R., Hodgson, A., Binka, F. & Greenwood, B. (2005). Cluster randomised trial of intermittent preventive treatment for malaria in infants in area of high, seasonal transmission in Ghana *BMJ*, *331*, 727-733.

[18] WHO: Update on Intermittent Preventive Treatment in infants. *Global Malaria Programme*, *World Health Organization* (WHO), *Geneva* 2006.

[19] ter Kuile, F. O. & Steketee, R. W. (2006). Intermittent Preventive Treatment in Infants-Adjusting Expectations and Seeing Opportunity: an editorial commentary. *Journal of Infectious Diseases*, *194*, 269-272.

[20] WHO: Implementation research: bridging the gap between efficacy trials and application. Special Programme for Research and Training in Tropical Diseases (*TDR*), 9th February 2004, *Newsletter No. 71*.

[21] Egan, A., Crawley, J. & Schellenberg, D. (2005). Intermittent preventive treatment for malaria control in infants: moving towards evidence-based policy and public health action. *Tropical Medicine and International Health*, *10(9)*, 815-817.

[22] Yin, R. K. (1994). *Case Study Research: Design and Methods*. 2nd ed. Thousand Oaks, C.A ; London: Sage Publications.

[23] Mapping Malaria Risks in Africa (MARA) (2000). Tanzania Malaria Transmission Risk. *Ministry of Health in collaboration with Tanzania Essential Health Interventions Project and MARA*. http://www.malvacdecision.net/pdfs/overview%20Malaria%Control%20DMF.pdf (accessed on 18th July 2007). *MARA, Ministry of Health Dar Es Salaam, Tanzania Essential Health Interventions Project*

[24] Torell, E. & Mmochi, A. (2007). Mkuranga Governance: Baseline Coastal Resource Centre. *University of Rhode*, 2006 http://www.crc.uri.edu/download/Mkuranga_baseline.pdf (accessed 1 Aug) .

[25] Eisele, T., Hotchikiss, D., Bingham, A., Silvestre, E., Gueye, D., Banke, K., Mmbuji, P. & Mboera, L. E. G. (2006). Assessing the Effectiveness of an Intervention Package for

Improving Analysis and Response of the Infectious Disease Surveillance System in Tanzania. *Bethesda, MD: The Partners for Health Reform plus Project, Abt Associates Inc*.<http://www.phrplus.org/Pubs/WP004_fin.pdf.

[26] Mubyazi, G., Bloch, P., Kamugisha, M., Kitua, A. & Ijumba, J. (2005). Intermittent preventive treatment of malaria during pregnancy in Tanzania: a qualitative study of knowledge, attitudes and perceptions of district health managers, antenatal service staff and pregnant women in Korogwe district, north-eastern Tanzania. *Malaria Journal*, *4*, 31.

[27] Robson, C. (2000). *Real World Research: Analysis of Qualitative Data*. Cornwall: T.J International Ltd.

[28] Hosmer, D. W. & Lemeshow, S. (2000). *Applied Logistic Regression*. Second Edition. John Wiley & Sons, Inc.

[29] Greene, W. H. (2003). *Econometric analysis*. Fifth Edition. Pearson Education Inc., New-Jersey, USA.

[30] Pindyck, R. S. & Rubinfeld, D. L. (1981). *Econometric models and economic forecasts*: Second Edition. McGraw-Hill, Inc., USA.

[31] Barry, C. (1998). Choosing Qualitative Data Software: Atlas/ti and Nurdist Compared. Social Research Online 1998. (*http://www.socresonline.org.uk/3/3/4html.*

[32] Dawson, S., Manderson, L. & Tallo, V. (1993). Methods of Social Science Research in Disease: A Manual for the Use of Focus Groups. WHO Social and Economic Research (SER), UNDP/World Bank/WHO Special Programme for Research and Training in Tropical Diseases (TDR), World Health Organization, Geneva.

[33] Kruger, R. A. (1988). *Focus Groups: A Practical Guide for Applied Research*. Newbury Park, C.A. Sage Publications.

[34] CIOMS. (2002). *International Ethical Guidelines for Biomedical Research Involving Human Subjects*. Council for International Organisations of Medical Sciences (CIOMS), ISBN 92 9036 0755.

[35] Hill, J. & Kazembe, P. (2006). Reaching Abuja Targets for intermittent preventive treatment of malaria in pregnancy in African women: a review of progress and operational challenges. *Tropical Medicine and International Health*, *11(4)*, 409-418.

[36] Mockenhaupt, F., Reither, K., Zanger, P., Roepcke, F., Danquah, I., Saad, E., Ziniel, P. et al., (2007). Intermittent preventive treatment as a means for malaria control: a randomised, double-blind, placebo-controlled trial in Northern Ghana. *Antimicrobial Agents and Chemotherapy*, *51(9)*, 3273-3281.

[37] ter Kuile, F. O. & Steketee, R. W. (2006). Intermittent Preventive Treatment in Infants-Adjusting Expectations and Seeing Opportunity: an editorial commentary. *Journal of Infectious Diseases*, *194*, 269-272.

[38] Tenbensel, T. (2002). Interpreting public input into priority setting: the role of mediating institutions. *Health policy*, *62*, 173-94.

[39] Family Health International (2002). Behaviour change – A summary of Four Major Theories.
http://www.fhi.org/NR/rdonlyres/ei26vbslpsidmahhxc332vwo3g233xsqw22er3vofqvrfjvubwyzclvqjcbdgexyzl3msu4mn6xv5j/BCCSummaryFourMajorTheories.pdf

[40] Haraway, D. (1991). Situated knowledges: the science question in feminism and the privilege of partial perspective. In Haraway D. *Simians, cyborgs, and women: the reinvention of nature*. New York: Routledge: pp 183-201.

[41] Rosenstock, I., Strecher, V. & Becker, M. (2002). The Health Behaviour Model and risk behaviour change: In: R. J. DiClemente, & J. L. Peterson (Eds.), *Preventing AIDS: Theories and Methods of Behavioural Interventions*, pages 5-25; New York Plennum Press.

[42] Mubyazi, G. M. & Gonzalez-Bloch, M. A. (2005). The role of research in changing the first-line antimalarial drug policy in Tanzania. *Malaria Journal, 4*, 51.

[43] Nsimba, E. D. (2006). How sulfadoxine-pyrimethamine was perceived in some rural communities after phasing out chloroquine as a first-line drug for uncomplicated malaria in Tanzania: lessons to learn towards moving from monotherapy to fixed combination therapy. *Journal of Ethnobiology and Ethnomedicine, 2*, 3.

[44] Alexander, N., Sutherland, C., Roper, C., Cisse, B. & Schellenberg, D. (2007). Modelling impact of intermittent treatment for malaria on selection pressure for drug resistance. *Malaria Journal, 6*, 9.

[45] Wuensch, K. L. (2004). Stepwise multiple regression. http://core.ecu.edu/psyc/wuenschk/MV/MultReg/Stepwise.doc (accessed 8th September 2007).

[46] Rowe, M. L., Bijaya, K. T., LeVine, R., LeVine, S. & Tuladhar, S. K. (2005). How does schooling influence maternal health practices? Evidence from Nepal. *Comparative Education Review, 49*, 512-533.

[47] Nganda, R. Y., Drakeley, C., Reyburn, H. & Marchant, T. (2004). Knowledge of malaria influences the use of insecticide treated nets but not intermittent presumptive treatment by pregnant women in Tanzania. *Malaria Journal, 3*, 42.

[48] Woodridge, J. F. (2006). *Introductory econometrics: a modern approach:* Third Edition. Thomson, South-western, USA.

[49] The Lancet-Editorial (2004). Mexico, 2004: Global health needs a new research agenda. *The Lancet, 364*, 1555-1556.

[50] Ministry of Health-Tanzania (1994). *Proposals for health sector reform*. Dar Es Salaam, 1994.

[51] Munday, S. (2007). Review of intermittent preventive treatment for malaria in infants and children. *Journal of Paediatrics and Child Health, 43(6)*, 424-428.

In: Antimalarial Drugs: Costs, Safety and Efficacy
Editors: Emanuel Csizmadia and Istvan Kalnoky

ISBN: 978-1-60741-432-2

Chapter IV

Implementing Intermittent Preventive Treatment for Malaria in Pregnancy: Review of Prospects, Achievements, Challenges and Agenda for Research

[*]*Godfrey Martin Mubyazi*[1,2], *Pascal Magnussen*[3], *Catherine Goodman*[4], *Ib Christian Bygbjerg*[5], *Andrew Yona Kitua*[1], *Øystein Evjen Olsen*[6], *Jens Byskov*[6], *Kristian Schultz Hansen*[3] *and Paul Bloch*[6]

[1]National Institute for Medical Research, Dar Es Salaam, Tanzania, P.O Box 9653 Dar Es Salaam, Tanzania

[2]Amani Medical Research Centre, P.O Box 81 Muheza, Tanzania.

[3]Department of Health Services Research, Institute of Public Health, University of Aarhus, Aarhus, Denmark.

[4]London School of Hygiene and Tropical Medicine, London, United Kingdom.

[5]Institute of International Health, Immunology and Microbiology, Faculty of Health Sciences, University of Copenhagen, Copenhagen, Denmark.

[6]DBL - Centre for Health Research and Development, Faculty of Life Sciences, University of Copenhagen, Charlottenlund, Denmark.

[*] Corresponding author: National Institute for Medical Research (NIMR), Centre for Enhancement of Effective Malaria Interventions (CEEMI), P.O Box 9653, Dar es Salaam, Tanzania,
Emails: gmmubyazi@yahoo.co.uk;mubyazig@hotmail.com

Abstract

Introduction

Implementing Intermittent Preventive Treatment for malaria in Pregnancy (IPTp) with sulfadoxine-pyrimethamine (SP) through antenatal care (ANC) clinics is recommended for malaria endemic countries. The vast biomedical literature on malaria prevention focuses more on the epidemiological and cost-effectiveness analyses of the randomised controlled trials carried out in selected geographical settings. Such studies fail to elucidate the economic, psychosocial, managerial, organization and other contextual systemic factors influencing the operational effectiveness, compliance and coverage of the recommended interventions.

Objective

To review literature on policy advances, achievements, constraints and challenges to malaria IPTp implementation, emphasising its operational feasibility in the context of health-care financing, provision and uptake, resource constraints and psychosocial factors in Africa.

Results

The importance of IPTp in preventing unnecessary anaemia, morbidity and mortality in pregnancy and improving childbirth outcomes is highly acknowledged, although the following factors appear to be the main constraints to IPTp service delivery and uptake: cost of accessing ANC; myths and other discriminatory socio-cultural values on pregnancy; target users, perceptions and attitudes towards SP, malaria, and quality of ANC; supply and cost of SP at health facilities; understaffing and demoralised staff; ambiguity and impracticability of user-fee exemption policy guidelines on essential ANC services; implementing IPTp, bednets, HIV and syphilis screening programmes in the same clinic settings; and reports on increasing parasite resistant to SP. However, the noted increase in the coverage of the delivery of IPTp doses in several countries justify that IPTp implementation is possible and better than not.

Conclusion

IPTp for malaria is implemented in constrained conditions in Africa. This is a challenge for higher coverage of at least two doses and attainment of the Abuja targets. Yet, there are opportunities for addressing the existing challenges, and one of the useful options is the evaluation of the acceptability and viability of the existing intervention guidelines.

Keywords: Malaria, antenatal-care, intermittent-treatment, pregnancy, health services.

Introduction

Malaria in Pregnancy

Globally, malaria causes 300–500 millions cases of illness each year and is the leading cause of morbidity and mortality, especially among pregnant women and children under the age of five years, popular as *underfives* (Steketee et al., 2001; WHO 2002; Brabin 1995; Menendez 1995). Of the estimated 1–3 million malaria deaths recorded globally each year, 90% occur in sub-Saharan Africa (SSA) (Rugemalila et al., 2006; Snow 2004). About 30 million women in malarious areas of SSA get pregnant each year, and the majority live in relatively stable malaria transmission (WHO and UNICEF 2003a). Among other consequences, malaria in pregnancy can cause severe anaemia, stillbirths, spontaneous abortion, neonatal mortality, low child birth-weight, child's brain damage and inter-uterine growth retardation (Vallely et al., 2007; van Geertruyden et al., 2004; Menendez 2001; Phillip-Howard 1999; Mutabingwa et al., 1993).

Intermittent Preventive Treatment of Malaria in Pregnancy (IPTp)

The World Health Organization (WHO) has recommended the malaria-endemic countries to implement *sulfadoxine-pyrimethamine* (SP) for intermittent preventive treatment for malaria during pregnancy (IPTp) as one of the essential services under the focused antenatal care service package (WHO 2004a). The recommendation specifies at least two doses to be administered, the first one during the second trimester and the second dose during the third trimester of pregnancy (WHO and UNICEF 2003ab). To ensure compliance in uptake of IPTp doses by the pregnant women attending antenatal care clinics (ANC), the guidelines emphasise direct observed treatment (DOT) by a qualified health worker (HW) (Vallely et al., 2007; D'Allessandro et al., 2003). Responding to WHO's call, SSA heads of state through the Abuja Declaration commonly agreed that each pregnant woman attending ANC clinics should receive two doses of IPTp during her pregnancy period and a subsidised insecticide treated net (ITN) (Guyatt et al., 2004; Holtz et al., 2004; WHO 2006). While many countries have recommended two doses of SP for IPTp, there is still debate about giving three doses or more, particularly to pregnant women who book early and continue attending ANC regularly (White 2005), and to those who are HIV positive (Filler et al., 2006; Holtz et al., 2004). Owing to evidence that two doses of IPTp with SP are inadequate to HIV infected women (Mutabingwa 2002), multiple doses are recommended, especially in the primigravidæ (Greenwood 2004; Verrhoeff et al., 1998). As detailed below, the limiting factors include low ANC attendance behaviours, fears about HIV tests, attitudes towards SP, and growing parasite resistance to SP, as detailed further below.

Efficacy, Safety and Cost-Effectiveness of SP for Malaria Treatment

There are fears that SP may induce side-effects in areas with high prevalence of human immunodeficiency virus (HIV) infection (Filler et al., 2008; Holtz et al., 2004). This being the case from a biological perspective, it should be understood that the programmatic effectiveness of an anti-parasitic drug is determined by the efficacy of that drug against the parasite and by the drug's characteristics, including affordability, availability, acceptability to the target population, and deliverability in terms of dosing requirements and incorporation into existing ANC delivery systems (WHO 2001). Alarming resistance to SP in some parts of East Africa has been reported many years ago (Goodman et al., 2003; Phillip-Howard et al., 2003 EANMAT 2001; Mutabingwa et al., 2001 Rønn et al., 1996), and this contributed to current concerns about its effectiveness for IPTp (White 2005). Although P.*falciparum* strains contribute to SP resistance (Phillip-Howard et al., 2003), poor prescription and consumption practices in the health-care system lowers the effectiveness of malaria interventions, including IPTp (Phillip-Howard et al., 2003; Menendez 2003). So far, there is a lack of evidence on: how IPTp-SP works in areas of low and seasonal malaria transmission areas especially in areas where SP has lost its efficacy (White 2005); added benefit of giving more than two doses of IPTp to each pregnant woman regardless of their HIV or gravidity status, as already this has been noted of being less advantageous (Goodman et al., 2001); perceived and real benefits and acceptability of SP to the target populations given in the existence of parasite resistance to SP especially in East and Southern Africa (Vallely et al., 2007; Greenwood 2004; Murray and Nyambo 2003); the use of artemisinin-based combination therapies (ACTs) for IPTp considering costs and risks (Vallely et al., 2007 Brieger 2007 Dellicour et al., 2007), and acceptability of SP for IPTp following replacement of SP by ACT in several countries (e.g. Tanzania) as the first-line drug for the treatment of uncomplicated malaria (Anders et al., 2008; Mubyazi et al., 2008).

Objective and Scope of This Review

ANC clinics are the most common entry points for IPTp implementation (WHO and UNICEF 2003ab). IPTp implementation through community-based HWs and traditional birth attendants (TBAs) has been considered and tried out in Malawi (Hill and Kazembe 2006) and Uganda (Mbonye et al., 2006ab) as a way of increasing coverage of IPTp and compliance. Experience from these two countries has shown that there have been some notable successes. Logically, integrating IPTp into ANC structures is highly advantageous, but the effects of one on the other are often underestimated (Ribera et al., 2007). The factors influencing IPTp implementation including the operational feasibility of IPTp and use of ANC services in general may be numerous and mutually non-exclusive (Hill and Kazembe 2006; White 2005; Mubyazi et al., 2005a). Factors such as the perceived cost, quality and benefits of ANC, and social values on pregnancy that makes women feel discriminated and humiliated in some ways, gender relations in the society may influence the outcome, although they are rarely analysed and documented empirically partly due to methodological difficulties (Ribera et al., 2007). Understanding the socio-cultural determinants of the use of malaria preventive services including those delivered through ANC clinics and of the compliance with drug uptake by the target populations is imperative (Menendez 2003). So far, studies on social perceptions of health and disease, cultural values and people's ability to cope with the existing malaria interventions in constrained socio-economic and health system contexts are inadequate (Breman et al., 2004; WHO 2004b; Breman 2004). Other authors have suggested the following:

- evaluations of malaria prevention and treatment strategies should consider the broad health service delivery contexts, including the motivation and behaviour of health service providers and the target service users (Hanson et al., 2004; Malaria Consortium 2004);
- research-based evidence on how the recommended intervention is implemented is crucial to enable elucidation of the specific underlying obstacles which policy decision authorities need to know in order to take appropriate policy actions (Walley et al., 2007).

This paper is a review focusing on the policy advances, constraints and challenges to malaria IPTp implementation, with emphasis on its operational feasibility in the context of health-care financing, provision and uptake, resource constraints and diverse psychosocial factors in SSA. Broad contextual factors currently affecting (or with potential effect on) women's perceptions, attendance to, and use of ANC including IPTp, as well as health service providers' attitudes, motivation and practice on ANC (and IPTp), are highlighted and discussed. Experiences from developing countries outside Africa on ANC provision, uptake and coverage similar to those of SSA, are cited, and lessons are drawn from programmes across Africa to feed into the current policy and inform the research agenda. The paper is based on peer-reviewed and non-peer reviewed articles, including grey literature and official working papers published by various agencies/authorities.

Review Methods

The articles reviewed in this paper were searched from the Internet, based on the application of key words to make important downloads from the PubMed. Sometimes the search was done by typing the key words in Google first. The articles reviewed were downloaded selectively based on the contents of the information displayed. If the full articles could not be accessed directly, WHO HINARI system was consulted as done by other authors (Vallely et al., 2007). The search words mostly used in relation to IPTp are: pregnancy, perceptions, malaria, treatment, chemoprevention, intermittent, and prevention, while those used for searching for the broad aspects concerning ANC are: antenatal, provision, utilisation, demand, cost, supply, quality, Africa, developing countries. The word AND was sometimes used to combine two or more search words so as to display the article(s) needed. Additional literature was obtained using email alerts from BioMed Central for online full published articles, unpublished reports (some of which are accessible online), and hard copies of some articles found in journals documented at the local libraries, particularly at the

National Institute for Medical Research (Tanzania), London School of Hygiene and Tropical Medicine (UK), DBL Centre for Health Research and Development and Faculty of Health Sciences at the University of Copenhagen (Denmark). Some articles were requested directly from the original authors. Although efforts were made to ensure that all articles relevant for this review were considered without restriction on the dates of their publication, most of the articles cited have been published between 2000 and 2007. In some parts of the results section, the present paper begins by presenting an overview of the themes related to ANC or IPTp. Then, it goes down to specific issues addressing the determinants of ANC and IPTp service supply and demand, before the general discussions and conclusions.

Results

Accessibility, Acceptability and Practicability of ANC and IPTp

Accessibility and coverage of malaria interventions in SSA are constrained by poverty, limited health infrastructure, ineffective drug policy regulations and other health-care market imperfections (Pokhrel 2006; Guyatt et al., 2004; Hanson et al., 2004). Strategies towards attaining the Millennium Development Goals (MDGs) through scaling-up malaria control interventions are constrained by, among other factors, weak health systems, unclear and disputed solutions weakly supported by evidence (Mills 2005). In 1996 WHO reported that at least 40% pregnant women in developing countries receive no ANC and that nearly 31% deliver at home (Adam and Salihu 2002). Coverage of IPTp in SSA varies from modest to low, as it is the case with ITNs (Ribera et al., 2007). In Blantyre (Malawi), it was found that 75.7% of 391 pregnant women who still were having ANC cards at household level had received at least one dose of IPTp, but only 36.8% received the second dose (Holtz et al., 2004). In the latter country, a previous study found that 24% of the women were not prescribed SP and only 30% received at least two IPTp doses (Rogerson et al., 2000). In rural Kenya, only 19.1% of 635 study participating women reported having received SP for IPTp while only 6.8% had received two doses, despite 89.9% of the women having attended ANC (Eijk et al., 2004). At the Tanzanian National Malaria Control Program (NMCP) level, records on IPTp showed that by March 2007 the coverage of the first and second doses (based on sentinel survey of 21 districts) were 67% and 45%, respectively (Mubyazi et al., 2008).

Contextual factors play a significant role in facilitating or constraining the effectiveness of any health intervention from the operational perspective. For instance, the effectiveness of any malaria intervention depends on consumer and provider acceptance and compliance, safety, cost, integration with other interventions, local health care delivery system and the degree of combination of all these (Robb 2002). Institutionalisation of public health interventions within constrained infrastructure, other supply and demand conditions is critical to the effectiveness of such interventions, and this has raised much concern in health policy programmes targeting the services to the populations in need (Hill and Kazembe 2006; Puska 2006; Ensor and Cooper 2004; Hanson et al., 2004).

Accessibility Barriers

In SSA, women's late presentation at ANC is common, with nearly 25% of them presenting for the first time in the second trimester and for the second time during the third trimester, and this has contributed to lowering the effectiveness of ANC and IPTp related services (WHO and UNICEF 2003a; Goodman et al., 2003; Holtz et al., 2004; Magnussen 2003). Rural residents are relatively more disadvantaged than their urban counterparts in terms of geographical and financial accessibility to ANC (WHO and UNICEF 2003b; Adam and Salihu 2002), and generally the poorer women whether in rural or urban areas are more disadvantaged (WHO and UNICEF 2003b).

Travel distance has continued being reported as one of the major challenges to women's access to and utilisation of reproductive and child health (RCH) services (van Eijk 2006; WHO 2005ab). Even if the RCH services were provided free of charge, the long travel distance leads to additional time cost, and in many cases, financial expenditures that overburden the poorer women who ultimately are dissuaded to attend clinics for ANC or childbirth (Borghi 2006; Barat et al., 2004; Hanson et al., 2004; Wagle et al., 2004; Magadi et al., 2000; Friedrickx 1998; Fantahun 1995; Thadeus and Maine 1994). The timing of ANC attendance is considered to increase the opportunity for the pregnant women to receive IPTp. However, a recent study in northern Tanzania found no association between early ANC attendance and uptake of IPTp, this suggesting that the efforts to foster timely attendance alone are unlikely to improve uptake of IPTp where other contextual barriers exist (Anders et al., 2008).

Travel distance to ANC clinics by the target populations

Due to delays in contacting clinics for ANC, a large proportion of SSA countries recommended four ANC visits and increased the spacing between them in conformity to WHO protocol (Overbosch et al., 2004). The optimal number of ANC visits for countries with limited resources is still debated at policy and programme levels (WHO 2005a). Sometimes the target ANC women show more concern with the quality of care than the number of ANC visits (Overbosch et al., 2004; Langer et al., 2005). Basically, the four ANC visits were mainly suggested in consideration of women residing far from health facilities (HFs) (WHO and UNICEF 2003a). However, having physical access to HFs is not enough in the acute and persistent shortages of drugs, medical equipment, other basic supplies, and HWs who are humane, skilled and motivated (Hanson et al., 2004; Adam and Salihu 2002; Acharya and Clerand 2000). HFs may be closer, but the target users bypass them by consulting the providers perceived as being more skilled for delivering better services (Leonard et al., 2002). Attendance to ANC gives the pregnant women an opportunity for accessing health education (including counselling) related to their pregnancy and their children/babies (WHO 2005a). None-regular ANC clinic attendees for various reasons (including long travel distance) have limited accessibility to IPTp services in the right time such as during the early stages of pregnancy (Anders et al., 2008), including RCH education in general (Nganda et al., 2004; van Eijk et al., 2004).

User charges in general and in relation to ANC services

Experience from SSA shows that real or perceived existence of user-fees is a stumbling block to pregnant women's contact of RCH clinics (Priya 2002). In some areas of Tanzania (Marchant et al., 2002), Uganda (Ndyomugyenyi et al., 1996), Zimbabwe (Kambarami et al., 2004), Nigeria (Okonofua et al., 1992), and South Africa (Wilkinson et al., 2001) user-fees have discouraged pregnant women with limited cash to attend ANC clinics. IPTp services are not necessarily free of user-fee barriers (Ribera et al., 2007), especially at private HFs (Mubyazi et al., 2005b; Malaria Consortium 2004), as studies in several districts in Tanzania (Mubyazi et al., 2005b)], Malawi (Hill and Kazembe 2006) and Kenya, have elucidated. In Kenya, Lynm and Munguti found that even in government clinics the ANC clients were often asked to pay for SP, leading to lower uptake of the IPTp doses recommended for such clients (Hill and Kazembe 2006).

Implementing exemption policies for RCH services in SSA is hampered by the low translation of the exemption guidelines into practice at HF levels. For example, in Uganda (Mbonye et al., 2006a), Ghana (Nyonator and Kutzin 1999) and Tanzania (Mubyazi et al., 2007a; Mubyazi et al., 2006; Boller et al., 2003; Murray and Nyambo 2003), pregnant women sometimes paid formally for laboratory tests, registration and an initial consultation fee, which were perceived as a heavy burden to such women. Outside the user-fee structure, there are other informal charges and other indirect cost hindering pregnant women's health service utilization (Borghi et al., 2006). Misunderstanding or ignorance of the user-fee structure and exemption policy contributes to lowering health service utilisation. For example, sometimes user-fee exemption guidelines are in place but the target populations do not use their opportunity to ask/claim for exemptions, as they do not know that they are eligible (Mubyazi 2004). In Korogwe district, Tanzania, the community was unhappy with pregnant women being required to pay for some RCH services contrary to what was believed to be the government policy entitling such women to be among the exempted vulnerable population groups (Mubyazi et al., 2006).

Socio-cultural barriers

The extent to which socio-cultural determinants of compliance with drugs also play a role in the optimal utilisation of existing HF based services has not been adequately studied, especially in a problem solving approach to improve facility utilisation and women's participation in the IPTp strategy (Mutabingwa 2002). Along with the financial barriers, it is widely evident that women in most developing countries are facing social-cultural barriers to their access to HFs delivering RCH services (Priya 2002). Such barriers have strong roots into gender imbalances beyond the HF settings limiting their autonomy and power to attend ANC clinics and use IPTp services (Brieger 2007; Ribera et al., 2007), among other RCH services (Creel et al., 1996). Shying away or fearing to reveal one's pregnancy in the early stage is one of the barriers (Ribera et al., 2007), as validated by findings from Tanzania (Mubyazi et al., 2008). Sometimes women delay to attend ANC clinics due to lack of permission from their spouses (Adam and Salihu 2002). Studies in Tanzania (Centre for Enhancement of Effective Malaria Interventions 2006, unpublished Research Report) and

The Gambia (Gates Malaria Partnership-DBL 2005, unpublished Consultancy Report) found that teenagers feared the severe legal and social implications of getting pregnant while schooling or before marriage. The two studies also found that delay in contacting ANC clinics also occurred in (a) married women who carried pregnancies outside the wedlock or did not have socially recognised partners (b) women aged from 35 years and above who shied away to be accompanied or seen by much younger pregnant women. Consequently, the pregnant women concerned did not access either one or both doses of IPTp and other ANC services.

Age may influence pregnant women prefer particular service providers. A study on the determinants of pregnant women's use of IPTp services in Mufindi district, Tanzania (Mubyazi, unpublished PhD Thesis officially submitted, August 2008) noted some older women disliking to be attended by the nurses whose ages were as low as the ages of such women's daughters. Myths and unfound beliefs may also negatively affect ANC attendances. In Mukono district, Uganda, women delayed attending ANC clinics and lowly utilised ITNs and IPTp due to the prevailing community myth and belief that adolescent girls and primigravidæ were at low risk (Mbonye et al., 2006ab).

Provider-client interactions and Perceptions of quality of ANC in generals

Supply and demand related factors in a general or the broad health service situation contribute influencing the target clients' choice of the service. Women may delay or completely decline to attend clinic because they appreciate comparative better service they received from the TBAs who may also portray better attitude of friendliness and devoting more time for listening to their clients about their health and social problems. Also, by experiencing frequent shortages of needed medication at ANC clinic, women find such services unreliable while they do not suffer such experience at TBAs (Ndyomugyenyi et al., 1998). Women are disappointed when: they wait longer at the service delivery point, are mishandled by nurses, and lack of diagnostic facilities (Mbonye et al., 2006a; Mubyazi et al., 2007a; Mubyazi et al., 2005a), avoid contacting clinics for ANC in fear of the lack of privacy at the consultation or bad language of the nurses (Murira et al., 2003), face unfriendly opening hours and/or unfair and unexpected costs (WHO 2005b). The need for the skilled ANC staff in the health-care system is one of the prerequisites for attracting women to clinics (WHO 2005b). Moreover, lack of- or shortage of the essential utilities such as cups at ANC level for use by the patients taking SP under DOT has constrained IPTp implementation in Tanzania, Uganda and Malawi (Hill and Kazembe 2006). Not all the ANC clients feel comfortable when they are required to share cups when taking the drugs under DOT for IPTp (Mufubenga 2003). Generally, analysis of trends and levels of ANC service provision in Africa and other developing countries has revealed that the ANC service provided are substandard, therefore, significantly contributing to lower the uptake of such services (Hill and Kazembe 2006; WHO 2005ab; Overbosch et al., 2004; WHO and UNICEF 2003b; Leonard et al., 2002). Vast literature documents the concern raised about the factors hindering pregnant women to attend clinics, but as Fathalla (1988) argued, the key question service providers must ask themselves is, "*do we offer the service that the women will accept*?, instead of asking "why do women not accept the service we offer?" (WHO 2005b).

Perceptions and Acceptability of SP

Psychological barriers: Perspective of pregnant women and the society around them concerning SP

Findings from SSA show pregnant women and the society associating SP with severe adverse outcomes such as abortion, skin reaction and lack of anti-fever effect (Brieger 2007; Irshad 2007; Hill and Kazembe 2006; Mbonye et al., 2006ab; Mubyazi et al., 2006; Nsimba 2006; Guyatt et al., 2004; Mwenesi 2003). Truly, SP can cause effects such as Stevens-Johnson syndrome in people who are allergic to sulfa with possible dramatic and potentially fatal effects (Adams et al., 2003; Phillip-Howard et al., 1989; Lenox-Smith 1987; Miller et al., 1986). However, such side-effects are rare and in most cases exaggerated (Phillip-Howard et al., 2003; Phillip-Howard 1999; Bjorkman and Phillip-Howard 1991). The perception people have on a drug may significantly determine their acceptance of that particular drug (Ribera et al., 2007). A drug that is bitter or associated with abortion in some cultures is likely to be less complied with by the target population (Newman et al., 2003). The situation is worse when health service providers share such sentiments and hence are unable to provide service users with correct information about the drug. In Tanzania, some health professionals expressed their doubts about the rationale for recommending SP for malaria treatment in areas where drug resistance is already high (Mubyazi and Gonzalez-Block 2005). In Malawi, some HWs believed that SP was not appropriate to be taken by a person with an empty stomach (Hill and Kazembe 2006).

Health care workers' knowledge and administration of IPTp-SP

It is important that health-care providers know well the health problems against which the services are provided. This includes knowledge on the causes, management and prevention of such problems (including diseases like malaria), which is essential for their own motivation and confidence in managing or giving advice to their clients (Mansfield et al., 2006). One study in Kenya found that IPTp was not administered at some clinics due to HWs being unaware of the guidelines (Guyatt et al., 2004). Similarly in Tanzania, HWs in two districts reported confusion they faced regarding timing of the doses and the number of the doses to be administered for IPTp (Mubyazi et al., 2008). In this circumstance of limited knowledge among the HWs, the effectiveness and coverage of health interventions remain to be undermined, and may expose the target populations to the risk of being attended by uninformed HWs (Snow 2004). A number of malaria control programmes deliberately emphasise initial training of HWs in order to improve their communication skills and prevent this negative effect (Hill and Kazembe 2006).

Health service providers' morale at their workplaces, perceptions on SP and its implications on ANC-IPTp

Reducing poverty by preventing malaria in pregnancy is among the MDGs (DCP 2007; Sachs 2005). But serious shortage of skilled and motivated staff in SSA and other developing countries' health sectors, is a conundrum (Wyss 2005). The working environment may affect

HWs' morale and performance of different health interventions including IPTp. In Tanzania, Uganda and Zambia, HF understaffing contributed to HWs' perceived overwork, affecting the quality of care and HWs, adherence to IPTp-DOT guidelines (Hill and Kazembe 2006). Also, poor infrastructural status and low staff remuneration have demoralized HWs and lowered the general quality of care in SSA (Hanson et al., 2004; Hongoro and McPake 2003). A recent review of country experiences indicated the shortage of water and cups at HFs having affected HWs' adherence to DOT for IPTp in Tanzania and Uganda (Hill and Kazembe 2006). Several HWs in Dar es Salaam and Mkuranga district, Tanzania, reported the inconvenience faced due to wasting time and occasionally spending their out-of-pocket money finding water for use at clinic level (Mubyazi, PhD Thesis, submitted). Most studies report the low quality of the health-care given by the nurses to discourage women in utilising RCH services. This is a reality, although it is important to consider the reasons for such HWs to behave/practice in the way they do rather than only accusing them. For instance, studies in Zimbabwe (Mathole et al., 2005; Mathole et al., 2004) and Tanzania (Mubyazi et al., 2007b) found nurses complaining to have been working under pressure and with little sympathy from their clients.

The issue of unofficial user-fees on the fee-empted RCH services discussed before can be connected to health service providers' working condition. There is evidence that even when the HWs are informed of the exemption policy, they may still charge their clients due to poor remuneration and economic pressures to maintain their own good living (Priya 2002). ANC staff may also fail to administer SP not necessarily due to loss of interest, but pregnant women may hate taking SP, or due to drug shortages as noted in Tanzania (Anders et al., 2008), Kenya (Guyatt et al., 2004) and Malawi (Hill and Kazembe 2006).

In areas where there is no service, outreach clinic services are crucial to ensure physical accessibility (WHO 2005b). Although mobile clinics have been implemented in attempt to increase coverage of the remote and difficult-to-reach communities, they are hampered by low morale of the HWs who dislike travelling to remote places. So far evidence shows that the IPTp strategy like other drug-based malaria interventions is constrained by low outreach coverage (Mutabingwa 2002). In Korogwe district (Tanzania) district health management team (DHMT) reported lack of transport occasionally limiting the DHMT,s ability to reach remote HFs for health service supervision as planned. Therefore, it was suggested that concerted efforts for improving HWs' morale (including the issue of transport and number of HF staff) are necessary if compliance with IPTp service provision has to be realized (Mubyazi et al., 2005b).

Achievements and Opportunities for IPTp-SP and ANC Services

Despite the constraints mentioned above, IPTp implementation in SSA in SSA is happening and there are indications that it is possible to attain the Abuja target of the 60% coverage of pregnant women receiving IPTp (WHO and UNICEF 2003ab). Recently, countries such as Kenya, Malawi and Tanzania have reached and even passed the 60% coverage of women attending ANC clinics for two or more times and in some districts IPTp coverage have reached >60% for the first dose (Worrall et al., 2007; Hill and Kazembe

2006). There is also an encouraging trend in the coverage for the second dose although still less than 50% in Tanzania (Mubyazi et al., 2008), as in many other countries in southern Africa (Worrall et al., 2007; Hill and Kazembe 2006). The IPTp coverage records are encouraging, though not much, from a policy and programme perspective. However, good access to ANC does not warrant high uptake of IPTp-SP, since quality of care delivery factors, HWs, knowledge and motivations, and target population's knowledge, attitudes towards IPTp and practices remain important (Anders et al., 2008; Mubyazi et al., 2008; Hill and Kazembe 2006).

Discussion

Importance of IPTp: There has been a common appreciation on importance of malaria IPTp in SSA. However, based on different authors' observations, special consideration should be given to possible factors that may hinder the achievement of the desired level of coverage.

Socio-Economic and Systemic Considerations

Service provision/supply issues: Advocacy for critical and broad analysis of factors affecting malaria interventions (Hanson et al., 2004) is supported by evidence elucidated regarding the understaffing, shortage of utilities and drugs at a number of HFs. Low knowledge especially on the rationale and benefits of interventions may remain critical to IPTp implementation if concerted efforts are not made to overcome the challenges. It is still critical as it allows low adherence to IPTp, false beliefs and perceptions, and may even bias the performance of the HWs. Informal visits to TBA is unlikely to cease in SSA communities, and despite the need for involving the TBAs in malaria prevention strategies, such providers should consider themselves as replacement of the formal ANC system, rather than complementing it. Also, any view that the target service users are most likely to be less aware of a new intervention is not supported by evidence on the low knowledge on IPTp guidelines from a study of HWs (Mubyazi et al., 2008; Hill and Kazembe 2006). This suggests that policy and programme authorities should continue considering the building the capacity of the existing HWs by allocating additional resources for training and emphasising on regular supervision and periodically monitoring their performances.

Although some of the factors identified to lead to the low HWs' morale, including understaffing, poor infrastructural facilities and unsatisfactory salaries may not be removed overnight, efforts are required towards improvement. Working on some of these problems may not only (and necessarily) need additional financial resources, but (also) an improved management system that allows responsiveness to local needs and accountability. HWs may not necessarily claim for increased salaries rather than needing timely remuneration packages.

Service demand issues: User-fees may remain as a crucial health care financing mechanism both in the public and private sectors. Nevertheless, their implementation without affecting RCH services is questioned considering resource-poor settings where already pregnant women are constrained by other social-cultural gender biased conditions (Priya 2002). It should be remembered that poverty is rampant and both the pregnant women and the HWs are under undue economic pressures. Anything that may be used as an excuse to evade the pregnant women to attend HFs implementing user-fees will sound well to such women and add to reduction of the many roadblocks towards achieving the Abuja targets. Wrong beliefs about the intervention may be minimised through equipping the HWs with current knowledge and improving their working conditions so that they can be better advocates for health interventions (including IPTp). To most of the service clients and even some health service providers, prevention benefits are not seen immediately.

Even in conditions where there might be an adequate supply of drugs, the target users may still hate taking it as reported above. The Health Belief and Behavioural Theories assert that people may only adapt a disease preventive measure if they believe that they are either susceptible to or threatened by the disease with perceived consequences, and in the case of prevention they weigh the benefits of adapting the recommended method against the undesirable risks, costs and other consequences (Family Health International 2002; Becker 1974). Therefore, the reported delay by women to attend clinics and their negative attitudes towards SP may also be rooted from their disregard of malaria prevention through IPTp-SP, besides other reported barriers concerning imbalanced gender relations and poverty conditions facing most women in SSA.

Conclusion

The implementation of IPTp in SSA is undoubtedly done in multifaceted socio-economic and ANC resource constrained settings, this having an impact on the achievement of the Abuja targets. However difficult it might be, it is crucial to get prepared for the challenges in an attempt to minimise their impacts. As long as it is acknowledged that the benefits outweigh the costs or risks, scaling-up IPTp to increase coverage is crucial, considering the severe consequences to the mother and offspring of malaria in pregnancy. Establishing and using a wider evidence-base may help to arrive at informed policy and management decisions related to IPTp implementation. Currently, the evidence available regarding the determinants of ANC provision, utilisation and coverage is vast for decision makers to capitalise on the strengths and work on the existing challenges. The scaling-up of IPTp would benefit from applying knowledge acquired through research on the real situation and how to improve it. Yet, political will and taking action to provide moral and financial support on operational research are crucial. This would help monitoring what works and what does not in relation to ANC (Marchant et al., 2002). In principle, educating the general population is desirable to bring everybody to a good level of understanding, hence enhancing compliance and coverage. Education and advocacy efforts must be continuous and their emphasis must be maintained at all times. This requires a strong health system and revealed by this review, a robust health system is required for effective implementation of the IPTp strategy. The healthcare system must be strengthened by adequate staffing levels, sharpening staff skills and motivating them by improving the general staff working conditions. IPTp programme managers and frontline implementers at district level should be aware that not all HWs on malaria control services are fully knowledgeable about the intervention strategy (Mubyazi et al., 2008). Special attention should therefore be paid to instill such knowledge and to monitor its implementation. Improving HWs' morale to ensure durable effects requires the training of such workers and regularly supervising them, increasing the number of HWs, improving health infrastructure and working tools, and building trust and confidence among such workers and their service users. To make an important difference, operational health service and policy research should be an integral part of the intervention programme (Walley et al., 2007). Researchers should ensure that the translation of research evidence into systemic action requires timely conduction of research, submission of the research reports and in a form that can be easily used by decision makers (Mubyazi and Gonzalez-Block 2005).

Research Agenda

This review suggests the need for understanding the (a) perceptions and attitudes of pregnant women, the general public and health service providers concerning IPTp-SP; (b) the risk of ANC clients missing SP or getting it in a sub-standard way; (c) effect of user-fees on general services or ANC and indirect cost, e.g. travel, waiting time on IPTp delivery and coverage; (d) acceptability and practice of IPTp-SP in countries which have replaced SP with ACTs as the first-line drug for uncomplicated malaria as some people may have now preferred drugs other than SP which may be seen to be no longer beneficial (e) the feasibility and viability of IPTp in the existence of other malaria preventive methods that are promoted and implemented in different socio- cultural and health care delivery settings (Brieger 2007; Greenwood et al., 2007), (f) implications of HIV counselling and screening services on ANC attendances and delivery/uptake of IPTp-SP. We observe that in situations whereby women have to pay for the screening services or are stigmatised by HIV screening services at ANC clinics, the delivery of IPTp may be lowered by decreased women's attendances. This observation is supported by other authors (Baiden et al., 2005) who argue that in societies where women suffer abuse, social inequality and injustice, screening them for HIV at ANC clinics has both socio-cultural and ethical implications, which means ANC attendance may be reduced. The morbidity and mortality effects of malaria in pregnancy remain to be experienced if the apparently persistent and increasing trend of P.*falciparum* resistance to the recommended drugs is not reversed. This is a challenge, calling for the biomedical researchers to continue investigation towards discovery of alternative more effective drugs (Schultz et al., 2004; WHO 2004b).

Authors' Contributions

As part of his PhD study, GMM conceived the study, undertook the major review and drafted the manuscript. Invaluable comments and suggestions were made by CG and AYK.

CG also provided some articles for reference. Other co-authors co-supervised GMM,s PhD study under coordination by PB and ICB, besides their great comments on this paper. All the authors read and approved the MS for publication.

Acknowledgements

Professor Brian Greenwood (LSHTM, UK) commented on the earlier draft of the manuscript. Also, useful advice was obtained from Prof. Wen L. Kilama (AMANET, Tanzania) and Drs. Don de Savigny (STI, Switzerland) and Jasper N. Ijumba (University of Dar es Salaam, Tanzania). The study was funded by the Bill and Melinda Gates Foundation through Gates Malaria Partnership (GMP) coordinated by the London School of Hygiene and Tropical Medicine (UK) in collaboration with DBL-Centre for Health Research and Development, University of Copenhagen (Denmark), and NIMR (Tanzania). All the authors whose papers have been cited as reference materials in this paper.

Conflict of Interest

All the authors declare non-existence of conflict(s) of interest in this paper.

References

Acharya, LB; Cleland, J. Maternal and child health services in rural Nepal. *Health Policy & Planning*, 2000, 15(2), 223-229.

Adam, YM; Salihu, HM. Barriers to antenatal and obstetric care services in rural Kano. *Journal of Obstetric Gynaecology*, 2002, 6(22), 600-603.

Adams, SJ; Broadbent, J; Clayden, LM; Ridley, M. Erythema multiforme (Stevens-Johnson) precipitated by fansidar. *Postgrad. Med. J.*, 1985, 61(713), 263-4.

Anders, K; Marchant, T; Chambo, P; Mapunda, P; Reyburn, H. Timing of intermittent preventive treatment for malaria during pregnancy and the implementation of current policy on early uptake in north-east. *Tanzania. Malaria Journal*, 2008, 7, 79.

Baiden, F; Baiden, R; Williams, J; Akweongo, P; Clerk, C; Philips, DJ; Hodgson, A. Review of antenatal-linked voluntary counselling and HIV testing in sub-Saharan Africa: Lessons and Options for Ghana. *Ghana Medical Journal*, 2005, 39(1), 8-13.

Barat, LM; Palmer, N; Basu, S; Worrall, E; Hanson, K; Mills, A. Do malaria control interventions reach the poor? A view through the equity lens. *Am J. Trop. Med. Hyg.*, 2004, 71(Suppl 2), 174-178.

Becker, MH. The health belief model and personal behaviour. *Health Education Monographs*, 1974, 2(4), 409-19.

Bjorkman, A; Phillip-Howard, PA. Adverse reaction to sulfa drugs: implications for malaria chemotherapy. *Bull WHO*, 1991, 69, 297-304.

Boller, C; Wyss, K; Mtasiwa, D; Tanner, M. Quality and comparison of antenatal care in private and public providers in Dar Es Salaam, United Republic of Tanzania. *Bull WHO*, 2003, 81(2), 116-122.

Borghi, J; Ensor, T; Somanathan, A; Lissner, C; Mills, A. Mobilizing financial resources for maternal health. *Lancet*, 2006, 368, 1457-1465.

Brabin, BJ. An analysis of malaria in pregnancy in Africa. *Bull WHO*, 1983, 61, 1005-1016.

Breman, JG; Alilio, MS; Mills, A. Conquering the intolerable burden of malaria: What is needed: A summary. *Am. J. Trop. Med. Hyg.*, 2004, 71(Suppl 2), 1-15.

Brieger, B. Treating Malaria in Pregnancy: Searching for an Answer. *Malaria Matters*: 2007 [cited 2007 October 16]. Available from: http://www.malariafreefuture.org/blog/?cat=3.

Creel, LC; Sass, JV; Yinger, N. New perspectives on Quality of Care, No 2, 1996, pp1-8. Population Reference Bureau, Washington. [cited 2007 June 10]. Available from: http://www.prb.org/pdf/NewPerspQOC-Clients.pdf.

D'Alessandro, U; Brabin, B. Verhoeff. Malaria in pregnancy receives more attention. In: PREMA-EU Newsletter No 2, March 2003. [cited 2007 October 12]. Available from: http://www.prema-eu.org/.

DCP. Achieving the Millennium Development Goals for Health: So far progress is mixed-can we achieve our targets? *Disease Control Priorities Project* (DCP). The World Bank Group, 2006 and 2007. [cited 2007 November 10]. Available from: http://www.dcp2.org/pubs/DCP/Section/940.

Dellicour, S; Hall, S; Chandramohan, D; Greenwood, B. The safety of artemisins during pregnancy: a pressing question. *Malaria Journal*, 2007, 6(1), 15-17 DOI 300719.

EANMAT (East African Network on Malaria Treatment): Monitoring antimalarial drug resistance within national malaria control programmes: the EANMAT experience. *Tropical Medicine & International Health*, 2001, 6(10), 1-8.

Eijk, AM; Blokland, IE; Slutsker, L; Odhiambo, F; Ayisi, JG; Bles, HM; Rosen, DH; Adazu, K; Lindblade, KA. Use of intermittent preventive treatment for malaria in pregnancy in a rural area of western Kenya with high coverage of insecticide treated bednets. *Trop. Med., Int. Health*, 2005, 10(11), 1134-1140.

Ensor, T; Cooper, S. Overcoming barriers to health service access and influence on the demand side through purchasing. Health and Nutrition Discussion Paper, International Bank for Reconstruction and Development, Washington DC, September 2004.

Family Health International. Behaviour change – A summary of Four Major Theories, 2002. [cited 2007 November 10]. Available from: http://www.fhi.org/NR/rdonlyres/ei26vbslpsidmahhxc332vwo3g233xsqw22er3vofqvrfjvubwyzclvqjcbdgexyzl3msu4mn6xv5j/BCCSummaryFourMajorTheories.pdf.

Fantahun, M; Olwit, G. Factors related to Antenatal Clinic Choice and reported activities by pregnant women in Gulele district, Addis Abeba. *Ethiopian Medical Journal*, 1995, 33(1), 51-8.

Fathalla, M. Preface. *Paediatric and Perinatal Epidemiology*, 1988, 12(Suppl 2), vii-viii.

Filler, S; Kazembe, P; Thigpen, M; Macheso, A; Parise, ME; Newman, RD; Steketee, RW; Hamel, M. Randomized Trial of 2-Dose versus Monthly Sulfadoxine-Pyrimethamine Intermittent Preventive Treatment for Malaria in HIV-Positive and HIV-Negative Pregnant Women in Malawi. *Journal of Infectious Diseases*, 2006, 194(3), 286-93.

Frederickx, I. Health in rural Tanzania: the determinants of health status, health care demand and health care choice: *Discussion Paper Series DPS 98.03*. Katholieke Universiteit Leuven, Centre for Economic Studies, 1998.

Goodman, C; Coleman, P; Hanson, K; Meek, S; Mills, A. Economics of Malaria Control in sub-Saharan Africa. *Global Forum for Health Research*, WHO, Geneva, 2003.

Goodman, C; Coleman, P; Mills, A. The cost-effectiveness of antenatal prevention in sub-Saharan Africa. *Am. J Trop. Med. Hyg*., 2001, 64(1 Suppl), 45-56.

Greenwood, B; Alonso, P; ter Kuile, F; Hill, J; Steketee, R. Malaria in Pregnancy: priorities for Research. *Lancet Infect Dis.*, 2007, 7(2), 169-74.

Greenwood, B. The use of antimalarial drugs to prevent malaria in the populations of malaria endemic countries. *Am. J. Trop. Med. Hyg*., 2004, 70(1), 1-7.

Guyatt, HL; Noor, AM; Ochola, SA; Snow, RW. Use of intermittent presumptive treatment and bed nets by pregnant women in four Kenyan districts. *Trop. Med. Int. Health*, 2004, 9(2), 255-261.

Hanson, K; Goodman, C; Lines, J; Meek, S; Bradley, D; Mills, A. The economics of malaria control interventions. *Global Forum for Health Research*, WHO Geneva, 2004.

Hill, J; Kazembe, P. Reaching Abuja Targets for intermittent preventive treatment of malaria in pregnancy in African women: a review of progress and operational challenges. *Tropical Medicine and International Health*, 2006, 11(4), 409-418.

Holtz, TH; Kachur, SP; Roberts, JM; Marum, LH; Mkandala, C; Macheso, A. Use of antenatal services and IPT for malaria among pregnant women in Blantyre, Malawi District. *Trop. Med. Int. Health*, 2004, 9(1), 77-82.

Hongoro, C; McPake, B. Editorial: Human resources in health: putting the right agenda back to the front. *Trop Med Int. Health*, 2003, 8(11), 965-6.

Irshad, O. Intermittent treatment of malaria in pregnancy in Somalia. Presentation at the Roll Back Malaria Meeting in Muscat, 2002. [cited 2007 September 17]. Available from: http://www.emro.int/RBM/Meetings/Muscat02/Presentations.

Kambarami, RA; Chirenje, MZ; Rusakaniko, S. Antenatal care patterns and risk factors associated with perinatal outcome in two rural districts in Zimbabwe. *Central African Journal of Medicine*, 1999, 45, 294-9.

Langer, A; Villar, J; Romero, M; Nigenda, G; Piaggio, G; Kuchaisit, C; Rojas, G; Al-Osimi, M; Miguel, BJ; Al-Mazrou, Y., et al., Are women providers satisfied with antenatal care? Views on a standard and simplified, evidence-based model of care in four developing countries. *BMC Women's Health*, 2002, 2, 7.

Lenox-Smith, I. Fatal Stevens-Johnson syndrome associated with Fansidar and Chloroquine. *J. Infect*., 1987, 14(1), 90-2.

Leonard, KL; Mliga, GR; Haile Mariam, D. Bypassing health centres in Tanzania: revealed preferences for quality. *J Afr Econ*., 2002, 11(4), 441-471.

Magadi, MA; Madise, NJ. Rodrigues. Frequency and Timing of Antenatal Care in Kenya: Explaining variations between women in Different Communities. *Social Science and Medicine*, 2000, 51, 551-61.

Magnussen, P. Antimalarial intermittent treatment during pregnancy: how do we ensure coverage and compliance in Africa? In: PREMA-EU Newsletter No 2, pp 4-6, March 2003. [cited 2005 April 14]. Available from: www.prema-eu.org.

Malaria Consortium. Tanzania Roll Back Malaria Consultative Mission Report. Malaria Consortium, London, UK, 17 February 2004.

Mansfield, PR; Lexchin, J; Wen, LS; Grandori, L; McCoy, CP; Hoffman, JR; Ramos, J. Educating Health Professionals about Drug and Device Promotion: Advocates' Recommendations. *PLoS Medicine*, 2006, 3(11), e451.

Marchant, T; Armstrong Schellenberg, JRM; Edgar, T; Ronsmans, C; Nathan, R; Abdulla, S; Mukasa, O; Urasa, H; Lengeler, C. Anaemia during pregnancy in southern Tanzania. *Annals of Tropical Med. Hygiene. Parasit.*, 2002, 96(5), 477-487.

Mathole, T; Lindmark, G; Ahlberg, BM. Dilemmas and paradoxes in providing and changing antenatal care: a study of nurses and midwives in rural Zimbabwe. *Health Policy and Planning*, 2005, 20(6), 385-393.

Mathole, T; Lindmark, G; Majoko, F; Ahlberg, BM. A qualitative study of women's perspectives of antenatal care in a rural area of Zimbabwe. *Midwifery*, 2004, 20(2), 122-32.

Mbonye, AK; Neema, S; Magnussen, P. Malaria in pregnancy, risk perceptions and care seeking practices among adolescents in Mukono district, Uganda. *International Journal of Adolescent Medicine and Health*, 2006a, 18(4), 561-573.

Mbonye, AK; Neema, S; Magnussen, P. Perceptions on use of sulfadoxine-pyrimathamine in pregnancy and the policy implications for malaria control in Uganda. *Health Policy*, 2006b, 77(3), 279-89.

Mbonye, AK. *A new approach to deliver malaria prevention interventions to pregnant women at community level in Uganda*. PhD Thesis, University of Copenhagen, Denmark, 2006.

Menendez, C. Malaria during pregnancy: a priority area of malaria research and control. *Parasitology Today*, 1995, 11(5), 178-83.

Menendez, C. Strategies for scaling up intermittent presumptive treatment for malaria and anaemia in pregnant women and children. Report of the Scientific Working Group on Malaria, WHO 2003, 83-132.

Menendez, C. The effect of Malaria during Pregnancy on Infant Mortality in an area of Low Malaria Transmission. *Am. J. Trop. Med. Hyg.*, 2001, 15(5), 459-465.

Miller, KD; Lobel, HO; Satriale, RF; Kuritsky, JN; Stern, R; Campbell, CC. Severe cutaneous reactions among American travelers using sulfadoxine-pyrimethamine (fansidar) for malaria prophylaxis. *Am J Trop. Med. Hygiene*, 1986, 35(33), 451-58.

Mills, A. The challenges of scaling up malaria control. *Acta Tropica* 2005, Fourth MIM Pan-African Conference Abstract No. O-75, S47.

Mubyazi, G; Bloch, P; Byskov, J; Hansen, K; Olsen, Ø; Magnussen, P. Economic and other contextual determinants of the acceptability and viability of intermittent preventive treatment of malaria during pregnancy in Tanzania. *Acta Tropica, MIM Conference Abstracts*, 2005b, 95S(2005), S1-S506 p252.

Mubyazi, G; Bloch, P; Kamugisha, M; Kitua, A; Ijumba, J. Intermittent preventive treatment of malaria during pregnancy in Tanzania: a qualitative study of knowledge, attitudes and perceptions of district health managers, antenatal service staff and pregnant women in Korogwe district, northeastern *Tanzania. Malaria Journal*, 005a, 4, 31.

Mubyazi, G; Massaga, J; Kamugisha, M; Mubyazi J-Nyangoma; Gesase, S; Magogo, GC; Mdira, K; Sukwa, T. Effects of user charges on revenue collections, quality of care and patient attendances for malaria at government dispensaries and health centres in Korogwe district, *Tanzania. Health Service Management Research*, 2006, 19(1), 23-35.

Mubyazi, GM; Bygbjerg, IC; Magnussen, P; Olsen, ØE; Byskov, J; Hansen, K; Bloch, P. Opportunities, achievements and challenges for scaling-up malaria chemoprevention in pregnancy in Tanzania: perspectives of national level officers. *Malaria Journal*, 2008, 7, 135.

Mubyazi, GM; Gonzalez-Block, MA. Research influence on national antimalarial drug policy in Tanzania: case study of changing from chloroquine to sulfadoxine-pyrimethamine. *Malaria Journal*, 2005, 4, 51.

Mubyazi, GM; Mushi, A; Kamugisha, M; Massaga, J; Mdira, KY; Segeja, M; Njunwa, KJ. Community views on health sector reform and their participation in health priority setting: case of Lushoto and Muheza districts, Tanzania. *Journal of Public Health*, 2007, 29(2), 147-156, doi:10.1.1093/pubmed/fdm016.

Mubyazi, GM; Mushi, AK; Shayo, E; Mdira, K; Ikingura, J; Mutagwaba, D; Malecela, M; Njunwa, KJ. Local Primary Health Care Committees and Community-Based Health Workers in Mkuranga District, Tanzania: Does the Public Recognise and Appreciate Them? *Ethno-Medicine*, 2007, 1, 27-35.

Mubyazi, GM. The Tanzanian policy on health care fee waivers and exemptions in practice as compared with other developing countries: evidence from recent local studies and international literature. *East African Journal of Public Health*, 2004, 1(1), 11-17.

Mufubenga, P. Prevention and control of malaria in pregnancy: The Ugandan experience. In: *PREMA-EU, Newsletter* No. 2, March 2003, 6-11. [cited 2005 April 14]. Available from: www.prema-eu.org.

Murira, N; Lutzen, K; Lindmark, G; Christensson, K. Communication patterns between health care providers and their clients at an antenatal clinic in Zimbabwe. *Health Care for Women International*, 2003, 24(2), 83-92.

Murray, SF; Nyambo, M. Exploring the role of private maternity services in India, Nepal and Tanzania. Final Report. Submitted to DFID by the Options Consultancy Services and King's College, London, 12 December 2003.

Mutabingwa, TK; Maxwell, CA; Sia, IG; Msuya, FH; Mkongewa, S; Vannithole, S; Curtis, J; Curtis, CF. A trial of proguinil-dapsone in comparison with sulfadoxine-pyrimethamine for the clearance of Plasmodium falciparum infection in Tanzania. *Trans. Roy. Soc. Trop. Med. Hyg*., 2001, 95, 433-438.

Mutabingwa, TK. Antimalarial Intermittent Treatment during Pregnancy in Africa. In: PREMA-EU Newsletter, Issue 1, November, 2002. [cited 2005 April 14]. Available from: www.prema-eu.org.

Mutabingwa, TK; Malle, LN; de Geus, A; Oosting, J. Malaria chemosuppression during pregnancy. II: Its effects on maternal haemoglobin levels, placental malaria and birth-weight. *Tropical and geographical medicine*., 1993, 45, 49-55.

Mwenesi, HA. Sociocultural and behavioural issues in the treatment and prevention of malaria. *Report of the Scientific Working Group on Malaria*, WHO 2003, 126-132.

Ndyomugyenyi, R; Neema, S; Magnussen, P. The use of informal services for antenatal care and malaria treatment in rural Uganda. *Health Policy & Planning*, 1996, 13(1), 94-102.

Newman, RD; Parise, ME; Slutsker, L; Nahlen, B; Steketee, RW. Safety, efficacy and determinants of effectiveness of antimalarial drugs during pregnancy: implications for prevention programmes in *Plasmodium falciparum-endemic* sub-Saharan Africa. *Tropical Medicine and International Health*, 2003, 8(6), 488-506.

Nganda, RY; Drakeley, C; Reyburn, H; Marchant, T. Knowledge of malaria influences the use of insecticide treated nets but not intermittent presumptive treatment by pregnant women in Tanzania. *Malaria Journal*, 2004, 3, 42.

Nsimba, ED. How sulfadoxine-Pyrimethamine was perceived in some rural communities after phasing out chloroquine as a first-line drug for uncomplicated malaria in Tanzania: lessons to learn towards moving from monotherapy to fixed combination therapy. *Journal of Ethnobiology and Ethnomedicine*, 2006, 2, 5.

Nyonator, F; Kutzin, J. Health for some? The effects of user-fees in the Volta Region of Ghana. *Health Policy and Planning*, 1999, 14(4), 329-341.

Okonofua, FE; Feyiseteam, BJ; Dvies-Adetugbo, Sanusi, YO. Influence of socio-economic factors on the treatment and prevention of malaria in pregnant and no-pregnant adolescent girls in Nigeria. *J. Trop. Med. Hyg*., 1992, 95(5), 309-15.

Overbosch, GB; Nsowah-Nuamah, NNN; van den Boom, GJM; Damnyag, L. Determinants of antenatal care use in Ghana. *Journal of African Economies*, 2004, 13(2), 277-301.

Phillip-Howard, P. Epidemiological and control issues related to malaria in pregnancy. *Annals of Tropical Medicine and Parasitology*, 1999, 93(Suppl. 1), 11-17.

Phillip-Howard, PA; Behrens, RH; Dunlop, J. Steven-Johnson syndrome due to pyrimethamine/sulfadoxine during presumptive self therapy of malaria. *Lancet*, 1989, 2(8666), 803-4.

Phillip-Howard, PA; Wennemuehler, KA; ter Kuile, FO; Hawley, WA; Kolczak, MS; Odhacha, A; Vulule, JM; Nahlem, B. Diagnostic and prescribing practices in peripheral health facilities in rural Kenya. *Am J Top Med Hyg*., 2003, 68(Suppl 4), 44-49.

Pokhrel, S. Scaling up interventions in resource-poor countries: what role does research in stated-preference framework play? A commentary. *Health Research Policy and Systems*, 2006, 4, 4.

Priya, N. Gender Dimensions of User fees: Implications for Women's Utilisation of Health Care. *Reproductive Health Matters*, 2002, 10(20), 127-134.

Puska, P. WHO Director General election: public-health infrastructures: Comment. *Lancet*, 2006, 368, 1400-1403.

Ribera, MJ; Hausmann-Muela, S; D'Alesaandro, U; Grietens, PK. Malaria in Pregnancy: What can Social Sciences Contribute? *PLoS Medicine*, 2007, 4(4), e92 pp 0001-0005.

Robb, A. Malaria in pregnancy: Implementation of Interventions. *Ann. Trop. Med. Par*., 2002, 93(1), Suppl. 1, 67-70.

Rogerson, SL; Chaluluka, E; Kanjala, M; Mkundika, P; Mhango, CG; Molyneux, ME. Intermittent sulfadoxine-pyrimethamine in pregnancy: effectiveness against malaria morbidity in Blantyre, Malawi, in 1997-1999. *Trans. R. Trop. Med. Hyg*., 2000, 94, 549-553.

Rønn, A; Msangeni, H; Mhina, J; Wernsdorfer, W; Bygbjerg, I. High level of resistance of *P. falciparum* to sulfadoxine-pyrimethamine in children in Tanzania. *Trans. R. Soc Hyg. Trop. Medicine*, 1996, 54, 179-181.

Rugemalila, JB; Wanga, CL; Kilama, WL. Sixth African Malaria day in 2006: how have we come after the Abuja Declaration? *Malaria Journal*, 2006, 5, 102.

Sachs, JD. Achieving the Millennium Development Goals- The Case of Malaria. *The New England Journal of Medicine*, 2005, 352(2), 115-117.

Schultz, L; Steketee, RW; Parise, M; Wirima, JJ; Oloo, A; Nahlen, B. A selection of Essays: Malaria During Pregnancy: An antenatal Intervention Strategy Whose Time Has Come. [cited 2004 August 26]. Available from: IRDC 2001, http://web.idrc.ca/en/ev/28394-201-1-DO_TOPIC.html.

Snow, RW. The invisible victims: A special supplement Issue. *Nature*, 2004, 430, 934-935.

Steketee, RW; Nahlen, BL; Parise, ME; Menendez, C. The burden of malaria in pregnancy in malaria-endemic areas. *Am. J. Trop. Med. Hyg*., 2001, 64 (Supple 1–2), 28-35.

Tanner, M; Vlassof, C. Treatment seeking behaviour for malaria: a typology based on endemicity and gender. *Social Science and Medicine*, 1998, 46, 523-532.

Thaddeus, S; Maine, D. Too far to walk: maternal mortality in context. *Social Science and Medicine*, 1994, 38, 1091-110.

Vallely, A; Vallely, L; Changalucha, J; Greenwood, B; Chandramohan, D. Intermittent preventive treatment for malaria in pregnancy in Africa: what's new, what's needed? *Malaria Journal*, 2007, 6, 16.

van Eijk, AM; Ayisi, AG; tel Kuile, FO; Otieno, JA; Odondi, MJO; Rose, DH; Kager, PA; Steketee, RW; Nahlen, BL. Implementation of intermittent preventive treatment with sulfadoxine-pyrimethamine for control of malaria in pregnancy in Kisumu, western Kenya. *Trop Med Int. Health*, 2004, 9(5), 630-7.

van Eijk, AM; Bles, H; Odhiambo, F; Ayisi, JG; Blokland, EI; Rosen, DH. Use of antenatal services and delivery among women in rural western Kenya: a community based survey. *Reproductive Health*, 2006, 3, 2.

van Geertruyden, JP; Thomas, F; Erhart, A; D'Alesandro, U. The contribution of malaria in pregnancy to perinatal mortality. *Am J Trop Med Hyg*., 2004, 71(Suppl 2), 35-40.

Verhoeff, FH; Brabin, BJ; Chimsuku, L; Kazembe, P; Russel, WB; Broadhead, RL. An evaluation of effects of intermittent sulfadoxine-pyrimethamine treatment in pregnancy on parasite clearance and risk of low birth-weight in rural Malawi. *Ann. Trop. Med. Parasit*, 1998, 92(2), 141-50.

Wagle, RR; Sabroe, S; Nielsen, BB. Socio-economic and physical distance to maternity hospital as predictors for place of delivery: an observation study from Nepal. *Pregnancy and Child Birth*, 2004, 4, 8.

Walley, J; Khan, AM; Shah, KS; Witter, S; Xiaolin, W. How to get practice into research. *Bulletin of the World Health Organization*, 2007, 85(6), 424-5.

White, N. Intermittent Presumptive Treatment for Malaria. *PLoS Medicine*, 2005, 2(1), e1/e3, pp 0028-0033.

WHO, UNICEF. Africa Malaria Report on Malaria in Pregnancy. World Health Organization, Geneva 2003a. [cited 2007 June 2]. Available from: http://www.rbm.who.int/amd2003/amr2003/ch4.htm.

WHO, UNICEF. Antenatal Care in Developing Countries: Promises, Achievements and Missed Opportunities: Analysis of Trends, levels and differentials. World Health Organization, Geneva, 2003b.

WHO. Implementation research: bridging the gap between efficacy trials and application. *TDR Newsletter* No. 71, 9 February 2004b.

WHO. Provision of effective antenatal care: Standards for maternal and neonatal care: *Doc. No 1.6: Integrated Management of Pregnancy and Childbirth* (IMPAC). World Health Organization, Geneva, 2005a. [cited 2005 April 14]. Available from: http/www.who.int/making_pregnancy_safer/publications/standards1.6N.pdf

WHO. Realizing the potential of antenatal care. In: *The World Health Report*, 2005b. WHO Geneva. [cited 2007 August 12]. Available from: http://www.who.int/whr/2005/chapter3/en/index2.*html.*

WHO. WHO renews call for effective malaria treatment. World Health Organization, 2004b, [cited 2007 November 17]. Available from: News-Medical.net, at www.newsmedical.net/

WHO: The Abuja Declaration and the Plan of Action: An extract from The African Summit on Roll Back Malaria, Abuja 25 April 2000. WHO/CDC/RBM/2000.17.

WHO: The use of antimalarial drugs: chemoprophylaxis treatment of malaria in special groups. WHO 2001; [cited 2007 January 12]. Available from: http://www.rbm.who.int/cmc_upload/0/000/014/923/am_3.htm#p3.1).

Wilkinson, D; Gouws, E; Sach, M; Karim, SS. Effect of removing user fees on attendance for curative and preventive primary health care services in rural South Africa. *Bulletin of the WHO Organization*, 2001, 79(7), 665-71.

Worrall, E; Morel, C; Shunmay, Y; Borghi, J; Webster, J; Hill, J; Wiseman, V; Mills, A. The economics of malaria in pregnancy – a review of the evidence and research priorities. *The Lancet*, 2007, 7, 156-168.

Wyss, K. An approach to clarifying human resources constraints to attaining health-related Millennium Development Goals. *Human Resources for Health*, 2005, 2, 11.

In: Antimalarial Drugs: Costs, Safety and Efficacy
Editors: Emanuel Csizmadia and Istvan Kalnoky
ISBN: 978-1-60741-432-2

Chapter V

SFC-MS Analysis of Contaminants in Primaquine Diphosphate Tablets and Spectral UV and NMR Characterising of Primaquine and Quinocide

Ilia Brondz*
Department of Biology, University of Oslo, P.O. Box 1066,
Blindern, 0316 Oslo, Norway

Abstract

In the *Pharmacopoeias*, characterization of the toxic contaminant in primaquine is not described. The *Pharmacopoeias* require chromatographic separation Rs greater than 2 between the contaminant and API peak, based on separation using HPLC. The United States Pharmacopeia (USP) and The National Formulary (NF) seek submission of a monograph proposing an improvement of analysis of primaquine phosphate tablets.

In this study, resolution based on supercritical fluid chromatography (SFC) and supercritical fluid chromatography-mass spectrometry (SFC-MS) satisfy the *Pharmacopoeia* standards.

Primaquine diphosphate 7.5 mg tablets were analyzed. Separation Rs greater than 2 was achieved between the major contaminant peak and the peak of the API in less than 15 minutes. The novelty of this work is the determination of the main contaminant in medical form primaquine diphosphate tablets.

Keywords: SFC-MS, Primaquine; Quinocide; Anti-malaria drug; Contaminations in primaquine tablets.

* Corresponding author: Department of Biology, University of Oslo, P.O. Box 1066, Blindern, 0316 Oslo, Norway, Phone: +47 22 85 73 53, Mobile: +47 93 81 48 64, E-mail: ilia.brondz@bio.uio.no

1. Introduction

Primaquine (CAS 90-34-6) is used as a treatment of malaria. It has recently been shown that unprocessed primaquine used in the pharmaceutical industry is contaminated with the positional isomer quinocide (CAS 525-61-1) [1–9]. Currently, *Pharmacopoeias* [10] allow primaquine purity from 98.5% to 101.5%. The nature of contaminants in this drug does not require a description, despite the high level of contamination allowed. In 2003 [1], evidence for the nature of the contaminant in primaquine diphosphate was first publicly presented. Since presentation at international meetings in 2003–4 [1, 2] and a paper published in J. Chromatography B in 2004 [3], very little has been done to develop analytical procedures to verify the quinocide in primaquine for inclusion in the *Pharmacopoeias*. The United States Pharmacopeia (USP) seeks submission of a monograph proposal for improvement of analysis of primaquine phosphate tablets. Quinocide, a highly toxic substance, is a principal contaminant in the drug primaquine diphosphate. The toxicological properties of quinocide and the tolerances of animals to the drug, and the metabolism are presented in [11–14]. The acute toxic effects of combinations of quinocide with other antimalarial drugs are presented in [15]. The conclusion is that quinocide caused either additive or synergistic toxic effects; similar observations were seen using a unicellular model [3].

Primaquine and quinocide can have a number of side effects, such as inducing methemoglobinemia [16–20], effects on the red blood cell membrane [21], and hemolytic effects [22, 23]. The neurotoxicity of the 8-aminoquinolines [24, 25] is well known. Polyamines may be involved in the development of hepatic encephalopathy and cerebral edema [26]. Neuropsychiatric manifestations after therapy with the quinoline derivative *mefloquine* [27] and cases showing the carcinogenicity of primaquine have also been reported [28]. Cardiotoxicity in patients undergoing malaria therapy with aminoquinolines due to blockade of Na^+ channels is discussed in [29].

Malaria is one of the most widely spread and deadly diseases on the planet. Primaquine has high antiparasitic effects against gametocytes and thus the ability to prevent the spread of the parasite from patients by mosquitoes. It is also used in radical cures and prevents relapses. Consequently, primaquine is a frequently used drug.

The aim of this study was to achieve chromatographic resolution between the principal substance and the major contaminant demanded in the *Pharmacopoeia* [10] and to record the presence of the toxic contaminant quinocide in pharmaceutical products such as medical form tablets.

In 2003 [1, 3], evidence of the nature of the principal contaminant in primaquine diphosphate was presented by using HPLC-MS, in 2004 the same was done by using GC-MS [2, 4], the results were supported by SFC-MS [6, 9].

The use of GC-MS with supersonic molecular beam (SMB) was performed to study the possible fast analysis of contaminants in pharmaceutical products such as medical form tablets.

SMB was used for interfacing the GC to the MS [30-32] and as a medium for ionization of sample compounds while in the SMB by electron ionization [33-35]. The technology of GC-MS with SMB is reviewed in reference [36]. SMBs are characterized by intra-molecular vibrational supercooling of its seeded compounds due to relatively low collision energies of sample compounds and carrier gas species during the supersonic expansion. Extended range of thermally labile molecules are amenable for analysis due to the use of high column flow rate and contact free fly-through ion source [36, 37].

2. Materials and Methods

2.1. Sample Preparation SFC-MS

Primaquine diphosphate p.a. (Sigma-Aldrich, Steinheim, Germany), and standard quinocide dihydrochloride, were used [3]. The standard solutions were prepared in 10 mL of ethanol (Arcus, Oslo, Norway) containing 0.4% (v/v) of diethylamine (Merck, Darmstadt, Germany). Thirty primaquine diphosphate 7.5 mg tablets purchased from the Norwegian Medical Depot (NMD, Oslo, Norway) batch No. 2080222 were used. Nine groups of three tablets were pulverized in an agate mortar with an agate pestle. Each group of tablets was quantitatively transferred to a glass centrifuge tube and extracted with 3 mL of ethanol containing 0.4% (v/v) diethylamine.

Extraction was performed with vigorous shaking, followed by centrifugation for 15 min at 4 °C at 5000 rpm. The procedure was repeated three times and the extracts combined. An additional round of extractions from each group of three tablets was performed to collect extracts for a control series for measuring the levels of any remaining substances. The final volume of extracts from tablets was justified to10 mL by adding some μL of respective extract from control series.

2.2. Sample Preparation for GC-MS with SMB

Three 7.5 mg primaquine diphosphate tablets were pulverized in agate mortar 5 mg of the pulverized mass was used in analysis. Primaquine diphosphate and quinocide dihydrochloride were used as standards. Each sample was dissolved in 1 mL of purified water grade I and 0.1 mL of concentrated ammonium hydroxide p.a. grade (Merck, Darmstadt, Germany), was added. The base was extracted in 1 mL of p.a. quality hexane (Merck).

2.3. Supercritical Fluid Chromatography (SFC) and Supercritical Fluid Chromatography-mass Spectrometry (SFC-MS)

The following instruments were used: a MiniGram SFC (Berger Instruments Inc., Newark, DE, USA) running under ProNTo software (Berger Instruments Inc.) and equipped with a K-2501 UV detector (Advanced Scientific Instruments, Dr. Knauer, Berlin, Germany) set at a wavelength of 261 nm. A part of the flow stream was diverted with a 10/1 fixed splitter (UV/MS) to feed a Micromass PLCZ 4190 mass spectrometer equipped with a pneumatically assisted electrospray ionization source (ESI) running under MassLynx 4.0 (Waters-Micromass, Manchester, UK). The connecting line to the MS was through T-form tubing equipped with a manually operated microvalve and capillary restrictor. The MS conditions were: cone voltage 60 V, extractor voltage 12 V, capillary voltage 4.5 kV, ion energy 1.0 V, multiplier at 400 V, analyzer vacuum of 2.6 kPa, and a desolvation gas flow of 495 L x hr^{-1}. The mass-to-charge ratio was scanned automatically in the range from 80 to 400. The MS was operated in the positive charge mode. The instrument was previously calibrated with sodium iodide. Isocratic chromatography was performed using CO_2 in a supercritical state with ethanol containing 0.4% diethylamine. At the end of the analysis, the manually operated microvalve was closed, thus closing the flow of effluent to the MS, and tubing directing the effluent to the waste through a capillary restrictor. The percentage of modifier in the effluent was elevated to 50% at a rate of 10% per min and held at 50% for 3 min, then lowered to the level required for analysis at a rate of 10% per min and held for 3 min to stabilize the column. The manually operated microvalve was then reopened to direct effluent to the MS for 3 min before analysis.

2.3.1. SFC-MS analysis of primaquine diphosphate 7.5 mg tablets

A Discovery HS F5 column 250 mm × 4.6 mm i.d. comprising 6 μm particles from Supelco (Supelco, Bellefonte, PA, USA) was converted to SFC. The column was converted as described previously [7]. Isocratic chromatography was performed using CO_2 in a supercritical state with 15% ethanol containing 0.4% diethylamine. The conditions for SFC-MS are described in section 2.2. Separation and the detection of analytes by UV are shown in the chromatogram in Figure 1 and the TIC in Figure 2. Three analyses were conducted for every extract.

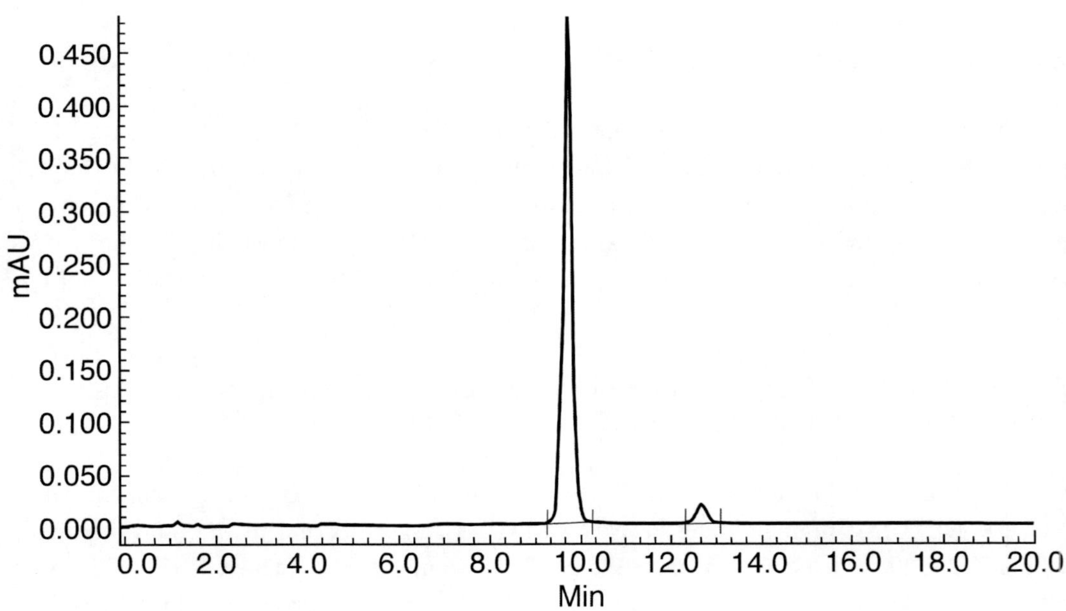

Figure 1. Chromatogram is showing the content of primaquine tablet resolved by SFC. There are two peaks on chromatogram, the primaquine is the major peak and the quinocide is the moderate peak. The details of the conditions described in the text.

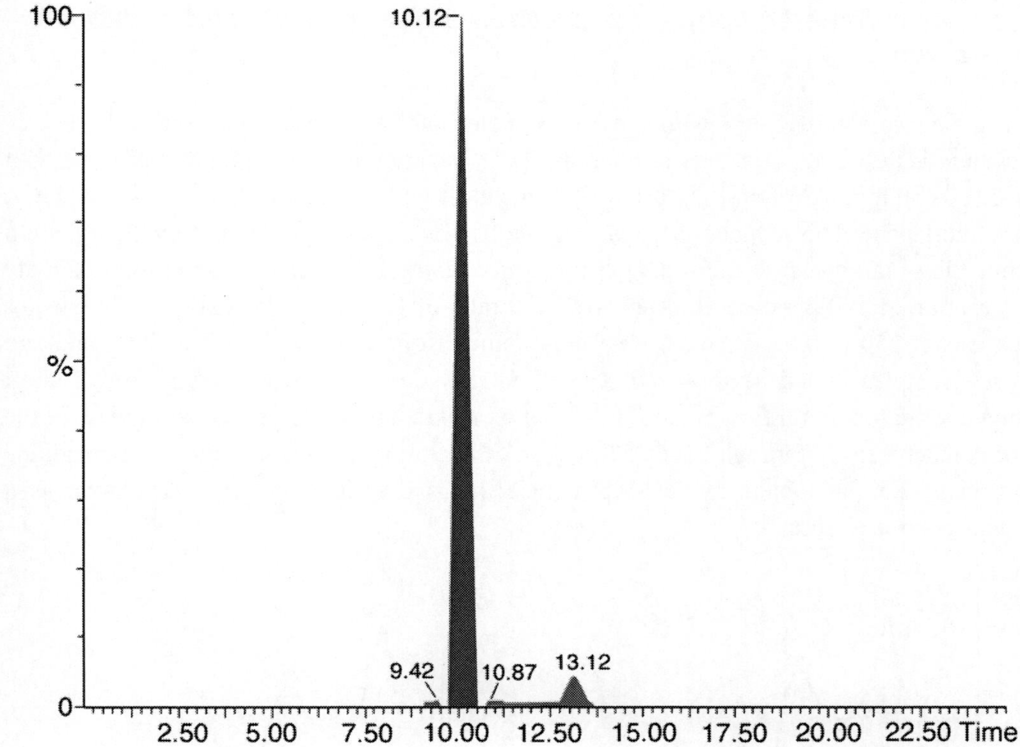

Figure 2. Total ion current (TIC) indicating content primaquine diphosphate tablets.
The analysis using UV detection shown in Fig 1 was monitored by MS. There are four peaks. The first is a minor peak with an R_t of 9.42 min is unidentified. The second peak is a major peak with an R_t of 10.12 min is primaquine. The third peak is minor one with an R_t of 10.87 min is unidentified. The fourth peak, with an R_t of 13.12 min, is quinocide.

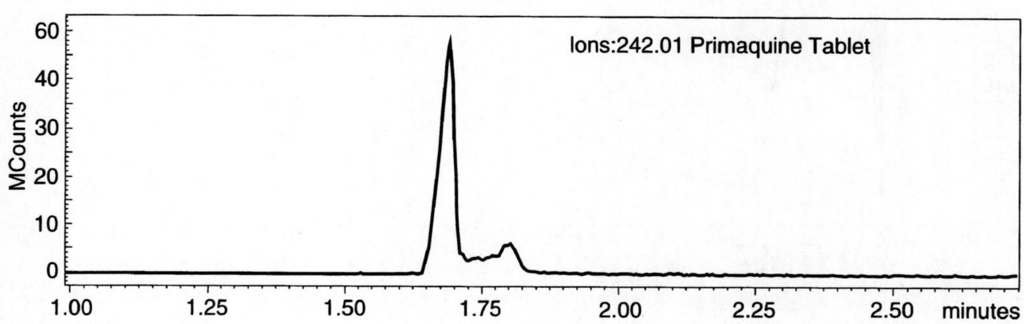

Figure 3. GC-MS with supersonic molecular beam (SMB) shows analysis of primaquine diphosphate 7.5 mg tablets. The tablets extract in hexane was analyzed at the conditions described in text above. The full scan (TIC) of the drug tablet in the mass spectral range 50-400 amu, shows the RSIM on *m/z* = 242. The major peak is the primaquine and the minor peak is the quinocide.

2.3.2. Gas chromatography-mass spectrometry with supersonic molecular beam

The experimental GC-MS with supersonic molecular beam based on a Varian 1200 GC-MS system is described in details in reference [32]. Separation of compounds was done with a VF-5HT column, 0.25 mm I.D., 0.1 μ film thickness and 4 m length (Varian, Middleburg, The Netherlands). The reduction of column length was done in the laboratory. The helium column flow rate was 8 ml/min. 1 μL sample extract in hexane at an approximate concentration of 200 ppm was injected with split ratio of 10:1 using the Varian 1079 injector which was at 250°C. The GC oven was programmed from 120°C to 300°C at 30°C/min and the drug samples eluted at about 165°C without any degradation due to the use of short column and high column flow rate [37]. Ion source degradation was prevented in view of the use of contact free fly-through EI ion source [36]. Separation and the detection of primaquine diphosphate 7.5 mg tablets by GC-MS with SMB is described in [38] and shown as a chromatogram in Figure 3.

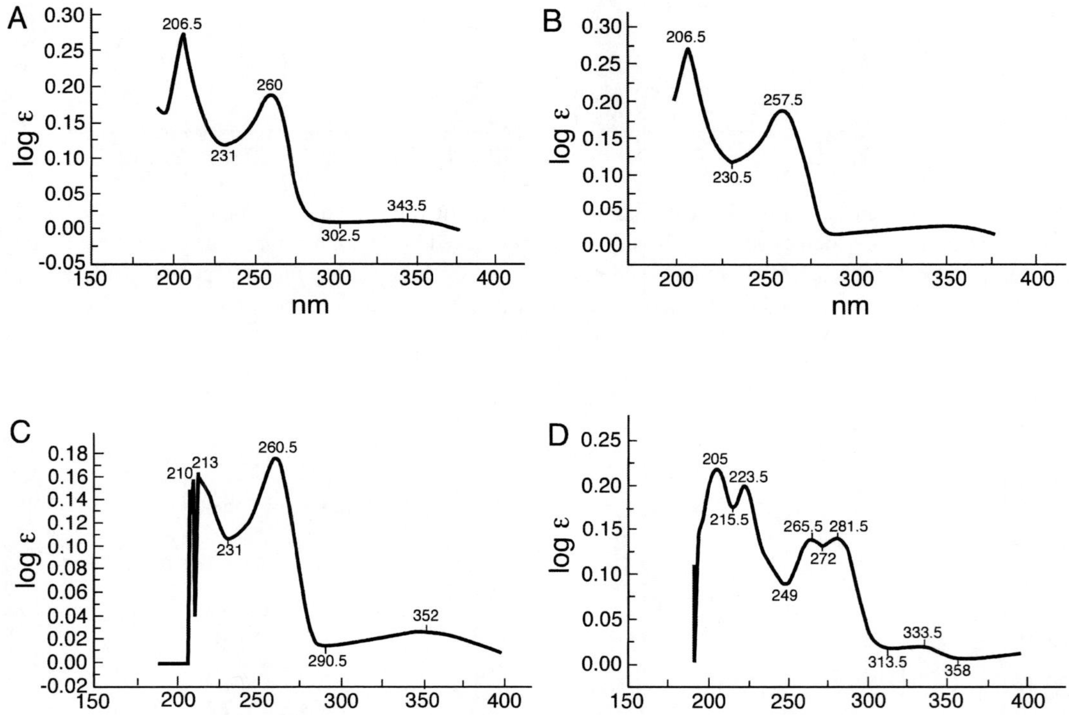

Figure 4. The UV spectra of primaquine batch 16039 [3] analyzed by using a Jasco J-810 spectrometer. The details described in the text.

A. Primaquine in deionized water.

B. Primaquine in a 0.01 N NH3OH.

C. Primaquine in a 0.01 N NaOH.

D. Primaquine in a 0.01 N HCl.

2.3.3. UV spectrometry

The UV spectra of primaquine and quinocide in p.a. quality hydrochloric acid (Merck) diluted to 0.01 N with deionized water, in p.a. quality ammonium hydroxide (Merck) diluted to 0.01 N with deionized water, in p.a. quality sodium hydroxide (Merck) diluted to 0.01 N with deionized water, and in deionized water were recorded using a Jasco J-810 spectrometer (Jasco International, Tokyo, Japan). Measurements were performed at 23 °C using a quartz cell with a path length of 1.0 cm. All measurements were performed at 0.04 mg mL^{-1} with respect to the primaquine or quinocide base. Samples were scanned five times at 50 nm min^{-1} with a bandwidth of 1 nm and a response time of 1 s over the wavelength range 190–400 nm. The data were averaged and the spectrum of a respective sample-free control sample (0.01 N HCl, 0.01 N NH_3OH, 0.01 N NaOH, and deionized water) was subtracted respectively. The resultant spectra were then smoothed using the means-movement method. All measurements were conducted twice. The UV spectra of primaquine in deionized water, NH_3OH, NaOH, and HCl are shown in Figure 4 A, B, C, and D, respectively, and the UV spectra of quinocide in deionized water, NH_3OH, NaOH and HCl are shown in Figure 5 A, B, C, and D, respectively.

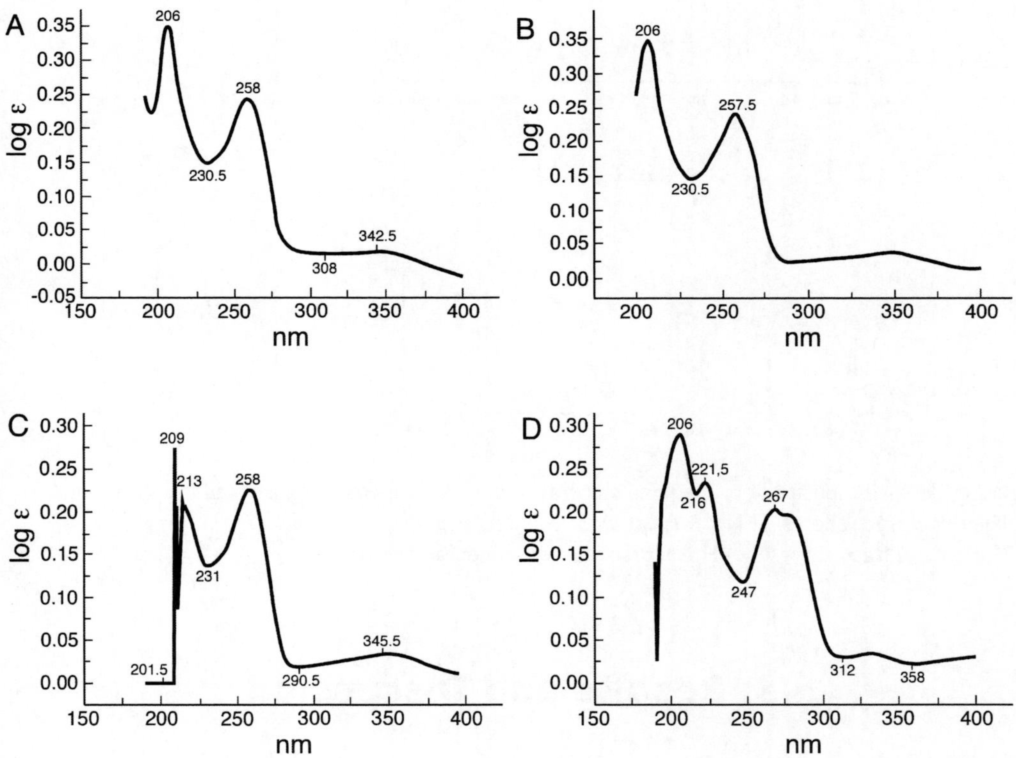

Figure 5. The UV spectra of quinocide batch 17172 [3] analyzed by using a Jasco J-810 spectrometer. The details described in the text.

A. Quinocide in deionized water.

B. Quinocide in a 0.01 N NH3OH.

C. Quinocide in a 0.01 N NaOH.

D. Quinocide in a 0.01 N HCl.

2.3.4. ^1H, ^{13}C, and ^{15}N NMR spectroscopy

The ^1H, ^{13}C, and ^{15}N NMR spectra of primaquine dichloride and quinocide dichloride in DMSO-d6 were recorded using a Bruker Avance 500 MHz instrument (Bruker BioSpin Gmb, Rheinstetten, Germany). The ^1H, ^{13}C, and ^{15}N chemical shift values are presented on a δ scale in ppm relative to DMSO-d6. The ^1H, ^{13}C, and ^{15}N chemical shift values were recorded on the δ scale in ppm relative to DMSO-d6 for ^1H and ^{13}C ref. 2.49 ppm and 39.5 ppm and for ^{15}N CH_2NO_2 in DMSO-d6 9:1 ref. 0.0 ppm. NMR ^1H spectra of primaquine dichloride and quinocide dichloride are shown in Figure 6 A and B and in Figure 7 and 8 shown chemical shift values including ^{15}N. NMR ^{13}C spectra of primaquine dichloride and quinocide dichloride are shown in Figure 9 A and B and in Figure 7 and 8 shown chemical shift values.

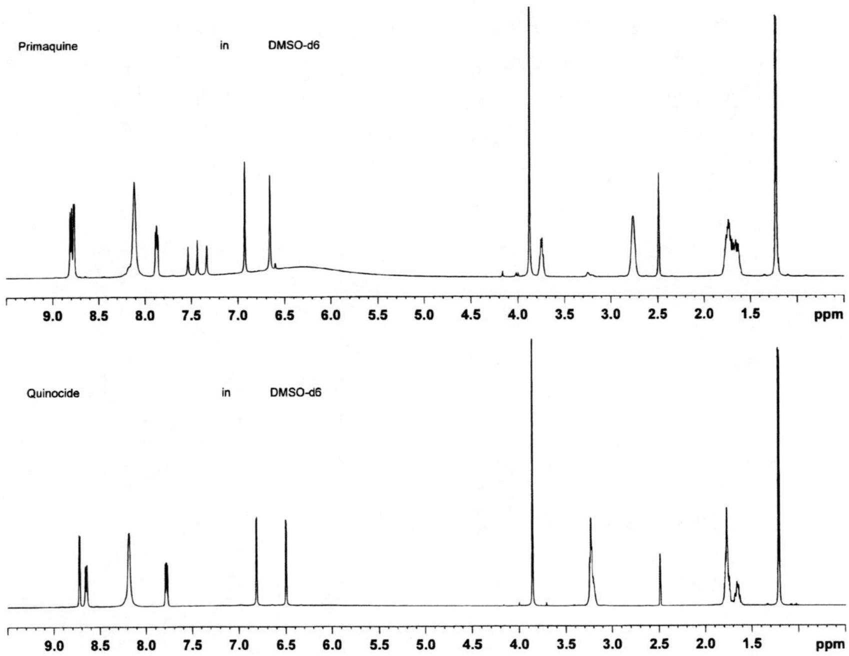

Figure 6. ^1H NMR spectra of primaquine chloride and quinocide chloride analysed in DMSO-d6.
A. The upper trace shows ^1H NMR spectra of primaquine chloride.
B. The bottom trace shows the ^1H NMR spectra of quinocide chloride.

3. Results and Discussion

3.1. The Nature of the Contaminant in Primaquine Diphosphate Tablets

Currently, the *Pharmacopoeia* [10] allows primaquine purity from 98.5% to 101.5%; however, the USP 31 [39] allows primaquine purity from 98.0% to 102.0% and primaquine phosphate tablets contain not less than 98.0 percent and not more than 107.0 percent of the labeled amount of $C_{15}H_{21}N_3O \cdot 2H_3PO_4$.

Used nomenclature:

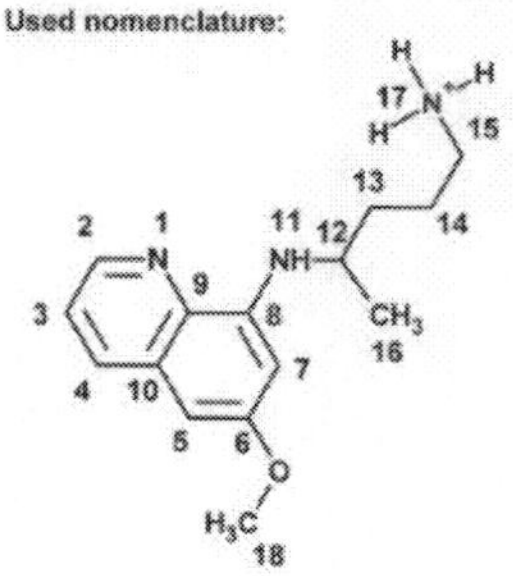

Primaquine

Atom	^{15}N	^{13}C	^{1}H		multiplicity
1	*				
2		139,5	8,77		d, J = 4.6
3		122,5	7,88		dd, J = 8.3 Hz 4.6 Hz
4		144,8	8,81		d, J = 8.3 Hz
5		94,8	6,93		d, J = 1.7 Hz
6		160,3			
7		102,5	6,66		s (d, J = 1.7 Hz [1])
8		139,8			
9		124,7			
10		131,8			
11	- 293,8		6,31		very broad
12		48,5	3,75		m
13		32,2	1,64	1,76	2 x m
14		23,9	1,74	1,74	m
15		38,8	2,76	2,76	m
16		19,6	1,23		d, J = 6.2 Hz
17	*		8,11		br s
18		56,1	3,88		s
Ref	0,0 ppm**	39,5 ppm	2,49 ppm		

* not observed

** CH_3NO_2 in DMSO - d_6 9:1

Figure 7. The molecule of primaquine with used nomenclature for C and N atoms is shown together with the table of chemical shift values including ^{15}N, ^{13}C and ^{1}H. The details described in the text.

The USP 31 [39] seeks submission of a monograph proposal for improvement of analysis for primaquine phosphate tablets "In an effort to improve drug product, drug substance, and excipient monographs to current scientific/regulatory standards, USP is seeking submission of proposals for improved methods for inclusion in the following USP-NF monographs to replace the current procedures that may be deficient, flawed, or unsafe".

The nature of the contaminant in unprocessed primaquine diphosphate was first publicly presented in 2003 [1] and later described in [2–9].

In this study, the toxic contaminant in tablets was characterized based on previous knowledge of MS spectra and by using authentic quality standard quinocide [1-9]. The new data gathered regarding the two minor contaminants of unknown nature using SFC-MS and GC-MS with SMB [38].

The novelty of this work is the determination of the main contaminant in the medical form of primaquine tablets.

Used nomenclature:

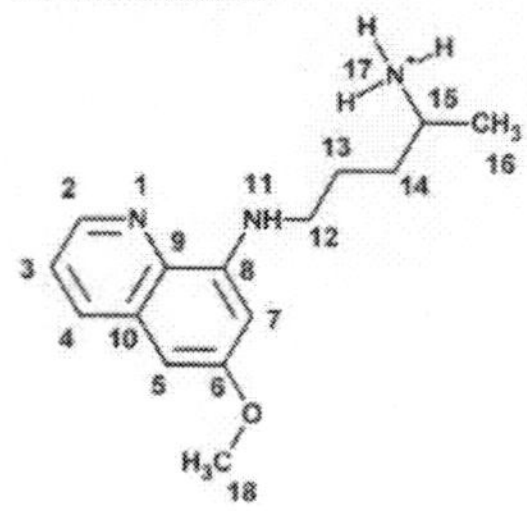

Quinocide

Atom	^{15}N	^{13}C	^{1}H		multiplicity
1	*				
2		140,4	8,73		dd, J = 5.0 Hz 1.4 Hz
3		122,2	7,79		dd, J = 8.4 Hz 5.0 Hz
4		142,2	8,65		br d, J = 8.4 Hz
5		93,8	6,81		d, J = 2.2 Hz
6		160,2			
7		100,5	6,50		d, J = 2.2 Hz
8		141,8			
9		126,9			
10		131,2			
11	- 308,7		6,54		very broad (3H) "double salt"
12		31,8	1,66	1,78	2 x m
13		23,7	1,77	1,77	m
14		42,9	3,23	3,23	m
15		46,6	3,20		m
16		18,2	1,21		d, J = 6.5 Hz
17	- 331,4		8,16		br s
18		55,6	3,86		s
Ref	0,0 ppm**	39,5 ppm	2,49 ppm		

* not observed

** CH_3NO_2 in DMSO - d_6 9:1

Figure 8. The molecule of quinocide with used nomenclature for C and N atoms is shown together with the table of chemical shift values including ^{15}N, ^{13}C and ^{1}H. The details described in the text.

3.2. UV spectrometry

The UV spectra of primaquine and quinocide are nearly identical [3, 9]. There is a tendency for a *hypsochromic shift* in λ max in the spectrum of quinocide in comparison with that of primaquine. In water, primaquine has λ max values of 206.5, 260, and 343.5 nm and λ min values of 231 and 302.5 nm, and quinocide has λ max values of 206, 258, and 342.5 nm and λ min values of 230.5 and 308 nm. In solutions of ammonium or sodium hydroxide, the spectra exhibit nearly the same patterns of λ max and λ min values. The maxima and minima recorded in alkaline solutions are near to the values seen in water solutions. In a solution of 0.01 N NaOH, the absorption by NaOH interferes with the measurement of the peak at 205 nm. In 0.01 N HCl, both substances undergo significant changes in their spectra pattern: primaquine has λ max values of 205, 223.5, 265.5, 281.5, and 333.5 nm and λ min values of

215.5, 249, 272, and 313.5 nm; quinocide has λ max values of 205, 221.5, 267, 278, and 332.5 nm and λ min values of 216, 247, 270, and 312 nm.

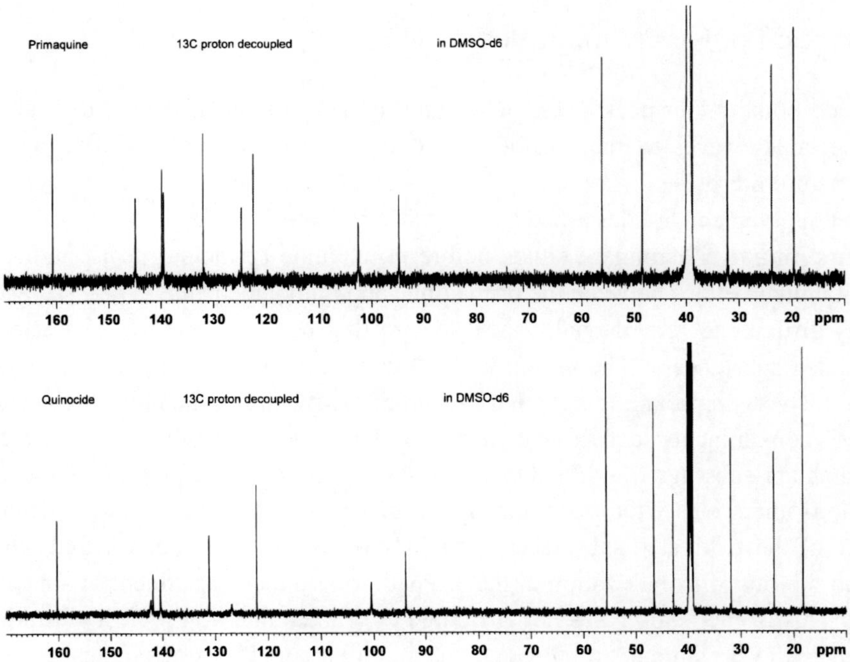

Figure 9. ^{13}C NMR spectra of primaquine chloride and quinocide chloride analysed in DMSO-d6.
A. The upper trace shows ^{13}C NMR spectra of primaquine chloride.
B. The bottom trace shows the ^{13}C NMR spectra of quinocide chloride.

From the spectra obtained (Figures 4 and 5), it is evident that optimal detection of primaquine in an alkaline environment should be at 261 nm, as described in the *Pharmacopoeia* [10]; however, our measurements of quinocide found a corresponding maxima at 258 nm in water and in NH_3OH and NaOH solutions. In USP 31 and NF 26 [39], detection at 254 nm is recommended. The maxima in the spectra of primaquine and quinocide depend on the pH of the solvent and are slightly different from each other.

3.3. ^{1}H, ^{13}C, and ^{15}N NMR Spectroscopy

In the ^{1}H spectra of primaquine, chemical shift at 3.75 ppm versus quinocide chemical shift at 1.66 and 1.78 ppm from C in position 12 as of primaquine chemical shift at 2.76 ppm versus quinocide chemical shift at 3.20 ppm from C in position 15 may be used for differentiation between isomers (Figures 6-9).

In the ^{13}C spectrum of primaquine, chemical shifts at 144.24, 95.83, 39.85, and 24.22 ppm are characteristic for this isomer. In the ^{13}C spectrum of quinocide, chemical shifts at 140.4, 142.2, and 100.5 ppm are characteristic for this isomer (Figures 6-9).

3.4. Extraction

The quality of extraction was judged by the absence of active API in the control extracts.

3.5. Detection of Minor Impurities by MS

Two additional minor peaks were detected using MS (Figure 2). SFC-MS analysis of the primaquine tablets revealed that besides quinocide, two other contaminating agents of an unknown nature are present. In the *Pharmacopeias* [10, 39], the nature of all contaminating agents are not given and are described as "related substances".

The first minor contaminant elutes before primaquine (principal peak) and the second minor contaminant elutes between the primaquine and quinocide peaks.

It was difficult to record quality MS spectra that could be used to characterize these minor "related substances". The reason is the low concentration of the minor contaminants. However, it is very important to note that in both of the spectra of the newly detected "related substances" contaminants; a fragment of m/z 175 is present, which may indicate that the contaminants are substituted quinolines. In GC-MS with SMB analysis the characteristic for primaquine isomers ions with m/z = 175, m/z = 187 and m/z = 242 also were detected [38]. The nature of these "related substances" or minor contaminants is not verified; however, in [40] the possibility of isomerization in the aromatic ring under attachment of substituent was described. This isomerization was not attributed to primaquine; however, it was attributed to compounds with very similar structure and under similar conditions of synthesis.

It was not possible to record peaks of these substances using UV detection (Figure 1), which may be because the peaks are irregular with very long tailing or because the concentrations and molar extinction coefficients of the analytes are low and thus below the level of detection. The characterization of these contaminants is in progress. The principal routs of fragmentation for primaquine and quinocide shown in Figure 10 and 11.

3.6. Regulation

Quinocide, a main contaminant in the drug primaquine diphosphate, is a highly toxic substance. The analysis of contaminants in drugs is an important and challenging subject for analysts in the pharmaceutical industry and health administration. The requirements for the validation of qualitative and quantitative parameters in new pharmaceutical products of impurities at the 0.05% level with respect to the main compound were discussed during the International Conference on Harmonization and the current Good Manufacturing Practice [41, 42]. In the Drug Quality and Information program (DQI) document published by USP [43], it was noted that in 2003 and 2004, 21% and 13%, respectively, of antimalarial drugs used were of poor quality. This is evidence that there are unprocessed primaquine and primaquine tablets with high concentrations of the toxic contaminant quinocide as "related substances"on the drug market.

3.7. Validation of Procedures

The method was validated in accordance with the terms of precision, accuracy, and linearity described in the International Conference on Harmonization of Technical Requirements for Registration of Pharmaceuticals for Human Use (ICH) guidelines [44].

3.8. Selectivity

The selectivity of the method is important for the differentiation and identification of the existing target analytes in primaquine diphosphate tablets. Analytes were identified by matching peak retention times (R_t) with the values of the corresponding standards in solutions analyzed under the same experimental conditions. For confirmation purposes, the specific fragmentation patterns of individual analytes were used to distinguish primaquine from quinocide. In addition, comparisons of MS spectra of peaks eluted with the spectra of authentic standards and comparisons with previously published spectra were conducted [1–9].

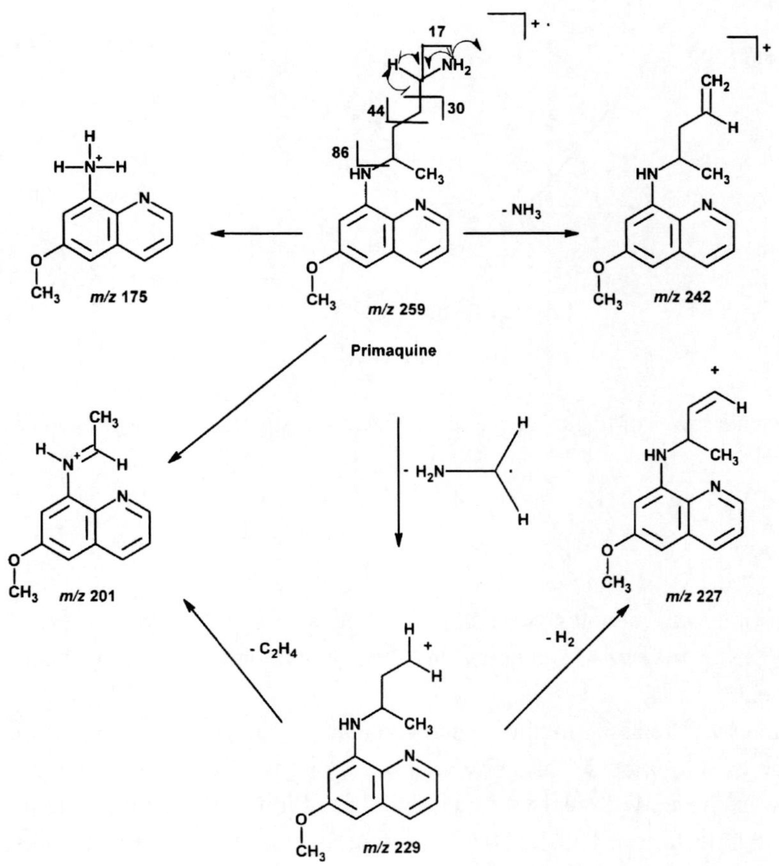

Figure 10. The main routes of fragmentation for primaquine, as suggested by electron ionization mass spectrometry [4].

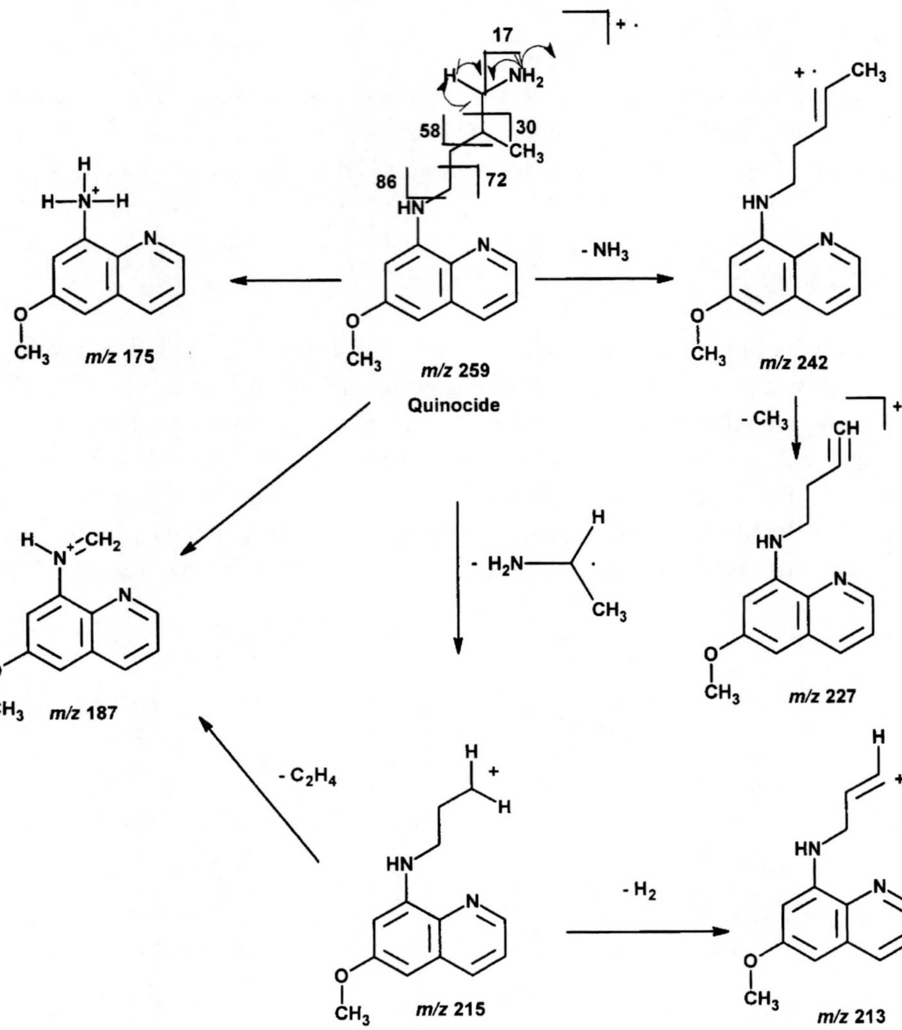

Figure 11. The main routes of fragmentation for quinocide, as suggested by electron ionization mass spectrometry [4].

3.9. Accuracy

The term *accuracy* denotes the nearness of measurement to its accepted value and is expressed in terms of *error*. Accuracy involves a comparison with respect to a true or accepted value.

The accuracy of the assay method was evaluated by carrying out analysis of the dilutions of primaquine and quinocide of known concentrations. The percentage composition of components was chosen with respect to data published in [1–9]. The individual compositions were analyzed nine times. The RSD of the experiments was within the limits of 2% for primaquine and 3% for quinocide for expected molar concentrations.

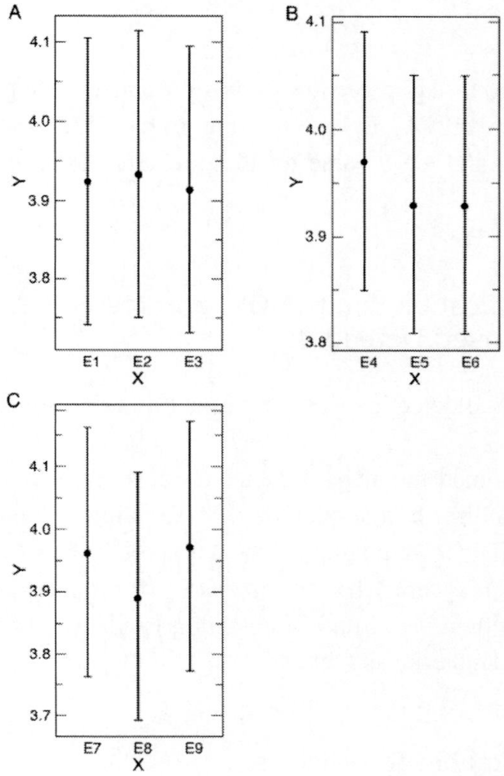

Figure 12. There are plots of means with 95% Confidence Intervals. Results of gropes analyzed in the same day.

A. Analyses are performed in day one.

B. Analyses are performed in day two.

C. Analyses are performed in day three.

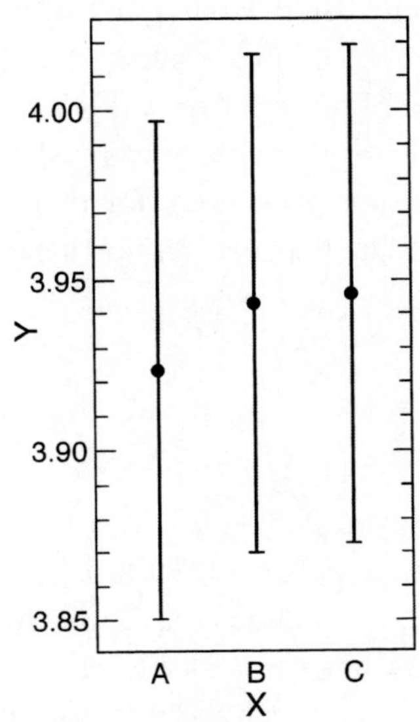

Figure 13. There is plot for day-to-day reproducibility with 95% Confidence Intervals. Groups analyzed in three different A, B and C days.

3.10. Precision

Both intraday and day-to-day precision studies presented very good results. The results are summarized in Figure 12 A, B, and C, and Figure 13. Day-to-day parameters are summarized in Figure 13, and the p value for these results, assuming the null hypothesis, is 0.889.

3.11. Method Quantification Limit (MQL) and Method Detectable Limit (MDL) of UV-Based Detection

The MDL for UV-based detection was established by using primaquine batch 16039 and quinocide batch 17172 [3].

The MDL was determined by analyzing analytes at levels that provided a signal at five times above background noise. In a similar way, MQL values were determined at signal-to-noise ratios of 10. The MDL for primaquine was 2.0×10^{-6} mM $\times$ L^{-1}, and 2.6×10^{-6} mM $\times$ L^{-1} for quinocide. The MQLs were 4.1×10^{-6} mM $\times$ L^{-1} for primaquine, and 5.5×10^{-6} mM $\times$ L^{-1} for quinocide. The method based on UV detection is adequately sensitive for monitoring the quality of unprocessed material and tablets.

3.12. Linearity and Calibration Curves

The external standard calibration method was employed on a series of individual standard solutions. The linearity of the UV detection was studied over a broad range of concentrations. Six-step dilutions of a linearity dilution series were used.

Dilutions were conducted on a molar basis because primaquine diphosphate and quinocide dichloride standards were used. Each point was determined nine times. The average values were used to construct calibration curves by plotting the corresponding peak areas versus the molar concentration of the analytes.

The linear regression parameters for primaquine were: slope = 7236, y-intercept = 13021, and $R^2 = 0.9998$; the linear regression parameters for quinocide were: slope = 11059, y-intercept = 14228, and $R^2 = 0.9985$. The linear regression parameters of both substances were better than 0.9900.

3.13. Statistics

Statistical analyses of results were conducted in accordance with [45]. The standard deviations for every series and the standard deviations between the series are presented. Three series were analyzed every day for three consecutive days. The variation between the different groups on day one (E1–E3), day two (E4–E6), and day three (E7–E9) are plotted in Figure 12 A, B, and C. The variation between the different days of analysis is presented in Figure 13. The results are presented as 95% confidence intervals.

4. Marketing and Publishing Ethics

4.1. Marketing

Quinocide, a main contaminant in the drug primaquine diphosphate [1-9, 38], is a highly toxic substance. Its use discouraged, even in its country of origin. However, the results of this study show that primaquine contaminated with quinocide and "related substances" is in use, this is in agreement with [43].

4.2. Publishing Ethics

Dongre et al. produced a publication [46] that contained no MS data or co-chromatography with authentic standards. The aim of publication [46] appears to be to demonstrate that primaquine was separated from quinocide. In the absence of quality standard quinocide, the authors presented questionable evidence of degradation and photo degradation to avoid questions about co-chromatography and spectral identity.

The authors of [46] stated "However, there are no reports available on stability indicating analytical method for primaquine phosphate API." How the authors of [46] could have dared to make this claim when there are numerous publications on the subject is beyond belief. Relevant publications are: S. Kristensen et al., Photochemical stability of biologically active compounds: V. Photochemical degradation of primaquine in an aqueous medium [47]; A. Brossi et al., Photooxidation products of primaquine, Structure, antimalarial activity and hemolytic effects [48]; and S. Kristensen et al. Photoreactivity of biologically active compounds, XIV: Influence of oxygen on light induced reactions of primaquine [49]. Moreover, S. Kristensen et al., [47] specifically stated that "Eight major and several minor decomposition products can be detected, many of which are oxygenated derivatives." How it was possible and why they claimed that there are no reports on the stability of primaquine?

Dongre et al. published [50]. The main and only reason presented by Dongre et al. to justify their investigation was that *"The first report published on this product by Elderfield* et al. [40] *suggested that one of the major impurities could possibly be its enantiomer. This reasoning appeared very unlikely and prompted us to investigate in details the structural elucidation of this impurity*." The cited publication makes no mention of the possibility of enantiomers of primaquine. Elderfield et al. never mentioned that primaquine is a racemate or a mixture of isomers. The truth is that Elderfield et al. [40] stated on p. 1525, lines 13–20: *"The drug prepared in experiment 32 was shown to be reasonably homogeneous by the 8-plate technique of Crag. However, when the 24-plate technique was applied, the substance appeared to consist of two components in approximately equal amounts. We interpret this to indicate a possible separation of the two racemates."*

What is the substance in experiment 32? On page 1526 of the same paper [40] is a list of experiments and products. Substance 32 is methoxi-8-aminoquinoline, with the substituteR_8-$NHCH(CH_3)(CH_2)_2CH(CH_3)N(C_2H_5)_2$. This is not the primaquine. The primaquine is described in experiment 24.

How could something that was not mentioned by Elderfield et al. [40] prompt Dongre et al. to investigate it?

5. Conclusion

A valid and easily performed *Pharmacopoeia*-based procedure is urgently needed because of the hundreds of millions of people who ingest primaquine as a drug containing significant amounts of contaminants [43]. The presented procedure for the qualitative analysis of the contaminant quinocide in primaquine tablets can be used as the basis for development of a USP monograph to analyze quinocide in primaquine tablets.

Acknowlegments

The author is grateful to Jon Reierstad, Technical Department and to Dirk Petersen Department of Chemistry, University of Oslo, Norway for technical assistance, to Professor Aviv Amirav, School of Chemistry, Sackler Faculty of Exact Sciences, Tel Aviv University, Tel Aviv, Israel, for cooperation with GC-MS SMB analysis. This research was financially supported by Jupiter AS, Ski, Norway, Sigma-Aldrich/Supelco Analytical, Bellefonte, PA, USA and Mettler-Toledo Berger SFC, Newark, DE, USA.

References

[1] Brondz, I; Mantzilas, D; Klein, U; Lebedeva, MN; Mikhailitsyn, FS; Souleimanov, GD; Ekeberg, D; 3rd Int. Symposium on Separation in BioSciences SBS 2003, A 100 Years of Chromatography, 13-18 May, Moscow, Russia, *Abstr.*, 2003, P-57, 165.

[2] Brondz, I; Klein, U; Ekeberg, D; Mantzilas, D; Hvattum, E; Schultz, H; Mikhailitsyn, FS. International Symposium Analytical Forum 2004, 4-8 July, Warsaw, Poland, *Abstr.*, 2004, P-119.

[3] Brondz, I; Mantzilas, D; Klein, U; Ekeberg, D; Hvattum, E; Lebedeva, MN; Mikhailitsyn, FS; Souleimanov, GD; Røe, J. *J. Chromatogr.*, 2004, B, 800, 211-223.

[4] Brondz, I; Klein, U; Ekeberg, D; Mantzilas, D; Hvattum, E; Schultz, H; Mikhailitsyn, FS. *Asian Journal of Chemistry*, 2005, 17(3), 1678-1688.

[5] Brondz, I; Klein, U. *TheReporter*, 2005, 23(4), 1-2.

[6] Brondz, I; Klein, U; Karaliova, L; Vlachos, V; Okley, P; Leideborg, R; Mikhalitsyn, FS. 29th International Symposium on High Performance Liquid Phase Separations and Related Techniques, June 26-30, 2005, Stockholm, Sweden, (2005) Abstr. P12:43.

[7] Brondz, I; Ekeberg, D; Karaliova, L; Jennings, I; Hustad, JA; Svendsen, R. *Trends in Chromatography*, 2005, 1, 77-81.

[8] Brondz, I; Klein, U. *TheReporter*, 2006, 19, 3 - 4.

[9] Brondz, I; Ekeberg, D; Bell, DS; Annino, AR; Hustad, JA; Svendsen, R; Vlachos, V; Oakley, P; Langley, GJ; Mohini, T; Amaury, CG; Mikhalitsyn, FS. *J. Pharmaceutical and Biomedical Analysis*, 2007, 43, 937-944.

[10] *European Pharmacopoeia* (2008) six ed., vol. 2, Council of Europe, Strasbourg, Germany, 2751-2752.

[11] Gladkikh, VF; Korogodina, IuV. *Meditsinskaia Parazitologiia I Parazitarnye Bolezni*, 1960, 29, 440-447.

[12] Gladkikh, VF; Kekllina, OI. *Meditsinskaia Parazitologiia I Parazitarnye Bolezni*, 1956, 25(4), 323-327.

[13] Soprunova, NYu. Meditsinskaia Parazitologiia I Parazitarnye Bolezni, 1962, 31:(6), 656-660.

[14] Soprunova, NYu. Meditsinskaia Parazitologiia I Parazitarnye Bolezni, 1963, 32:(4), 443-447.

[15] Lebedeva, MN; Brusilovskaya, VM. *Meditsinskaia Parazitologiia I Parazitarnye Bolezni*, 1980, 49:(6), 27-31.

[16] Sin, DD; Shafran, SD. *J. Acquir. Immune Defenc. Syndr. Hum. Retroviral.* 1996, 12, 477-481.

[17] Coleman, MD; Coleman, NA. *Drug Saf.*, 1996, 14, 394-405.

[18] Marrs, TC; Bright, JE; Morris, BC. *Toxicol. Lett.*, 1987, 36, 281-287.

[19] Kantor, GS. *N. Engl. J. Med.*, 1992, 327, 1462.

[20] Allahyari, R; Srtother, A; Tilton, BE; Fraser, IM. *Abstr. Am. Chem. Soc.*, 1986, 192, 86.

[21] Wed, R. Journal of Clinical Investigation, 1961, 40, 140-143.

[22] Kellermeyer, RW; Carson, PE; Schrier, SL; Tarlov, AR; Alving, AS. *Journal of Laboratory and Clinical Medicine*, 1961, 58, 715-24.

[23] Dern, RJ; Beutler, E; Alving, AS. *Journal of Laboratory and Clinical Medicine*, 1981, 97, 750-759.

[24] Schmidt, IG; Schmidt, LH. *J. Neuropathy Exp. Neurol.*, 1948, 7, 368-398.

[25] Schmidt, IG; Schmidt, LH. *J. Neuropathy Exp. Neurol.*, 1948, 8, 337-367.

[26] Bullimore, D. *Eur. J. Gastroenterol. Hepatol.*, 1993, 5, 63- 67.

[27] Rønn, AM; Rønne-Rasmussen, J; Gøtzsche, PC; Bygbjerg, IC. *Trop. Med. Int. Health*, 1998, 3, 83-88.

[28] El-Mofty, MM; Khudoley, VV; Skar, SA; Abdelgawad, HS. *Nutr. Cancer*, 1992, 18, 191-198.

[29] Orta-Salazar, G; Bouchard, RA; Morales-Salgado, F; Salinas-Stefanon, EM. *British Journal of Pharmacology*, 2002, 135:(3), 751-763.

[30] Dagan, S; Amirav, A. *Int. J. Mass Spectrom. Ion. Proc.*, 1994, 133, 187.

[31] Amirav, A; Gordin, A; Tzanani, N. *Rapid. Com. Mass Spectrom.*, 2001, 15, 811.

[32] Fialkov, AB; Steiner, U; Jones, L; Amirav, A. *Int. J. Mass. Spectrom.*, 2006, 251, 47.

[33] Amirav, A; Danon, A. *Int. J. Mass Spectrom. Ion. Proc.*, 1990, 97, 107.

[34] Amirav, A. *Org. Mass Spectrom.*, 1991, 26, 1.

[35] Dagan, S; Amirav, A. *J. Am. Soc. Mass Spectrom.*, 1995, 6, 120.

[36] Amirav, A; Gordin, A; Poliak, M; Fialkov, AB. *J. Mass Spectrom.*, 2008, 43, 141.

[37] Fialkov, AB; Gordin, A; Amirav, A. *J. Chromatogr. A.*, 2003, 991, 217.

[38] Brondz, I; Fialkov, AB; Amirav, A. *J. Chromatogr. A.*, 2008, submitted.

[39] The United Stats Pharmacopeia, Thirty-First Revision and The National Formulary, Twenty-Sixth ed., The United Stats Pharmacopeia Convention, 2008 Volume 3, Rockville, MD.

[40] Elderfield, RC; Gensler, WJ; Head, JD; Hageman, HA; Kremer, CB; Wright, JB; Holley, AD; Williamson, B; Galbreath, J; Wielderhold III, L; Flohardt, R; Kupchan, SM; Williamson, TA; Birstein, O. *J. Am. Chem. Soc.*, 1946, 68, 1524.

[41] Impurities in new drug substances; ICH-Q3A(R); International Conference on Harmonization: Geneva, Switzerland, October 2006.

[42] Impurities in new drug products; ICH-Q3B (R2); International Conference on Harmonization: Geneva, Switzerland, June 2006.

[43] United States Pharmacopoeia, Drug Quality and Information Program, Mekong Malaria Initiative. Antimalarial Drug Quality Monitoring and Evaluation (2004) U.S. Agency for International Development, Washington, 1-25.

[44] ICH topic Q2(R1), Validation of analytical procedures: text and methodology, (2005) version 4.

[45] De Muth, JE. Basic Statistics and Pharmaceutical Statistical Applications, 2006, second ed., CRC Press.

[46] Dongre, VG; Karmuse, PP; Rao, PP; Kumar, A. *J. Pharm. Biomed. Analysis*, 2008, 46:(4), 236-242.

[47] Kristensen, S; Grislingaas, AL; Greenhill, JV; Skjeten, T; Karlsen, J; Tønnesen, HH. *International Journal of Pharmaceutics*, 1993, 100, 15-23.

[48] Brossi, A; Gessner, W; Hufford, CD; Homo, JK; Millet, F; Landau, PI. *FEBS Lett.*, 1987, 223, 77-81.

[49] Kristensen, S; Nord, K; Orsteen, AL; Tønnesen, HH. *Pharmazie*, 1998, 53:(2), 98-103.

[50] Dongre, VG; Karmuse, PP; Nimbalkar, MM; Singh, D; Kumar, A. *J. Pharm. Biomed. Analysis*, 2005, 39, 111-116.

In: Antimalarial Drugs: Costs, Safety and Efficacy
Editors: Emanuel Csizmadia and Istvan Kalnoky
ISBN: 978-1-60741-432-2

Chapter VI

Artemisia Annua: A Program of Local Production for Treatment of Malaria in the Poorest Countries

M. Onimus[1], J. M. Vouillot and G. Clerc[2]
[1]Besançon University, France,
[2]Artemisine Contre Paludisme 7 Grande Rue F-25330 LONGEVILLE

It is well known that artemisinin-based combination therapy is the more effective way for fighting falciparum malaria [23], and this is the World Health Organization's recommended guideline for the treatment of malaria [24]. However the modern antimalarial preparations made from semi-synthetic derivatives (arthemeter, artesunate) are not routinely available in remote rural areas, and they are still expensive and very frequently not easily affordable for poor families. Meanwhile many studies have confirmed the immediate efficacy of artemisinin, which may be a solution for resolving the tragedy of malaria in young children in endemic areas.

Tea preparations from *Artemisia Annua*, used in traditional Chinese medicine for centuries, have proved to be effective and safe in treatment of all human malaria parasites, and notably multidrug-resistant plasmodium falciparum. Artemisinin clears peripheral parasitaemia more quickly than other antimalarial drugs. It is active on early trophozoïte and ring blood-stages of the parasite cycle [1], with a rapid in vitro effect suggesting a high parasitocidal action [2]. Administration of artemisinin prevents the development in the more mature trophozoïte stage with adherence of the parasite to the vascular endothelium, resulting in sequestration in the small blood vessels of vital organs: this sequestration stage is thought to be responsible for the complications of malaria or cerebral malaria.

The authors consider that, although not entirely satisfying, treatment of malaria by tea preparations from leaves of *Artemisia Annua* may be an alternative to modern antimalarial drugs. They have developed a program of cultivation of *Artemisia Annua*, the aim being to provide seeds to local populations in endemic areas of undeveloped countries, to favour local cultivation, to promote knowledge about *Artemisia Annua,* and to supply advice and documents. They have created an association entitled Artemisine Contre Paludisme, located in Longeville, Franche-Comté, East of France. The plant is cultivated there at 700 m above sea level, without fertilization.

Cultivation

Seedling: seeds are very thin (up to 10 000 seeds/gr) and should be mixed with fine sand (one spoon of seeds for 5 to 6 spoons of sand) before sowing. The mixture should be sown in a box filled with softened soil, and well-watered. Bedding out is necessary and should be performed when the seedling becomes too dense, usually after 3 – 4 weeks. It should be done in small pots or jars. Each young plant should be transferred to a pot.

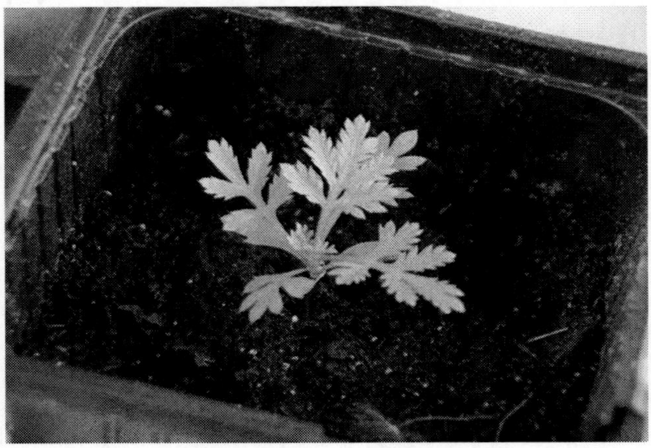

Figure 1. The plant was grown in a pot and has got 5 leaves. It may now be transferred to open soil.

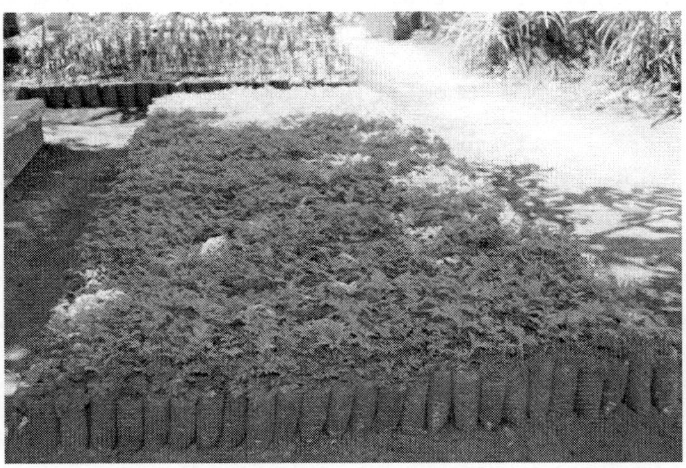

Figure 2. This cultivation was done in Madagascar. Plants were grown in small bags. They are ready for transferring.

When the plant has grown 15 cm or has got 5 to 6 leaves (Figure 1 and 2), it should be again transferred to open soil. This occurs about 3 weeks later. After softening the soil the whole content of the pot should be planted out, preserving a few centimeters interval between each plant. It takes several weeks for the plant to come up.

In the Longeville experience, with sowing during spring, at the beginning of April, bedding out is performed during the last week of April and the leaves are harvested at the end of August. In temperate climates, as in France, the plant may reach 1.5 to 2 m of height and it is necessary to plant out with 80 cm intervals. Five grams of seeds are sufficient for covering one hectare in open soil.

When days are invariably of the same duration, as in black Africa, maturation is rapid and the growth does not exceed 20 to 80 cm. In these areas cultivation may be simplified: broadcast sowing may be attempted without further planting. Seeds should not sink into the soil; they should be kept at the surface, in a humid atmosphere. After a slight raking the soil should be tamped with a roll or a plank. Then the seeds may be scattered, taking care to widely spread them out. A copious watering is mandatory. For retaining humidity, which is essential for germination, the sowed area may be covered with a fine coat of soft soil or sand. If bedding out is performed, a 30–60 cm interval only should be preserved between plants, as the growth potential is limited. Ideally the soil should be prepared with compost and termitary sand. In an attempt of cultivation made in Senegal, budding occurred 3 months after seeding; the height of the plant was 60 cm. In another cultivation in Benin, bedding out was performed 3 weeks after sowing (in January); the maximum height of the plant was 1 m. In Burkina Faso the obtained height was 20–30 cm. In African areas, sowing may be performed at any period in the year, taking care to generously bring water during the dry season until germination or until transferring the plants.

Harvesting

The date of harvesting the leaves is of great importance, as the concentration of artemisinin in the leaves is highest during budding and will rapidly decrease after flowering.

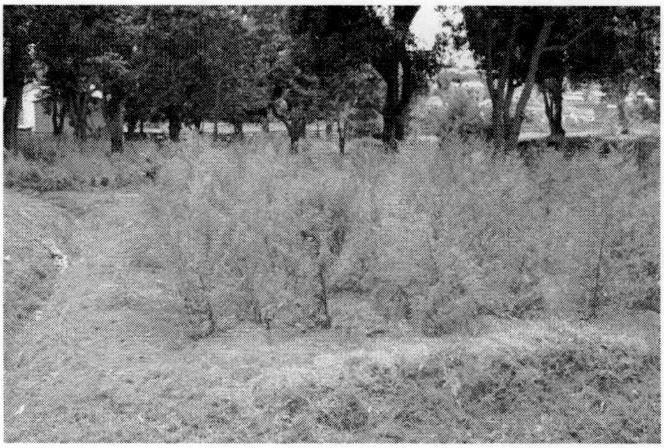

Figure 3. The plant is mature and leaves may be harvested

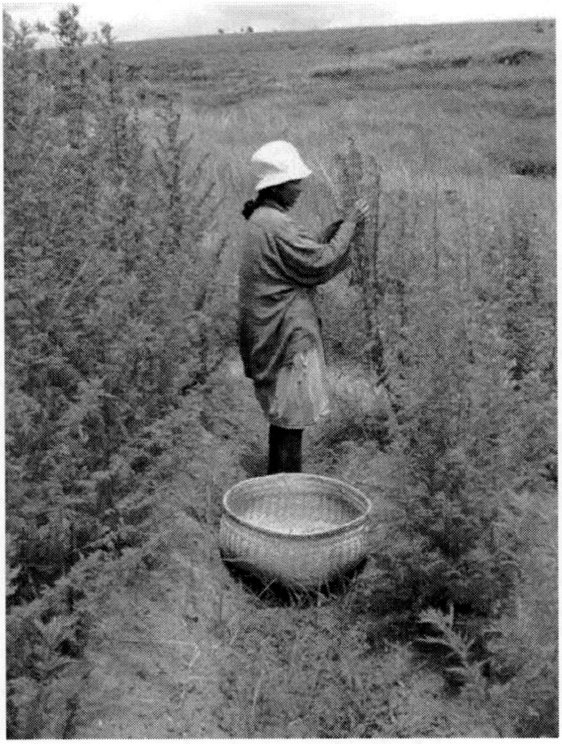

Figure 4. Harvesting green leaves is made one by one directly on the plant.

In a study performed in Longeville, with budding occurring during the last days of August, the artemisin content of the leaves was 0.13% on August 16th ; it was 0.31% on August 26th ; it was again 0.31% on September 2nd and it was 0.25% on September 9th. Ideally the leaves should be harvested just before flowering (Figure 3).

The simplest way for harvesting is to cut and collect the plants, then spread them out on mesh material for drying. During drying the plant should be protected from the sun and kept in a shady area in order to avoid reduction of the artemisinin concentration, light and heat being harmful for the artemisinin rate. When drying is completed (after 3–4 days), the leaves should be detached from the stems by grasping the branch at the foot and pulling the leaves with fingers from bottom to top.

Another way is to shake or thresh the plants, then sieve for eliminating the stems. However the disadvantage of this technique is to fragment or smash the leaves. A different way of harvesting is to avoid cutting the plant and to directly pull out the leaves one by one in the field (Figure 4), then dry them. This technique is more time-consuming, but the leaves keep a more normal appearance. Lastly, after drying leaves should be stocked in mesh bags in a shaded and fresh area.

Determining the exact moment of transition between leaves and flowering may be difficult as the leaves slightly vanish during budding; moreover the flowers are very small, yellowish coloured, and may be difficult to differentiate from leaves. Harvesting the seeds should not be done too early, as the seeds may not be mature enough, and should not be done too late as the seeds may fall down on the ground and be lost. In Longeville the best time for harvesting the seeds occurs in autumn just before the first frost. Lastly, one should remember that harvesting the leaves at the right time, before flowering, in order to have an optimal concentration of artemisinin, results in a reduction of the number of seeds, and when gathering the leaves one should preserve a part of the crop for later harvesting the seeds.

Artemisinin Efficacy

The results of the treatment of malaria with extracted artemisinin as well as artemisin tea preparation have been widely documented. The leaves' concentration of artemisinin depends upon many factors, including the time of harvesting, the method of drying, the method and duration of preserving the leaves, as well as the variety of *Artemisia Annua*. In an experience in Burkina Faso, we obtained 0.30% as an initial concentration just after harvesting; the rate dropped to 0.12% after one year. The commonly admitted content of artemisinin ranges from 0.10% to 1%. In Madagascar, we obtained 0.5%. In Senegal different varieties were studied, including Brasilean, Anamed and Mediplant. In all varieties the artemisin content was over 0.8%, up to 1.3% with the Mediplant variety. It was 0.63–0.70% in the Mueller study [17]. Hybridation of *Artemisia annua* may considerably improve the content. However hybridation may jeopardize the production of seeds. Phosphorus fertilizer may have a potential role in improving the concentration of Artemisinin [12].

The standard recommended amount of leaves for tea preparation is 9–10 grams of dryed leaves to be infused for 4–5 minutes in one liter of boiling water. However similar clinical results were observed with tea preparations containing 5g/l only [7,18]. In one liter of tea preparation made with 9 grams of leaves, Räth [20] measured 94.5 mg of artemisinin. Jansen [11] reported 24.2 mg/l, but the measurement was made with a questionable analytic method. According to Mueller [17] 40% of artemisinin contained in the leaves may be extracted by tea preparation, meaning 40 mg if we consider 1% content in 10 g of leaves. These figures may be matched with the usually recommended daily dose of extracted artemisinin, which is 500 mg. However there is no definite study to support this 500 mg dosage. Ashton [5] observed a similar efficacy of oral and rectal artemisin, although bioavailability after rectal relative to oral artemisinin was 30%, suggesting that a 500 mg initial dose may be unnecessarily too high. So one liter of tea preparation provides a substantial amount of artemisinin.

The maximum plasma concentration after intake of 500 mg of extracted artemisin ranges from 364 µg/l to 615 µg/l : it was 615 µg/l in the Alin study [3], 391 µg/l in the Duc study [8] and 364 µg/l in the de Vries study [22]. The maximum concentration after intake of a tea preparation with 9 grams of artemisinin leaves was 240 µg/l in Räth's study [20], suggesting a faster and better absorption of the artemisinin in tea preparation than the extracted artemisinin. Tea preparation contains other compounds than artemisinin, possibly improving the absorption rate. According to Alin [2] and Heide [10] the minimum artemisinin concentration required for growth inhibition of Plasmodium falciparum in vitro is 9 µg/l, therefore quite lower than the measured blood concentration.

The maximum plasma concentration of artemisinin is very rapidly obtained: 3 hours after absorption of 500 mg of extracted artemisinin in Alin's study [4] and 2 hours in Duc's study [8] after intake of tea preparation (9g/l), resulting in a rapid parasite clearance and clinical improvement. In vitro, Alin observed that the parasite growth was inhibited by 63% within 3 hours of artemisinin exposure [2]. Clinically the time for parasite clearance is about 36 hours: it was 26 h in Alin's study [4], 48 hours in Mueller's study [17], 36 hours in de Vries's study [22]. Meanwhile the mean half-life of artemisinin is short, averaging 2-and-a-half hours to 3 hours [3,8,22], potentially resulting in risk for recrudescence of the parasitaemia. Recurrence of the parasitaemia is usually considered as a treatment failure [7,18] and for this reason most of the authors consider that treatment by artemisin alone is unacceptable. However a persisting or recurrent low parasitaemia may be considered as not significant if not associated to recurrence of clinical symptoms: Silachamroon [21] observed in patients treated with artemisinin derivatives that early rising parasitemia occured in 25% of uncomplicated falciparum malaria.

The authors agree with Willcox's statement [26] "the aim of the treatment by artemisinin is not to definitively eradicate the disease, but to cure the malaria attack and to avoid its complications". Due to the short clearance of artemisinin the duration of the treatment should be at least 5 days [15]; the usual recommended duration is 7 days.

Artemisinin Administration

The artemisinin is well tolerated and no adverse effect has been observed. Tea is the simplest method for administration, but when oral anti-malarial therapy cannot be given, as in uncompliant patients or patients with cerebral malaria, rectal administration may be used. This has been investigated by the World Health Organization (25). Artemisinin by rectal administration has the advantage to avoid any of the complications commonly observed after parenteral quinine treatment (19). Many studies have confirmed the effectiveness of rectal artemisinin [5, 6, 9, 14, 16], rectal artemisinin initiating parasite clearance more rapidly than parenteral treatment (parasite clearance time is about 24h), and being more active and safer than parenteral quinine, even in severe illness. According to Koopmans [14] the artemisinin blood concentration after rectal administration is higher than after oral administration. According to the meta-analysis of Karunajeewa [13] on 39 studies, rectal preparations appear to have an acceptable therapeutic efficacy, even if their clinical outcome is not superior to that of conventional treatment. Thus, intrarectal artemisinin may be considered as a potential standard treatment which may replace conventional parenteral quinine. Suppositories of extracted artemisinin as well as its derivatives are currently available, but the cost may be prohibitive for poor families, and extracted artemisinin may be replaced by a tea preparation, with a protocol similar to oral tea preparation, i.e 9–10 grams of leaves infusing 5 minutes in one liter of boiling water, to repeat the following days. The tea preparation is available at an affordable price. It should be administered as a drop-by-drop, using a rectal cannula, resulting in a no-cost treatment.

Conclusion

Developing treatment of malaria by an artemisinin tea preparation has the advantage of being inexpensive and economically acceptable for most populations, and is easy to prepare and to take. Another advantage is the possibility of having locally grown herbs, avoiding the uncertainties of routing or dispatching and a shortage in supply. Either oral or rectal *Artemisia annua* tea preparations are acceptably effective for treatment of falciparum malaria, provided that the duration of treatment is convenient. This is an objection to be kept in mind as the necessary duration of the treatment may be poorly compatible with the frequent low compliance of the patients or families.

References

[1] Agtmael (van), MA; Eggelte, TA; Boxtel, (van) CJ. Artemisinin drugs in the treatment of malaria: from medicinal herb to registered medication. *Trends Pharmacol Sci*., 1999, 20, 199-205.

[2] Alin, MH; Bjorkman, A. Concentration and time dependency of artemisinin efficacy against Plasmodium falciparum in vitro. *Am J Trop Med Hyg*., 1994, 50, 771-16.

[3] Alin, MH; Ashton, M; Kihamia, CM; Mtev, GJ; Björkman, A. Clinical efficacy and pharmacokinetics of artemisinin monotherapy and in combination with mefloquine in patients with falciparum malaria. *Br J Clin Pharmacol*, 1996, 41, 587-92.

[4] Alin, MH; Ashton, K; Kihamia, CM; Mtey, GJ; Bjorkman, A. Multiple dose pharmacokinetics of oral artemisinin and comparison of its efficacy with that of oral artesunate in falciparum malaria patients. *Trans R Soc Trop Med Hyg*., 1996, 90, 61-5.

[5] Ashton, M; Nguyen, DS; Nguyen, VH; Gordi, T; Trinh, NH; Dinh, XH; Nguyen, TN; Le, DC. Artemisinin kinetics and dynamics during oral and rectal treatment of uncomplicated malaria. *Clin Pharmacol Ther*., 1998, 63, 482-13.

[6] Birku, Y; Makonnen, E; Bjorkman, A. Comparison of rectal artemisinin with intravenous quinine in the treatment of severe malaria in Ethiopia. *East Afr Med J*., 1999, 76, 154-9.

[7] Blanke, CH; Naisabha, GB; Balema, MB; Mbaruku, GM; Heide, L; Müller, SM. Herba *Artemisia annuae* tea preparation compared to sulfadoxine-pyrimethamine in the treatment of uncomplicated falciparum malaria in adults: a randomized double-blind clinical trial. *Trop Doct*., 2008, 38, 113-6.

[8] Duc, DD; Vries, (de) PJ; Nguyen, XK; Le Nguyen, B; Kager, PA; Boxtel (van), CJ. The pharmacokinetics of a single dose of artemisinin in healthy Vietmanese subjects. *Am J Trop Med Hyg*., 1994, 51, 785-90.

[9] Gomes, M; Ribeiro, I; Warsame, M; Karunajeewa, H; Petzold, M. Rectal artemisinin for malaria: a review of efficacy and safety from individual patient data in clinical studies. *BMC Infect Dis*., 2008, 28, 38-9.

[10] Heide, L. Artemisinin in traditional tea preparations of *Artemisia annua. Trans R Soc Trop Med Hyg*., 2006, 100, 802.

[11] Jansen, FH. The herbal tea approach for artemisinin as a therapy for malaria? *Trans R Soc Trop Med Hyg.*, 2006, 100, 285-6.

[12] Kapoor, R; Chaudhary, V; Bhatnagar, AK. Effects of arbuscular mycorrhiza and phosphorus application on artemisinin concentration in *Artemisia annua L. Mycorrhiza*, 2007, 17, 581-7.

[13] Karunajeewa, HA; Manning, L; Mueller, I; Ilett, KF; Davis, TM. Rectal administration of artemisin derivatives for the treatment of malaria. *JAMA*, 2007, 297, 2381-90.

[14] Koopmans, R; Ha, LD; Duc, DD; Dien, TK; Kager, PA; Khanh, NX; Boxtel (van), CJ; Vries (de), PJ. The pharmakinetics of artemisinin after administration of two different suppositories to healthy Vietnamese subjects. *Am J Trop Med Hyg.*, 1999, 60, 244-7.

[15] Le, NB; Pham, TY; Nguyen, BN; Dang, CT; Pham, TL; Le, DC. Efficacy and effectiveness of five days treatment of uncomplicated falciparum with artemisinin or artesunate in Vietnam. *Southeast Asian J Trop Med Public Health*, 1999, 30, 3-6.

[16] Mehta, SR; Das, S. Management of malaria: recent trends. *J Commun Dis.*, 2006, 38, 130-8.

[17] Mueller, MS; Karhabomga, IB; Hirt, HM; Wemakor, E. The potential of *Artemisia annua L.* as a locally produced remedy for malaria in the tropics: agricultural, chemical and clinical aspects. *J Ethnopharmacol*, 2000, 73, 487-93.

[18] Mueller, MS; Runyambo, N; Wagner, I; Borrmann, S; Dietz, K; Heide, L. Randomized controlled trial of a traditional preparation of *Artemisia annua L.* (Annual Wormwood) in the treatment of malaria. *Trans R Soc Trop Med Hyg.*, 2004, 98, 318-21.

[19] Onimus, M; Brunet, L; Gaudeuille, F; Issa Mapouka, A. Treatment of complications of intramuscular injection of Quinine in Africa. *Med Trop.*, 2007, 67, 63-75.

[20] Räth, K; Taxis, K; Walz, G; Gleiter, CH; Li, SM; Heide, L. Phamacokinetic study if artemisinin after oral intake of a traditional preparation of *Artemisia annua L.* (annual wormwood). *Am J Trop Med Hyg.*, 2004, 70, 128-32.

[21] Silachamroon, U; Phumratanaprapin, W; Krudsood, S; Treeprasertsuk, S; Budsaratid, V; Pornpininworakij, K; Wilairatan, P; Looareesuwan, S. Frequency of early rising parasitaemia in falciparum malaria treated with artemisinin derivatives. *Southeast Asian J Trop Med Public Health*, 2001, 32, 50-6.

[22] Vries (de), PJ; Tran, KD; Nguyen, XK; Le Nguyen, B; Pham, TY; Dao, DD; Boxtel (van), CJ; Kager, PA. The pharmacokinetics of a single dose of artemisinin in patients with uncomplicated falciparum malaria. *Am J Trop Med Hyg.*, 1997, 56, 503-7.

[23] White, NJ; Nosten, F; Looareesuwan, S; Watkins, WM; Marsh, K; Snow, RW; Kokwaro, G; Ouma, J; Hien, TT; Molyneux, ME; Taylor, TE; Newbold, CI; Ruebush II, TK; Danis, M; Greenwood, BM; Anderson, RM; Olliaro, P. Averting a malaria disaster. *Lancet*, 1999, 353, 1965-7.

[24] *WHO guidelines for the treatment of malaria*, World Health Organization, Geneva 2006.

[25] Use of rectal artemisinin-based suppositories in the management of severe malaria. *Report of a WHO Informal Consultation*, 27-28 March 2006, World Health Organization, Geneva 2007.

[26] Willcox, M; Rasoanaivo, P. Comment on: Randomized controlled trial of a traditional preparation of *Artemisia annua L.* (Annual Wormwood) in the treatment of malaria. *Trans R Soc Trop Med Hyg.*, 2004, 98, 755-6.

In: Antimalarial Drugs: Costs, Safety and Efficacy
Editors: Emanuel Csizmadia and Istvan Kalnoky
ISBN: 978-1-60741-432-2

Chapter VII

Quinine Toxicity and Cinchonism

Viroj Wiwanitkit
Wiwanitkit House, Bangkhae, Bangkok Thailand

Abstract

Quinine is a well-known antimalarial drug that is widely used in clinical practice. Although quinine is effective, it also poses a considerable toxicity. Quinine toxicity has been known for decades and the specific term "cinchonism" is used for describing the quinine toxicity. In this article, the author will review the cinchonism focusing on several aspects of this disorder. Important reports will be quoted and summarized in this article.

Introduction

Quinine is the drug of choice for treatment of severe malaria cases. A common side effect of quinine is headache induction. Although quinine is an effective, well-known antimalarial drug that is widely used in clinical practice, it poses a considerable toxicity. High concentrations of quinine are very toxic to the cardiovascular system, causing hypotension and abnormal myocardial conduction [1 - 2]. Auditory symptoms, gastrointestinal disturbances, vasodilatation, sweating, and headache can be seen in cases with moderately elevated plasma quinine concentration [3]. Quinine toxicity has been known for decades and the specific term "cinchonism" has been used to describe quinine toxicity. In this article, the author will review cinchonism focusing on several aspects of this disorder. Important reports will be quoted and summarized in this article.

Cinchonism in the Treatment of Malaria

As previously mentioned, quinine can cause cinchonism. The classic symptoms include acute bilateral blindness, nausea, vomiting, and tinnitus [4 – 11]. In general, quinine might cause cinchonism at standard therapeutic doses [10]. The toxic dose is 2 grams, and the lethal dose is 8 grams [4 – 11]. High-tone hearing loss occurs, but irreversible auditory or ocular effects are not common [10]. Parenteral quinine is more likely to cause toxicity than oral quinine [4]. Padmaja et al. said that 24 of 90 patients with falciparum malaria who received parenteral quinine developed quinine toxicity. They noted that quinine should be used cautiously in patients with impaired hepatic or renal function and in those with prolonged QTc as it could bring cardiotoxicity in the form of I0 AV block, prolonged Q-Tc, broad QRS tachycardai or fatal bradyarrhythmia [4]. They suggested a dosage reduction to 5 mg/kg body weight for prevention [4]. However, the variation in quinine's pharmacokinetics during the episodes of falciparum malaria can be seen and there are different therapeutic regimens proposed in different countries [5]. And they said that the quinine dose might be reduced on day 4 of treatment when asexual parasitemia disappeared [5]. Kofoed et al. reported that the recommended dose of 10 mg quinine/kg bodyweight 3 times a day for 7 days for treatment of malaria was so high that a number of patients could develop cinchonism [6]. Kofoed et al. said that 15 mg of quinine salt/kg bodyweight daily should be used for treatment of symptomatic Plasmodium falciparum malaria [6]. Metha et al. reported an experience on loading dose quinine therapy in cerebral malaria treatment [7]. According to their report [7], mild cinchonism occurred in two cases after the loading dose while this was observed only in one case in the conventional dose group implying the safety of the loading dose therapy for serious cerebral malaria conditions [7]. Wattangoon et al. reported that an intramuscular loading dose of quinine for falciparum malaria, an alternative mean of starting treatment in patients with moderately severe falciparum malaria who could not swallow tablets and intravenous administration could not be done, was safe and would cause only mild cinchonism [11]. Wienke et al. concluded that quinine was effective in the treatment of *P. falciparum* infection and is mandatory if the clinical condition required a fast-acting blood schizonticide, in cases of hyper-parasitaemia and if multi-drug resistance occurs [8]. Weinke also stated that quinine should also not be restricted by reversible side-effects such as cinchonism [8].

In addition to single drug administration, there are also reports on cinchonism in a combined quinine and other antimalarial drug regimen. Miller et al. reported on the combination azithromycin-quinine that cinchonism occurred in nearly all subjects [12]. However, they noted that this combination was safe, well tolerated, and effective in curing drug-resistant falciparum malaria [12]. Looareesuwan et al. reported on another combination—quinine and tetracycline [13]. Looareesuwan et al. found that nearly all subjects developed cinchonism [13]. Looareesuwan et al. concluded that the combination of mefloquine plus tetracycline was equally effective and less toxic than quinine plus tetracycline for treatment of acute uncomplicated falciparum malaria in areas requiring combination therapy for drug resistance [13]. Bunnag et al. also reported on this combination [14]. Bunnag et al. reported that although this regimen was effective and might be used as home treatment the patient compliance was usually not satisfactory due to cinchonism adverse effects [14]. Finally, Bich et al. reported on a regimen of single dose of 20 mg/kg of artemisinin followed by three days of quinine, 10 mg/kg three times a day and said that this regimen was effective but adverse effects mainly limited to cinchonism were seen [15].

Cinchonism Due to Other Conditions

In addition to quinine administration in malarial treatment, there are also other cases of cinchonisms. Those conditions are interesting. The author will hereby be quoted for some important reports on this topic.

A. Cinchonism in Quinine Administration for Abortion

Cinchonism in quinine administration for abortion is also mentioned in the literatures. Dannenberg et al. reported that quinine was available over-the-counter and could be misused for self-abortion [16]. Cinchonism is this scenario can be seen [16]. Newell et al. reported another case with cinchonism and an elevated anion gap in a case with self-abortion [17].

B. Cinchonism in Quinine Administration for Cramps

Quinine can be used as a drug for treatment for benign nocturnal cramps. Beyens et al. studied on the side effect of quinine usage as a regimen for cramp relief. They found that most involved hypersensitivity reactions, rash, pruritus, generalized anaphylaxis, thrombopenia and hepatitis while cinchonism was rarely observed at the usually low dose of quinine in this indication [18]. Barrocas and Cymet said that the use of quinine for this purpose was controversial with conflicting studies regarding its efficacy and the side effect profile, cinchonism, could not be ignored [19]. Warburton et al. noted that the simple expedient of increasing the nightly dose of quinine might bring the concomitant risk of cinchonism [20]. It was concluded that the risk-benefit ratio of quinine for cramps justified that it not be recommended due to common dose-dependent sensory manifestations of cinchonism [21].

C. Other Cases

There are also other sporadic rare cases of cinchonism. For example, Balfour reported on an interesting case in aviation medicine [22]. In this case, blood quinine about 0.2 mg/L was found at autopsy in pilots who died in aviation accidents and this suggested that quinine toxicity played a causative role [22]. Indeed, only 100 mg of quinine in tonic water is sufficient to produce positional abnormalities of the electronystagmograph [22]. Another example is the cinchonism in the psychiatric patient on lithium [23]. Additional side effects in this situation should be noted [23].

Treatment for Cinchonism

Most cases of cinchonism are usually mild and require only supportive treatment such as fluid care. Underdiagnosis should be avoided because it causes more unfavorable results [24].

References

[1] Jacqz-Aigrain, E; Bennasr, S; Desplanques, L; Peralma, A; Beaufils, F. Severe poisoning risk linked to intravenous administration of quinine. *Arch Pediatr*., 1994, 1, 14-9.

[2] Hachfi-Soussi, F; Coudert, V; Biron, R; Barois, A. Acute quinine poisoning treated with high dose of diazepam. *Arch Fr Pediatr*., 1993, 50, 485-8.

[3] Bateman, DN; Dyson, EH. Quinine toxicity. *Adverse Drug React Acute Poisoning Rev*., 1986, 5, 215-33.

[4] Padmaja, UK; Adhikari, P; Periera, P. Experience with quinine in falciparum malaria. *Indian J Med Sci*., 1999 Apr, 53(4), 153-7.

[5] Vieira, JL; Midio, AF. Drug monitoring of quinine in men with nonsevere falciparum malaria: study in the Amazon region of Brazil. *Ther Drug Monit*., 2001 Dec, 23(6), 612-5.

[6] Kofoed, PE; Lopes, F; Johansson, P; Dias, F; Sandström, A; Aaby, P; Rombo, L. Low-dose quinine for treatment of Plasmodium falciparum malaria in Guinea-Bissau. *Trans R Soc Trop Med Hyg*., 1999 Sep-Oct, 93(5), 547-9.

[7] Mehta, SR; Lazar, AI; Kasthuri, AS. Experience on loading dose--quinine therapy in cerebral malaria. *J Assoc Physicians India*, 1994 May, 42(5), 376-8.

[8] Weinke, T; Held, T; Trautmann, M; Rögler, G; Mravak, S; Alexander, M; Pohle, HD. Malaria therapy in 452 patients, with special reference to the use of quinine. *J Infect*., 1992 Sep, 25(2), 173-80.

[9] Wolf, LR; Otten, EJ; Spadafora, MP. Cinchonism: two case reports and review of acute quinine toxicity and treatment. *J Emerg Med*., 1992 May-Jun, 10(3), 295-301.

[10] Phillips-Howard, PA; ter Kuile, FO. CNS adverse events associated with antimalarial agents. Fact or fiction? *Drug Saf*., 1995 Jun, 12(6), 370-83.

[11] Wattanagoon, Y; Phillips, RE; Warrell, DA; Silamut, K; Looareesuwan, S; Nagachinta, B; Back, DJ. Intramuscular loading dose of quinine for falciparum malaria: pharmacokinetics and toxicity. *Br Med J (Clin Res Ed)*., 1986 Jul 5, 293(6538), 11-3.

[12] Miller, RS; Wongsrichanalai, C; Buathong, N; McDaniel, P; Walsh, DS; Knirsch, C; Ohrt, C. Effective treatment of uncomplicated Plasmodium falciparum malaria with azithromycin-quinine combinations: a randomized, dose-ranging study. *Am J Trop Med Hyg*., 2006 Mar, 74(3), 401-6.

[13] Looareesuwan, S; Vanijanonta, S; Viravan, C; Wilairatana, P; Charoenlarp, P; Lasserre, R; Canfield, C; Kyle, DE; Webster, HK. Randomised trial of mefloquine-tetracycline and quinine-tetracycline for acute uncomplicated falciparum malaria. *Acta Trop*., 1994 Jun, 57(1), 47-53.

[14] Bunnag, D; Karbwang, J; Na-Bangchang, K; Thanavibul, A; Chittamas, S; Harinasuta, T. Quinine-tetracycline for multidrug resistant falciparum malaria. *Southeast Asian J Trop Med Public Health*, 1996 Mar, 27(1), 15-8.

[15] Bich, NN; De Vries, PJ; Van Thien, H; Phong, TH; Hung, LN; Eggelte, TA; Anh, TK; Kager, PA. Efficacy and tolerance of artemisinin in short combination regimens for the treatment of uncomplicated falciparum malaria. *Am J Trop Med Hyg*., 1996 Oct, 55(4), 438-43.

[16] Dannenberg, AL; Dorfman, SF; Johnson, J. Use of quinine for self-induced abortion. *South Med J*., 1983 Jul, 76(7), 846-9.

[17] Newell, GC. Self-induced abortion and an elevated anion gap. *Hosp Pract* (Off Ed)., 1989 Apr 30, 24(4A), 33, 36.

[18] Beyens, MN; Guy, C; Ollagnier, M. Adverse effects of quinine in the treatment of leg cramps. *Therapie*, 1999 Jan-Feb, 54(1), 59-62.

[19] Barrocas, AM; Cymet, T. Cinchonism in a patient taking Quinine for leg cramps. *Compr Ther*., 2007 Fall, 33(3), 162-3.

[20] Warburton, A; Royston, JP; O'Neill, CJ; Nicholson, PW; Jee, RD; Denham, MJ; Dobbs, SM; Dobbs, RJ. A quinine a day keeps the leg cramps away? *Br J Clin Pharmacol*, 1987 Apr, 23(4), 459-65.

[21] Quinine and cramp: uncertainty efficacy, major risks. *Prescrire Int*., 2000 Oct, 9(49), 154-7.

[22] Balfour, AJ. The bite of Jesuits' bark. *Aviat Space Environ Med*., 1989 Jul, 60(7 Pt 2), A4-5.

[23] Rathbun, JM. Cinchonism in a patient for whom lithium was prescribed. *Am J Psychiatry*, 1978 Jul, 135(7), 874.

[24] Schonwald, S; Shannon, M. Unsuspected quinine intoxication presenting as acute deafness and mutism. *Am J Emerg Med*., 1991 Jul, 9(4), 318-20.

In: Antimalarial Drugs: Costs, Safety and Efficacy
Editors: Emanuel Csizmadia and Istvan Kalnoky
ISBN: 978-1-60741-432-2

Chapter VIII

Antimalarial Peroxides: From Artemisinin to Synthetic Peroxides

Jernej Iskra*
Laboratory of Organic and Bioorganic Chemistry,
Department of Physical and Organic Chemistry,
"Jozef Stefan" Institute, Jamova 39, Ljubljana, Slovenia

Abstract

Malaria remains on of the most prevalent and deadly of the insect-borne communicable diseases. Since the parasite *Plasmodium* developed resistance to classical drugs of quinine type, artemisinin-based peroxides have become the most important antimalarial drugs. Various artemisinin derivatives have been developed to improve the antimalarial performance, while insights into its mechanism of action reveal that the pharmacophore unit in artemisinin is a peroxide group bound to the 1,2,4-trioxane skeleton. However, it is not economical to synthesize artemisinin directly and currently, the global demand for artemisinin cannot be met by the low yield obtained from the cultivation of herb *Artemisia annua*. Therefore, current research focuses on the development of easily accessible, cheap and effective antimalarial drugs based on synthetic peroxides. The main synthetic analogues of artemisinin belong to a 1,2,4-trioxane type of organic peroxides, that together with structurally related 1,2,4,5-tetraoxanes and 1,2,4-trioxolanes constitutes the core of antimalarial synthetic peroxides, while various endoperoxides, cyclic and acyclic perketals are also active antimalarial agents. Another interesting concept in antimalarial chemotherapy are chimeric compounds or hybrids; these are composed of two different antimalarial agents joined in one molecule. The following chapter discusses synthetic antimalarial peroxides with an emphasis on the development of synthetic compounds from 2000 onwards.

* e-mail: jernej.iskra@ijs.si

1. Introduction

Protozoan parasites of the genus *Plasmodium* are pathogens of malaria, the most widespread and the deadliest of the communicable diseases transferred to humans by a mosquito vector. It may well be that humans and malaria parasites have co-existed during the whole era of *Homo sapiens*, in Africa the latest genetic evidence suggests that the parasite population rapidly increased 10,000 years ago.[1] Despite this lengthy coexistence, our immune system has no durable defense against malaria. Currently, 40% of world's population is at threat from malaria and it is estimated that there are over 500 million episodes of clinical *Plasmodium falciparum* malaria each year.[2] Malaria also kills one child every 30 seconds resulting in a cumulative human death toll of over 3 million annually.[3] Today, malaria is endemic in underdeveloped regions and is often linked with poverty, although it is also the cause of poverty. The poor economic strength of those countries where malaria is endemic means they are unable to invest in effective control measures.

Intensive development of antimalarial drugs began when malaria became a player in major wars including the American Civil War, the World Wars and Vietnam.[4] Today, globalization has increased the awareness that poorer regions, like Africa, need help in fighting malaria. The situation is further complicated by climate change, and its potential for allowing the spread of malaria to the central or even northern parts of Europe and large parts of North America.[5] More detailed calculations show that while some areas will become malarious others will become unsuitable for vectors and as a result less dramatic change in malaria distribution is predicted.[6] Nevertheless, there is a growing awareness for the need to act against tropical diseases and various programmes like the *Special Programme for Research and Training in Tropical Diseases* run by the World Health Organization (TDR), together with international, national agencies and philanthropic foundations are creating an improved environment for a stable pipeline of drug discovery and the development of candidate drugs through public-private partnerships.[7-9]

Despite malaria's long history it was not until the beginning of 20th century that science began to understand this disease. The milestones of malaria research are marked by two Nobel prizes in physiology or medicine; one awarded in 1902 to the Scottish physician Sir Ronald Ross who demonstrated that malaria is transmitted by mosquitoes and the other to a French army doctor - Charles Louis Alphonse Laveran in 1907, who identified that a protozoan parasite later named *Plasmodium* was the cause of the disease. Only four types of *Plasmodiums* are identified as a source of human malaria, *P. falciparum*, *P. vivax*, *P. ovale* and *P. malariae*, with the first two being the most important ones. The life cycle of the parasite is complex and this is one reason why malaria is difficult to eradicate. The female anopheles mosquito is the primary host transmitting sporozoites when biting to a human who then becomes the secondary host (Figure 1). Once in the body, it takes approximately one hour for the sporozoites to reach the cells of the liver. Once present, the pre-erythrocytic and exo-erythrocytic stages result in the development of schizonts. After 5-7 days these schizonts release thousands of merozoites which invade the host's red blood cells and begin the erythrocytic phase. Asexual reproduction produces schizonts through trophozoites and discharges merozoites into the blood within 48h. Alternatively, sexual reproduction occurs when some merozoites develop into male and female gametocytes that are ingested by the mosquito when it feeds on an infected human host's blood. These gametocytes fuse to produce sporozoites and the cycle starts over.[10]

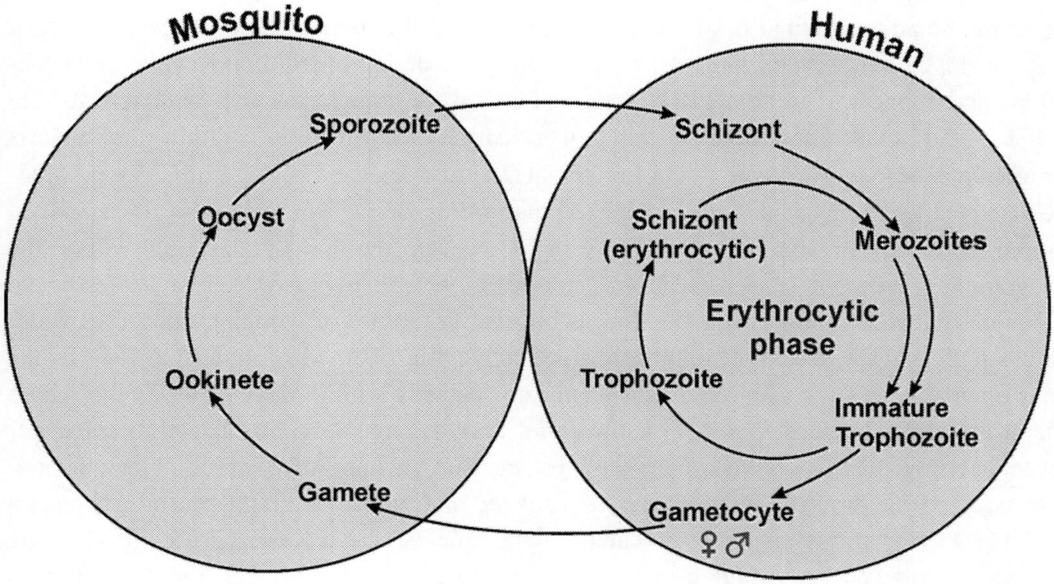

Figure 1. Life cycle of malaria parasite.

Despite this complex life cycle providing the parasite with a good defense system it does offer several possible targets for disease control. These include: vector control, immunotherapy, vaccination and drug therapy. Classical drugs of the quinine-type act on the asexual stage of parasite's life cycle. Unfortunately, the parasite has developed a resistance to these agents. This resistance requires a new approach to control malaria and various agents are in development that target parasite proteases, the mitochondrial system, parasite membrane synthesis, and parasite transporters.[10-15]

Among the agents that target the erythrocytic stage of *Plasmodium,* artemisinin and its derivatives and synthetic peroxides occupy an important position. These compounds are active against chloroquine resistant strains of *Plasmodium falciparum* and are the first line-of-defense for this type of malaria. In following sections the development of artemisinin and its derivatives will be discussed with an emphasis on recent advances in the field of synthetic peroxides from 2000 onwards. The synthetic peroxides are grouped according to structural similarities and key synthetic strategies are presented. Wherever possible the antimalarial activities are presented to show how the structure of peroxide effects the activity of peroxides of similar structural type. The *in vitro* activities against chloroquine-resistant strain of *P. falciparum* are given by the IC_{50} values while the *in vivo* activities of compounds administered by orally (po), subcutaneously (sc) or intraperitoneally (ip) to *P. berghei* infected mice are represented by their ED_{50} or ED_{90} values obtained using the Peters protocol.

2. Artemisinin

Traditional medicine contains a wealth of knowledge concerning the effect that herbs have on human health, and nowhere is this truer than in traditional Chinese medicine, which has developed over several thousand years. During the period of Cultural Revolution (1966-1976) practitioners of traditional Chinese medicine were brought together with scientists to subject traditional knowledge to modern scientific securitization. Within the malaria programme, *qinghao* was among the first ten herbs to be screened because of Ge Hong (284-363), a renowned physician, who suggested that a drug derived from *qinghao* or *Artemisia annua* be used for "intermittent fever".[16] However, the initial screening within the programme gave poor results and it was not until 1971, that a group led by Professor Tu Youyou, by carefully following Ge Hong's original procedure of wringing out a cold water infusion of *qinghao*, were able to prepare an effective drug. This was followed in 1972 by the first report of the successful treatment of malaria patients with *qinghao*. The finding had a major effect on the development of antimalarial drug therapy; *qinghao* (*Artemisia annua)* or sweet wormwood as it is known in the west became an important source of antimalarial agents. In 1973, the active compound was isolated and named as qinghaosu or artemisinin **1**.[4,16] Artemisinin is insoluble in water which explains why it was so difficult to prepare the herbal drug, but by wringing out a cold infusion of the herb an emulsion of flavonoids and aromatic oils present in the plant help to solubilise the artemisinin. A possible synergism among them could also not be excluded. This also explains why it is difficult to use traditional tea preparations of *Artemisia annua*.[17-20] Such encouraging initial results led to further research on artemisinin and its derivatives with pharmaceutical production of the drug beginning in 1986. By 2004, the World Health Organization WHO had changed its policy on malaria treatment and recommended that an artemisinin-based combination therapy – ACT (main combinations: artemether/ lumefantrine, artesunate/ amodiaquine, artesunate/ mefloquine, artesunate/ sulfadoxine/ pyrimethamine) should represent the first-line treatment for malaria. Then in 2006, WHO basing its argument on published research reinforced the statement[21] that monotherapy with artemisinin derivatives should be abandoned and it requested that pharmaceutical companies stop marketing "single-drug" artemisinin malaria pills in order to prevent the mosquito developing a resistance to it.[22] The importance of artemisinin to antimalarial chemotherapy and the scientific community's continued interest in its development is reflected in the many review papers dedicated to it and its derivatives.[23-28]

The structure of artemisinin 1 is impressive with a 1,2,4-trioxane ring incorporated into a sesquiterpene skeleton. The pharmacophore unit is a 1,2,4-trioxane ring or more precisely a peroxide bond (

Figure 2). Unfortunately, although artemisinin 1 is a very active compound its insolubility makes it unsuitable for therapeutic use. One solution is to transform artemisinin into dihydroartemisinin (DHA) 2; this was first prepared in 1973 by the group led by Tu Youyou while characterizing the structure of 1 without realising they had discovered an even more potent agent.[16] Etherification or esterification of the 10-hydroxy group produced the first generation of artemisinin derivatives, of which the most important are artemether 3 and artesunate 5 (

Figure 2).[24] These first generation artemisinin derivatives are fast-acting agents and have a high potency, but they have a short half-life in plasma as result of their rapid hydrolysis to DHA 2 leading to elimination via glucoronidation by Phase II metabolism.[27] Hence the need for their combination with a longer-acting drug (ACT) to prevent recrudescence of malaria.

To improve artemisinin derivatives further, development has focused on derivatives with a prolonged half-life in plasma (Figure 3).[11,24] Another important factor is the cost of preparation, which must be as low as possible as the drug is mostly destined for developing countries. Toxicity, in particular neurotoxicity is a key consideration in drug development and it is important that any newly developed compounds have a sufficiently low lipophilicity to prevent them crossing the blood-brain barrier.

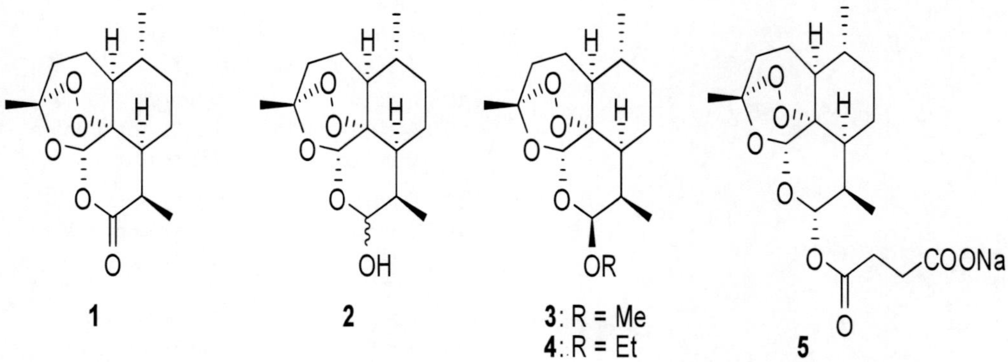

Figure 2.

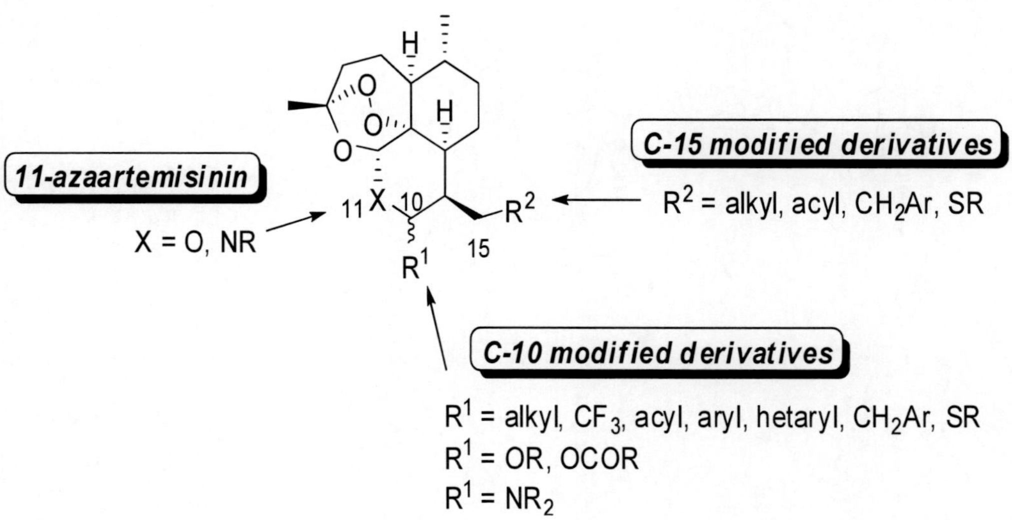

Figure 3.

The majority of derivatives belong to a group of artemisinins functionalized at the C-10 position. These are prepared from DHA 2 where the C-10 alcohol group is altered to give ether, ester or carbonate functionality. A recent example shows that the incorporation of biphenyl 6, fluorenyl 7, and adamantyl 8 scaffold through an ether linkage gives an orally active antimalarial agent that is more active against *P. yoelii* than β-arteether (Scheme 1).[29] Interestingly, stereochemistry plays an important role in these compounds and it is the α-isomers of the ethers that have the highest activity contrary to arteether 4, where the β-isomer is more active. These derivatives are quite lipophilic with a logP > 6, which according to the authors results in increased oral bioavailability. No toxicity data for these C-10 derivatized DHAs 6-8 are reported.

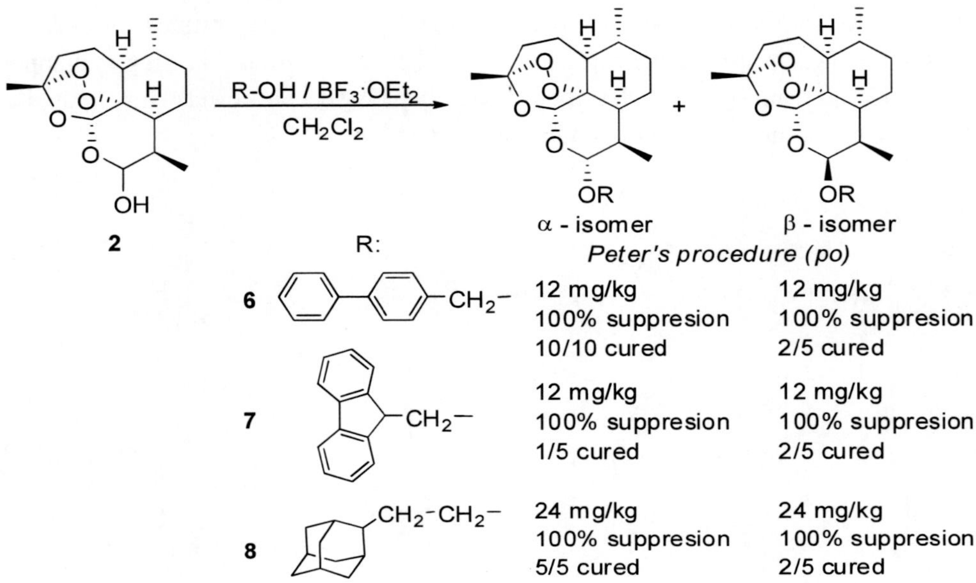

Scheme 1.

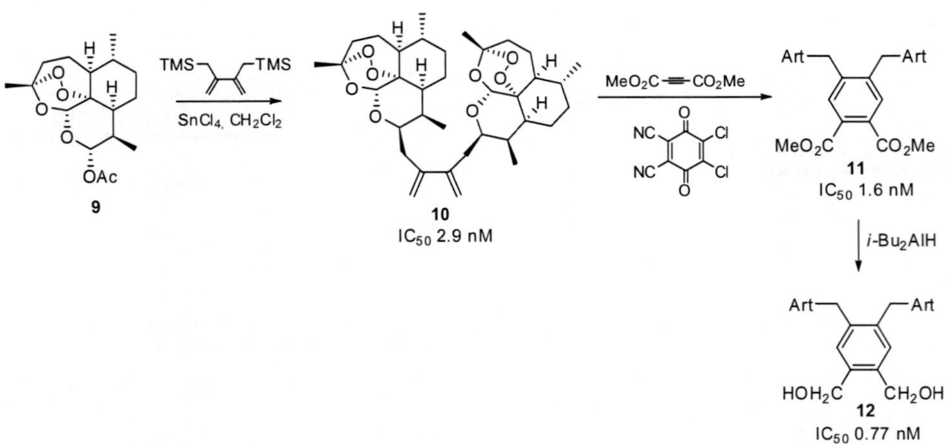

Scheme 2.

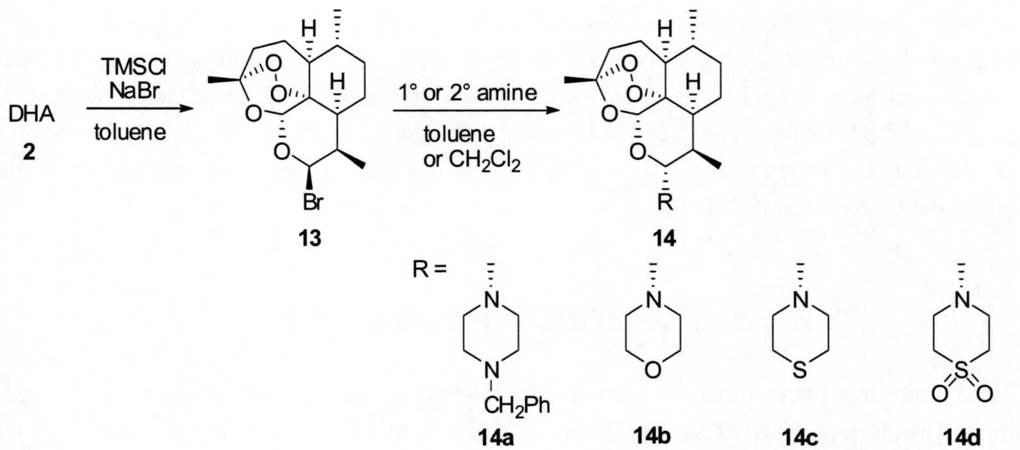

	14a	14b	14c	14d
logP	5.62	3.05	4.97	2.49
neurotoxicity	low	high	high	very low
ED90 (sc)	0.8 mg/kg	0.18 mg/kg	0.51 mg/kg	1.5 mg/kg
(po)	3.5 mg/kg	1.3 mg/kg	1.9 mg/kg	3.1 mg/kg

Scheme 3.

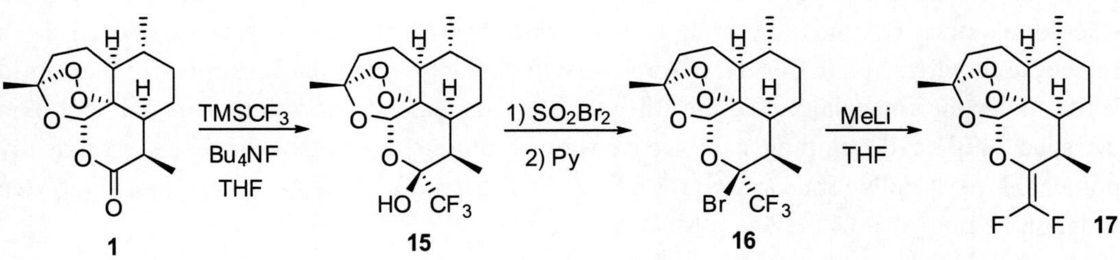

Scheme 4.

To prevent the hydrolysis of artemisinin to DHA 2 and consequently its elimination from the organism various C-10 alkyl and aryl derivatives have been synthesized. A recent example includes the use of artemisinin dimers 10-12 as longer-lived antimalarials that show curative activity after a single low parenteral dose (Scheme 2).[30,31]

Another possibility to prevent hydrolysis while at the same time incorporating a polar group to reduce lipophilicity and thus possible neurotoxicity is to introduce an alkylamino group at position 10 in artemisinin. 10-Alkylamino artemisinin derivatives 14 are very active, while neurotoxicity depends on the nature of the heteroatom or substituent in the alkylamino structure (Scheme 3).[32] Furthermore, lipophilicity is easily tuned by the correct choice of amine. The best candidate in this group - artemisone 14d, was prepared at a comparable price but with improved characteristics that allows a lower dosage. Preclinical screening showed that 14d has good properties with negligible cyto- and neurotoxicities making it a good candidate for clinical trials.

Another approach to turn artemisinin into a metabolically more stable compound is that described by the group of Bonnet-Delpon.[33] They substituted the 10-carbonyl group of artemisinin into the 10-*gem*-difluoroethylene group that sterically and electronically mimics the carbonyl group. In doing so were able to develop an artemisinin analogue 17 with improved stability, longer lasting antimalarial activity and a higher activity against *P. falciparum* FCB1 strain (IC_{50} 4.6nM) than its parent artemisinin 1 (IC_{50} 8.9nM). Despite these changes the structure of the derivative remains the same as does the recognition of the agent by the organism (Scheme 4).

3. Synthetic Peroxides

The main drawbacks of artemisinin and its first generation derivatives were successfully addressed by the creation of semisynthetic artemisinin derivatives, however their principle disadvantage *i.e.*, the necessity of artemisinin for their synthesis still remains. This is significant because the current demand for artemisinin globally exceeds supply, a fact made evident by the shortage in supply in 2004. Estimation for global demand in 2005 was 120 million of adult treatment courses.[34] The content of artemisinin in the leaves of *Artemisia annua* is low and is strongly dependent on growth conditions, region and strain.[35] After WHO recommended artemisinin-based combination therapy, the cultivation of *Artemisia annua* has expanded and hopefully the quantity and the yield will increase through improved agricultural practice and novel biotechnologies. An example of such approach is a collaboration between UC Berkeley, Amyris Biotechnologies and the Institute for One World Health under the financial aid of the Bill and Melinda Gates Foundation. This collaboration was successful in developing a low cost way of producing artemisinin using genetically engineered yeast cells (*Saccharomyces cerevisiae)* to produce artemisic acid in a three-step oxidation of amorpha-4,11-diene.[36]

An more obvious solution to produce large amounts of artemisinin is organic synthesis, however the 10 steps required to synthesise artemisinin makes it uneconomical.[37-39] An alternative approach includes the preparation of synthetic organic peroxides that can mimic the action and/or structure of artemisinin.[23,26,40-42] This methodology will be more fully addressed later.

Having established that the peroxide bond is essential to the antimalarial activity of artemisinin, its mode of action could then be linked with the parasite's digestion of haemoglobin. It was the elimination of the dangerous heme that led to the logical conclusion that it is the interaction with Fe(II) within the erythrocytes that generates poisonous radicals resulting in artemisinin's antimalarial action. This mechanism is supported by experimental data, but the actual mode of action of the artemisinin derivatives remains a hot topic of debate within the scientific community as new data shows that artemisinin inhibits enzyme PfATP6, a key metabolic enzyme of SERCA-type Ca^{2+} ATPase.[22,43,44] However, it does pave the way for the development of synthetic peroxides because it was believed that the most important thing is the interaction with heme. Of course, almost any peroxide, being an oxidant, can react with the iron(II) species. Even simple peroxides, like hydrogen peroxide and *tert*-butyl hydroperoxide, are antimalarial agents.[45,46] Therefore, the organic scaffold around the peroxide bond gives the agent its correct activity in the organism. A variety of structures of synthetic antimalarial peroxides show that there are many ways of wrapping a peroxide bond with an organic scaffold to produce an antimalarial effect. In the following sections, peroxidic antimalarials are organized according to the structural element of the basic peroxidic bond.

3.1. Trioxanes

Artemisinin has a very interesting tetracyclic structure with a 1,2,4-trioxane ring incorporated into a sesquiterpene core. Having in mind the synthesis of artemisinin analogues a question immediately arises, i.e., whether or not its complicated structure is essential for antimalarial activity. This is important because a simpler structure usually means a less complicated synthesis. The most evident structure in artemisinin is the peroxidic 1,2,4-trioxane ring and various synthetic trioxanes evolved directly from artemisinin and were studied as potential antimalarial agents.

3.1.1. Tricyclic 1,2,4- trioxanes

To simplify the structure of artemisinin it would be necessary to know which ring could be left out without affecting its antimalarial activity. Research has shown that the lactone ring in 1 is superfluous and that the tricyclic analogue 18 is active (Figure 4).[47] Furthermore, by changing the 7-membered ring in 18 into a 6-membered one 19 the antimalarial activity is lost.[48] Whereas, analogue 20 with its ABC ring combination and without the 7-cyclic ring was active.[47]

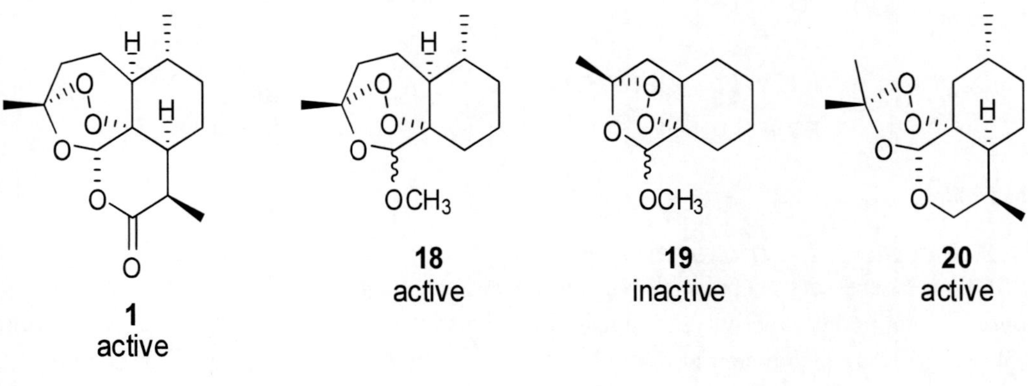

Figure 4.

Posner's group presented a series of tricyclic trioxanes with retained rings A, C and D of the parent artemisinin scaffold. Their synthesis started with cyclohexanone that was converted to the nitrile 21. Wittig methoxymethylenation and arylation by aryl lithium produced the precoursor 23. A peroxide group was introduced using a singlet oxygen oxygenation followed by an acid catalyzed rearrangement to give 3-aryltrioxane 24 (Scheme 5).[49-51] Studies on the antimalarial activity of 3-aryltrioxanes 24 show that they are promising drug candidates and have been found to show good activity *in vitro* and especially *in vivo* studies. Furthermore they are non-toxic in therapeutic doses. Development of water-soluble trioxanes 25 and 26 following a similar methodology produce even more efficient derivatives with enhanced bioavailability.[52-54] The multi step synthesis of these 3-aryltrioxanes 24 limits their development but research into these substrates does provide valuable information on the mechanism of action of artemisinin-like compounds. It has also been observed that chirality does not influence antimalarial activity as both enantiomers of 24d have a similar *in vitro* activity against the *P. falciparum*.[55,56]

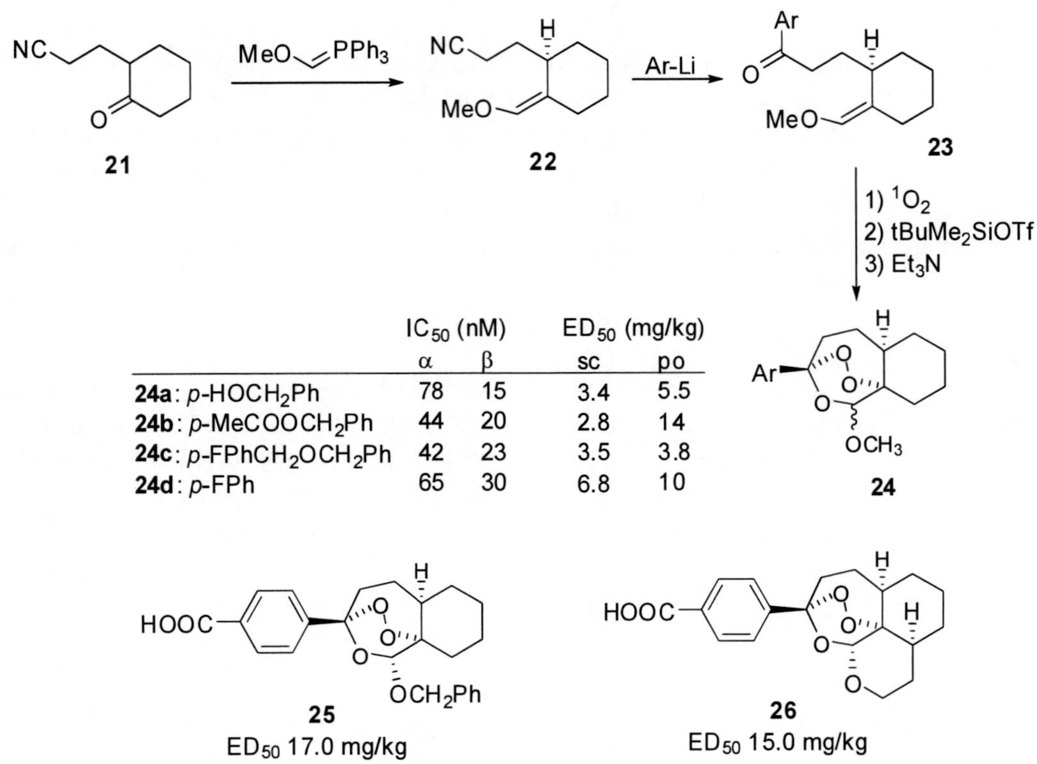

	IC_{50} (nM)		ED_{50} (mg/kg)	
	α	β	sc	po
24a: *p*-$HOCH_2Ph$	78	15	3.4	5.5
24b: *p*-$MeCOOCH_2Ph$	44	20	2.8	14
24c: *p*-$FPhCH_2OCH_2Ph$	42	23	3.5	3.8
24d: *p*-FPh	65	30	6.8	10

Scheme 5.

3.1.2. Bicyclic 1,2,4-trioxanes

It is not necessary to preserve the tetracyclic artemisinin skeleton for a compound to show good antimalarial activity. It appears that apart from the tricyclic trioxanes the bicyclic 1,2,4-trioxanes are also potent building blocks for antimalarial active compounds as indicated by the activity of 20 (Figure 4). *cis*-Fused cyclopenteno-1,2,4-trioxanes 29 are an example of bicyclic peroxides with potent antimalarial activity. They are synthesized from 1,4-diaryl-1,3-cyclopentadienes 27 by photooxygenation to introduce a peroxy function in the form of a 1,4-endoperoxide 28 that is transformed by acid-catalyzed ring-enlargement with either a ketone or aldehyde into 29 (Scheme 6).

Intensive research on these structures reveals an interesting effect that their structure has on their activity. A 3,3-spirocycloalkane substituent is important for the antimalarial activity, while the highest activity is observed for the cyclopentane ring 29a. On the other hand, the heteroatoms in the 3,3-cyclohexane ring does not influence to any great extent its activity, with the spiropyran analogue 29c having an even higher activity, while steric effects are more important – this can be judged from the lower activity of 29d. The most promising candidate among this family is Fenozoan 29e, which has all the important elements for good activity: 3,3-spirocyclopentane substituent, *cis*-fused 1,2,4-trioxane, cyclopentene ring and fluorine substituents on the *para* position in the aryl ring with the emphasized effect on *in vivo* activity. [57-59]

Singlet oxygen is the major source of peroxide functionality in the preparation of bicyclic peroxides containing the 1,2,4-trioxane structural unit. In a recently published synthetic strategy, ene-reaction was used to transform allylic alcohols 30 into unsaturated vicinal hydroperoxy alcohols 31 that were then transformed into various cyclic peroxides with a 1,2,4-trioxane ring in the bicyclic structure, as exemplified in 32a (Scheme 7).[60] Preliminary studies on the *in vitro* antimalarial activity against *P. falciparum* show that these bicyclic 1,2,4-trioxanes 32 posses moderate antimalarial activity and could serve as a skeleton for further derivatization.

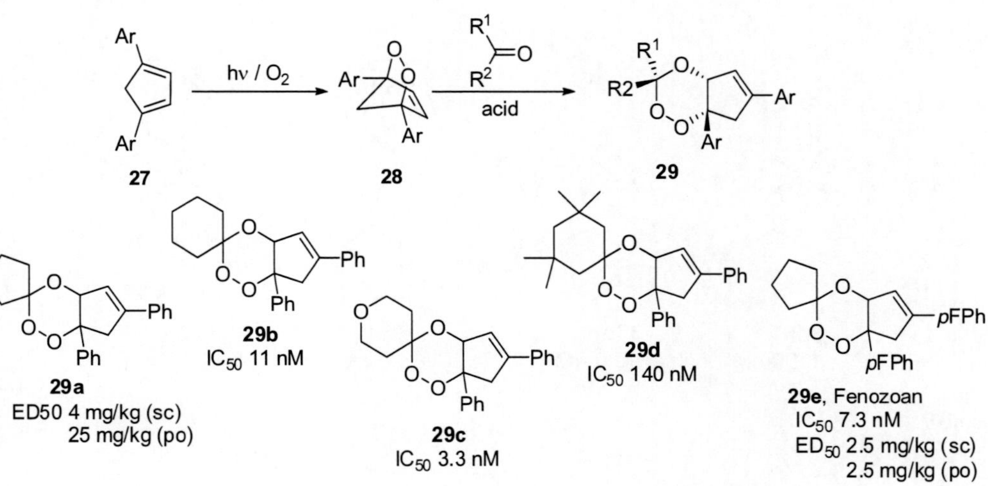

Scheme 6.

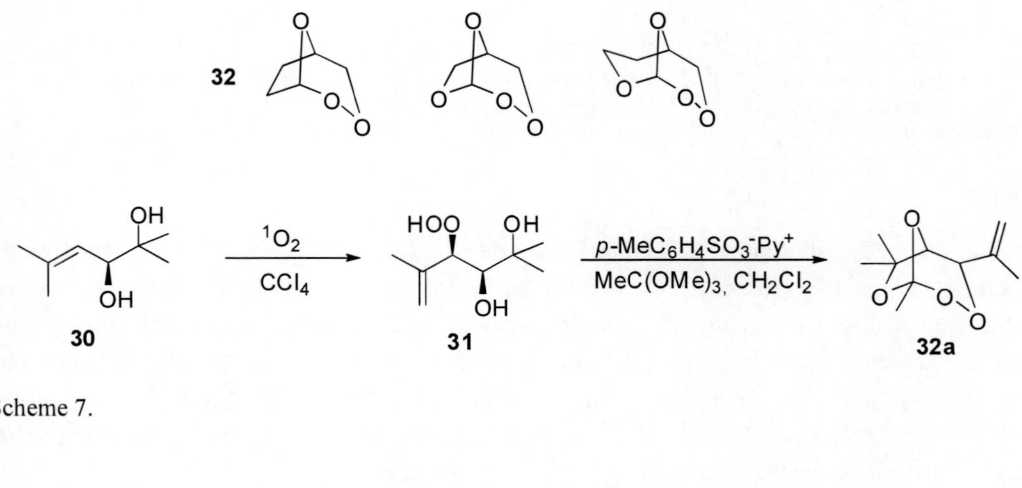

Scheme 7.

3.1.3. Spiro 1,2,4-trioxanes

Alternatively, O'Neill's group reports constructing a trioxane ring using Mukaiyama hydroperoxysilylation of allyl alcohols by molecular oxygen as a source of the peroxide bond with a subsequent cyclization by another carbonyl compound (Scheme 8).[61]

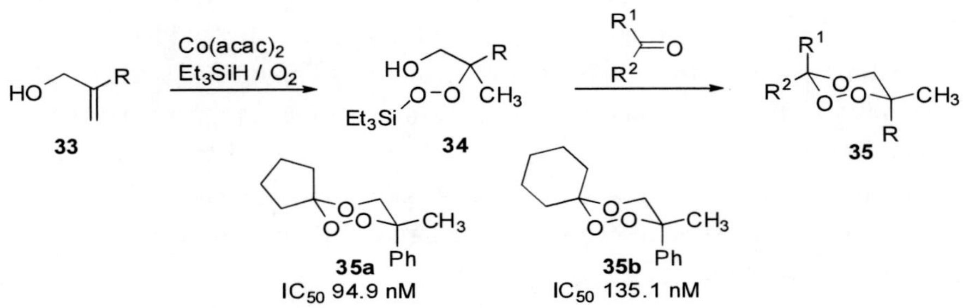

Scheme 8.

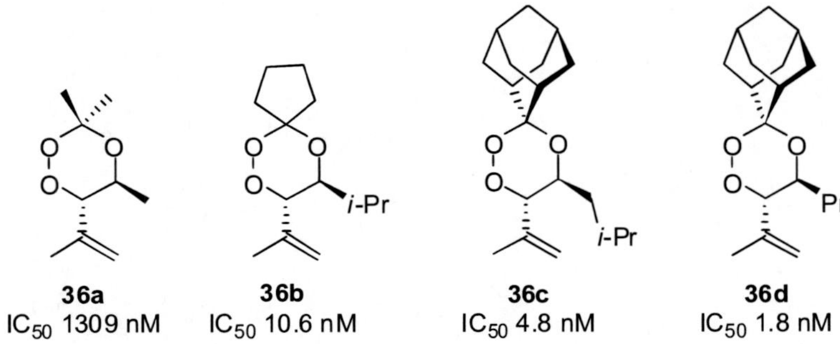

Scheme 9.

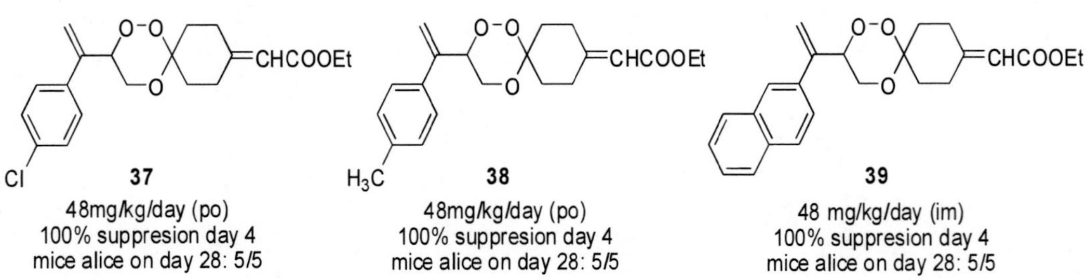

Figure 5.

The majority of synthetic methods include singlet oxygen for the construction of trioxanes. In a similar strategy to that outlined in Scheme 7, spiro-1,2,4-trioxanes 36 were synthesized from an ene-reacton of allylic alcohols with the subsequent cyclization of the previously formed *vic*-hydroperoxy alcohols with ketones (cycloalkanones, adamantanone) to prepare compounds 36. These compounds display antimalarial activity on the nanomolar scale with low toxicity (Scheme 9).[62-64] Results show the necessity for constructing spiro bicyclic trioxanes over the *gem*-dialkyl substituted trioxanes.

Spiro 1,2,4-trioxanes were prepared using a similar strategy to forming natural compounds and geraniol was used as replacement for allyl alcohol[65,66] or steroidal ketones were used for cyclization,[67] nevertheless natural compounds did not augment the antimalarial activity that remained moderate. Improved results were obtained by using 3-aryl substituted allyl alcohols for ene-reaction followed by cyclization using 1,4-cyclohexadienone to obtain spiro-1,2,4-trioxane with the carbonyl function on the cyclohexane ring that served as an entry point for further transformation.[68] Screening for oral *in vivo* activity delivered two compounds 37 and 38 that were orally active with a profile that is better than β-arteether against *P. yoelii* (Figure 5). The authors claim that by changing phenyl ring into a naphthyl ring 39 they obtained a compound whose activity resembles that of artemisinin against rodent and simian malaria.

3.2. Tetraoxanes

3.2.1. 1,2,4,5-Tetraoxanes

1,2,4,5-Tetraoxanes differ from 1,2,4-trioxanes in having an additional oxygen atom in the six-membered ring. This means that they have two peroxide bonds per molecule instead of one. The use of symmetrical dispiro 1,2,4,5-tetraoxanes 42 as potent antimalarial agents was studied by the group of Vennerstrom. These compounds have been examined in detail and various substitution patterns and substituents studied to identify a candidate with the best antimalarial properties (Scheme 10).[69-72] Tetraoxane 42a prepared from 2-methylcyclohexanone 40a was selected as the most promising agent amongst the tetraoxanes having a good *in vitro* activity against *P. falciparum* K1 strain. While *in vivo* activity against *P. berghei* on a day 3 post-infection was similar to artemisinin, survival time of mice was better.[71,73] The synthesis of these compounds should be straightforward requiring only the acid-catalyzed peroxidation of cyclohexanones with aqueous hydrogen peroxide. However, selectivity depends on the structure of the ketone and various peroxides are formed, with hexaoxonane 43 being the main byproduct.[74-76] For this reason, the actual synthesis is mainly performed by ozonolysis of O-methyl oximes 41 or enol ethers.

The use of 30% aqueous hydrogen peroxide would be more desirable than ozone. Using fluorinated alcohols (2,2,2-trifluoroethanol - TFE or hexafluoro-*iso*-propanol – HFIP) as solvents for acid-catalyzed peroxidative cyclization tetraoxanes were formed selectively from a variety of ketones without the formation of other peroxides. [74,77] The use of fluorinated alcohols enabled 3,3,6,6-tetraalkyl-1,2,4,5-tetraoxanes 44 to be synthesized. These were studied because of the ease by which small variations in polarity and structure of tetraoxanes could be achieved by changing the length and branching of alkyl chains (Scheme 11).[78] The steric effects play an important role on the *in vitro* antimalarial activity as is indicated by the lower activity of tetraoxane that have the *i*-Pr 44b and *t*-Bu 44c groups on the tetraoxane scaffold in relation to 44a. Furthermore, polarity, as expressed by the length of alkyl chains, influences activity *i.e.*, smaller chains results in improved activity (44a *vs*. 44d), but the effect is not so clear as a significant difference in activity exists between methyl/ethyl substituted tetraoxane (44e/44d) albeit their polarity is similar.[78]

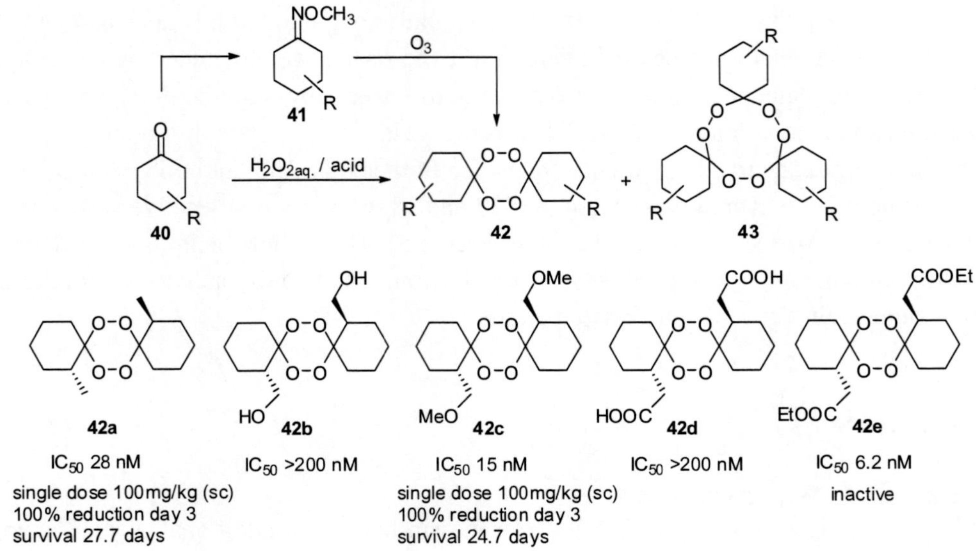

Scheme 10.

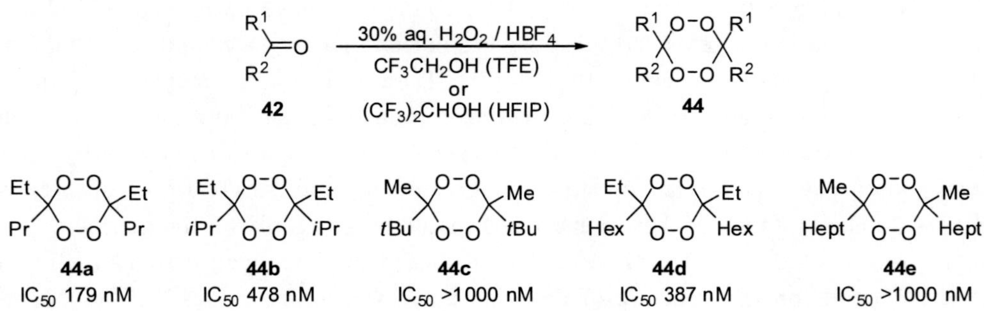

Scheme 11.

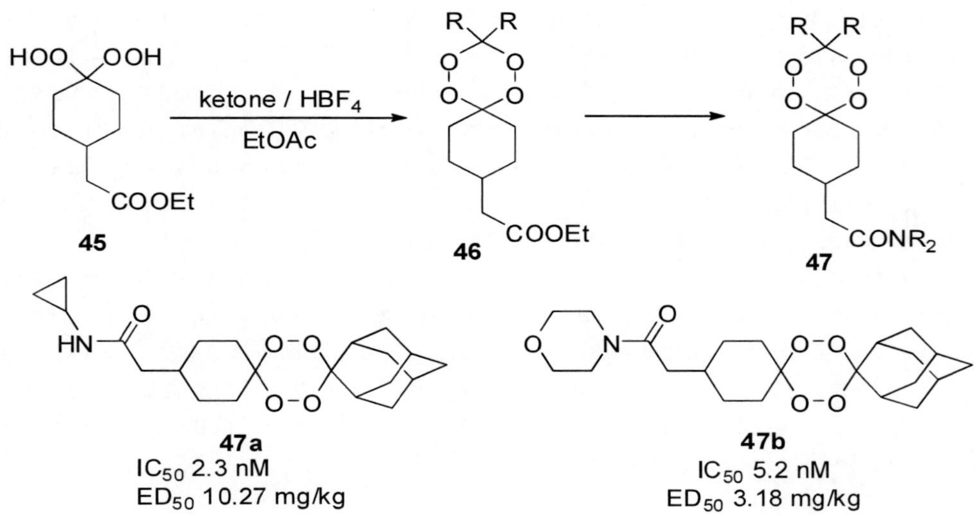

Scheme 12.

Further advances were made by O'Neill's group by developing a second generation of tetraoxanes with improved stability and oral bioavailability.[79] Important was the introduction of the amino and amido polar groups into the tetraoxane skeleton to increase water solubility and therefore bioavailability (Scheme 12). Different strategies were taken to obtain targeted compounds with excellent in vitro antimalarial activity against P. falciparum with the best of them having an activity better than that of artemisinin. Similar observations were also observed during in vivo experiments against P. berghei, where oral activity was enhanced by the presence of a cyclododecane or a adamantane ring in the dispiro tetraoxane structure. This confirms that dispiro tetraoxanes are more active than spiro analogues. Two particularly interesting facts are their relatively simple synthesis from simple starting compounds and that they are achiral. Nevertheless, it is that 47a and 47b have an activity equivalent to artemisinin should be emphasized.

Non-symmetrical tetraoxanes offer the possibility to incorporate two different structures on each side of the tetraoxane ring. This makes it possible to obtain compounds with the desired properties that can be tuned by each of the substituents on the tetraoxane scaffold. Recently new methods for the preparation of non-symmetrical or mixed tetraoxanes have become available.[77,79-83] A group led by Solaja published an interesting approach for increasing the bioavailability of antimalarial tetraoxanes by attaching a tetraoxane ring to a natural steroid carrier. Moreover, by using cholic acid as a ketone, symmetrical steroidal tetraoxanes were synthesized with the carboxylic acid function on the side chain, which served as an entry point for further derivatization to various amides.[84,85] Their *in vitro* antimalarial activity against *P. falciparum* D6 clone matches almost that of artemisinin when the *n*-propylamido functional group was present on the side chain, while toxicity is low with the selectivity >10,000. Furthermore, these bis-steroidal tetraoxanes have antiproliferative activity and can induce apoptic cell death. This approach was upgraded to a second-generation of steroidal tetraoxanes consisting of mixed tetraoxanes to provide a selective and broad manipulation of the tetraoxane scaffold. The carrier properties of steroid was preserved, while additional activity was achieved by incorporating another smaller cyclic structure and at the same time the molecular mass of the active compound was reduced. [83,86,87] Synthesis consisted of preparing *gem*-dihydroperoxide of cholic or deoxycholic acid followed by acid-catalyzed cyclization with another ketone and the targeted derivatization of the ester in the cholic group (Scheme 13). Deoxycholic acid was introduced to increase metabolic stability, but despite this their antimalarial activity *in vitro* and *in vivo* was weaker than that of the corresponding cholic acid derivatives.[87] Derivatives with a secondary amido group on the steroid side chain have comparable *in vitro* activity to artemisinin against the multidrug resistant *P. falciparum* strain TM91C935. *In vivo* testing showed that compounds 50 are effective in curing mice infected with *P. berghei* without any observable toxic effects.

3.2.2. 1,2,4,5-Tetraoxacycloalkanes

gem-Dihydroperoxides are also the starting compounds for the preparation of 1,2,4,5-tetraoxacycloalkanes, macrocyclic analogues of a more elaborate group of 1,2,4,5-tetraoxanes. Silver(I) oxide or caesium hydroxide were used as a catalyst for the cyclization of *gem*-dihydroperoxides, prepared from ketones with hydrogen peroxide or ozonolysis of enol ethers, with 1,n-diiodoalkanes to obtain the 1,2,4,5-tetraoxacycloalkanes (Scheme 14). The influence of the peroxide ring structure on the activity is clear and can not be correlated just to the size of the ring. However, the *in vitro* activity of some compounds against *P. falciparum* is similar to artemisinin. The most active compound is 53. This compound together with its low toxicity has a selectivity index of 10,000. *In vivo* experiments against *P. berghei* pointed at 52a as the best candidate. Further tests have shown that 52a is also orally active and comparison with artemisinin proves it is a better agent.[88]

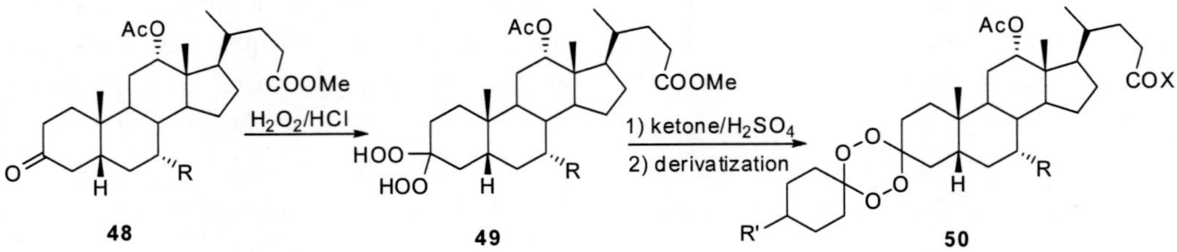

50a: R = H, R' = (R)-CH_3
X = $NHCH_2CH_2NMe_2$
IC_{50} 14.72 nM
160mg/kg/day
3/5 alive on day 31
survival 29 days

50b: R = OAc, R' = (R)-CH_3
X = $NHCH_2CH_2NMe_2$
IC_{50} 12.24 nM
40mg/kg/day
1/5 alive on day 31
survival 19 days

50c: R = OAc, R' = H
X = $NHCH_2CH_2NMe_2$
IC_{50} 19.65 nM
320mg/kg/day
5/5 alive on day 31
survival 31 days

40mg/kg/day
2/5 alive on day 31
survival 21 days

Scheme 13.

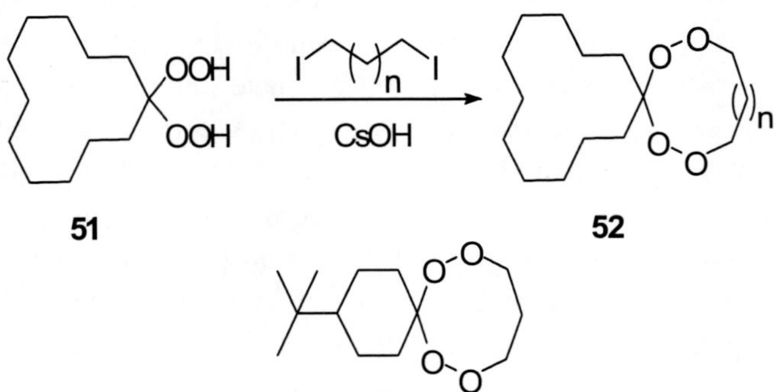

	EC_{50} (nM)	ED_{50} (ip) (mg/kg)
52a: n=1	25	12
52b: n=2	100	48
52c: n=3	280	
52d: n=4	10	160
52e: n=6	1700	
53	3	15

Scheme 14.

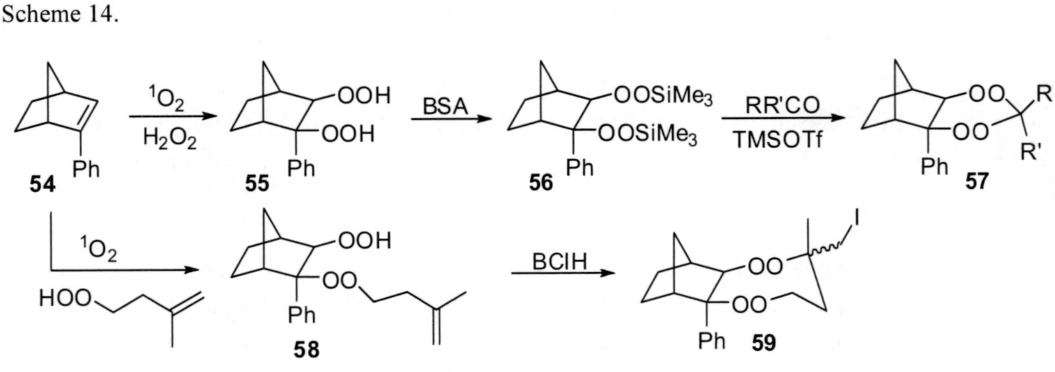

Scheme 15.

3.2.3. 1,2,5,6-Tetraoxacycloalkanes

Another variant of the peroxidic macrocycle *i.e.*, with four oxygen atoms is derived from the cyclization of *vic*-dihydroperoxide with a ketone or 1,*n*-diiodoalkane. *vic*-Dihydroperoxide 55 or 58 were prepared by a singlet oxygen oxygenation of 2-phenyl-norbornene 54 in the presence of hydrogen peroxide or alkenyl hydroperoxide, respectively (Scheme 15). Cyclization of 1,2-dihydroperoxides was performed according to Scheme 14 or alternatively both hydroperoxy groups were first trimethylsilylated and afterwards cyclized with a carbonyl compound catalyzed by a Lewis acid. The alkenyl perethers 58 were cyclized *via* the reaction with bis(collidine)iodine hexafluorophosphate (BCIH).[89] The antimalarial activity of these 1,2,5,6-tetraoxocycloalkanes is moderate.

3.3. Trioxolanes

Ozonolysis of alkenes forms 1,2,4-trioxolanes or secondary ozonides as intermediate products that are usually not stable. However, tetrasubstituted ozonides are stable due to the absence of α-hydrogen atoms. Grisbaum developed a method for the preparation of secondary ozonides by coozonolysis of O-alkyl oximes and carbonyl compounds.[90] The group of Vennerstrom used this to develop antimalarial 1,2,4-trioxolanes through an interesting approach.[91] They first selected a candidate that satisfied the essential characteristics for a trioxolane antimalarial drug: low product cost, good potency and pharmacokinetic properties for a maximum 3-day treatment regime with once-daily administration, low potential toxicity and no evidence for resistance development. To do this a candidate selection matrix was composed and subjected to further optimization and compound selection. Eventually, trioxolane 60 (OZ277 or Rbx-11160) was selected as a structurally simple drug development candidate with an economically feasible and scalable synthesis, with superior antimalarial activity and a biopharmaceutical profile (Figure 6). The development of this drug was taken further in a public-private partnership with the Medicines for Malaria Venture (MMV) and Ranbaxy Pharmaceuticals. According to a series of recommendation given by WHO for the usage of combined therapy, this drug is now undergoing clinical studies trials in combination with piperaquine. According to Ranbaxy Pharmaceuticals Inc. a new drug application for a combination of Rbx-11160 and PQP could be filed in early 2009.[92] This would be the first synthetic antimalarial peroxide on the market.

Ketone oxime ether 61 reacts with ozone at 0°C in the presence of a second ketone 62 and forms a stable tetrasubstituted secondary ozonide or 1,2,4-trioxolane 63.[91,93] Its antimalarial activity is derived from the trioxolane 63 structure, which incorporates a peroxide bond in the organic scaffold (Scheme 16). However, because the peroxide bond in diadamantyl 63a or dicyclohexyl 63c trioxolanes is sterically inaccessible or too exposed respectively, these compounds are inactive, while mixed trioxolane 63b has equilibrated both effects and is highly active. Evidence for the importance of the peroxide bond in determining the activity of the trioxolanes was confirmed by the synthesis of the inactive 1,3-dioxolane derivative.[94,95]

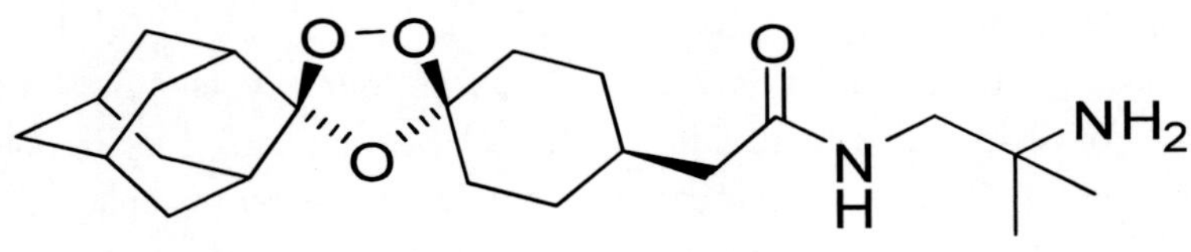

60, OZ227, Rbx-11160

Figure 6.

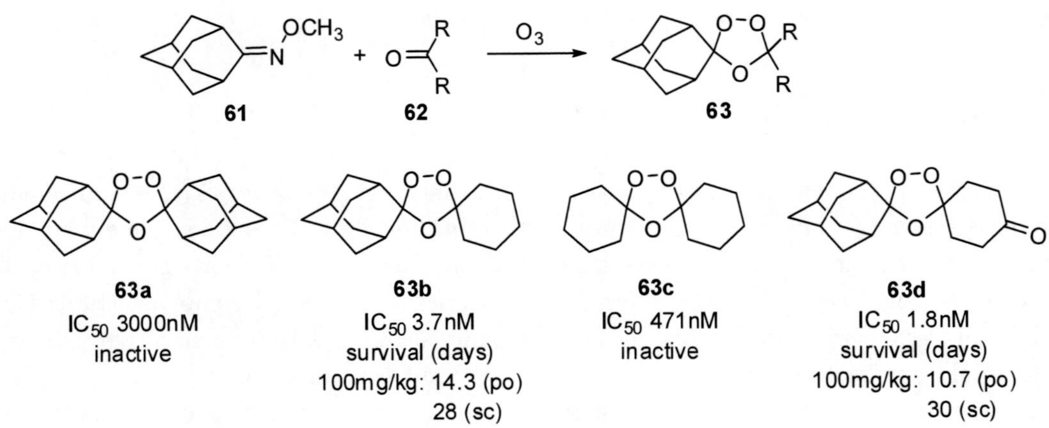

Scheme 16.

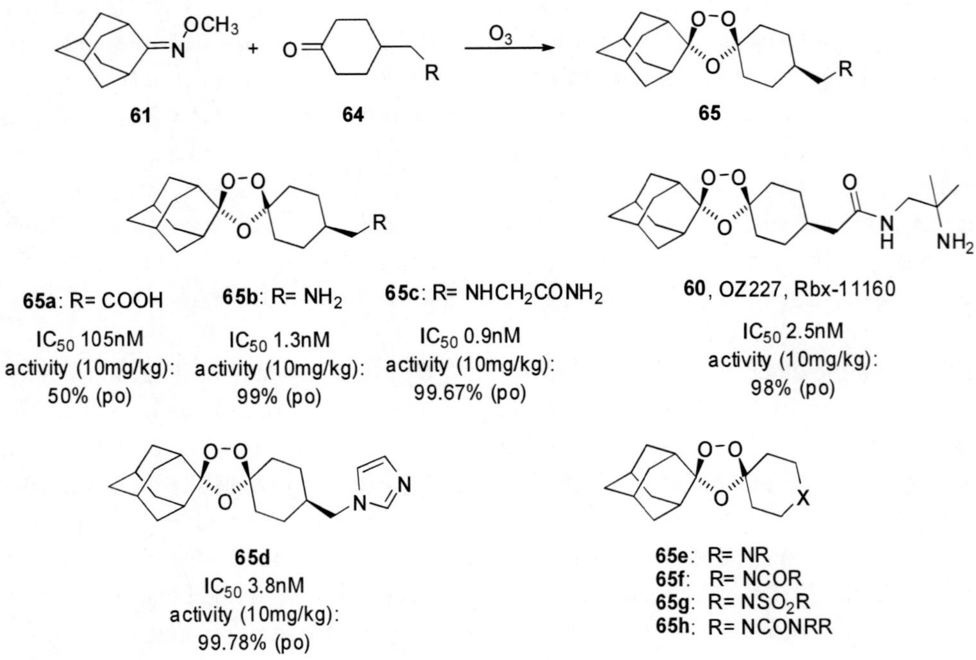

Scheme 17.

These substrates are however, too lipophilic and have low aqueous solubility and low oral bioavailability. Improved biopharmaceutical properties were expected from trioxolanes with polar functional groups. The best choice was deemed as having an adamantane structure on one side and a 4-substituted cyclohexane ring with functional groups that would allow further derivatization (R= OH, CH_2OH, COOH, CH_2COOH, NH_2, CH_2NH_2, =O) on the other side of the trioxolane ring. The structure of 65 excludes any problems associated with chirality and its diastereoselectivity is defined only by the substituent on the cyclohexanone ring. Ozonolysis occurs preferentially by forming the *cis*-isomer (Scheme 17).[93]

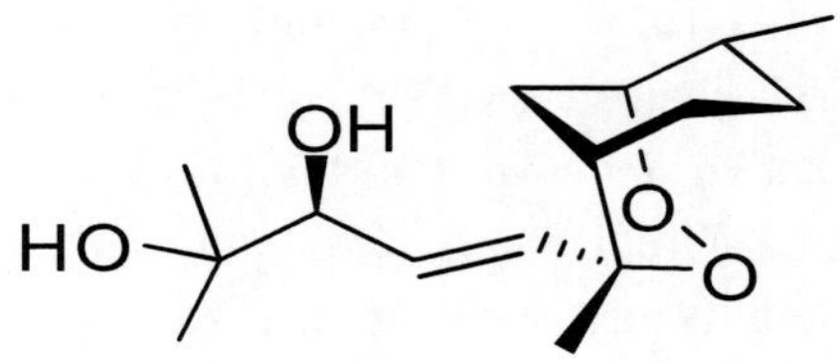

66, Yingzhaosu A

Figure 7.

Initially, three derivatives were targeted among which 60 had the best profile (OZ227, Rbx11160).[91,96] Later, new derivatives were synthesized to identify those substrates that have the optimum characteristics of lipophilicity and aqueous solubility and containing those functional groups linked with antimalarial properties. Analogues of 65 with a piperidine ring instead of cyclohexane and additionally functionalized into amines, amides, sulfonamides and ureas 65e-h possessed good *in vitro* activity but were less potent *in vivo*. Furthermore, products with acid functional groups are less potent than those with neutral or weak basic functional groups.[97,98] This led Vennerstrom and his team to prepare weak base trioxolanes with good oral activity, good biopharmaceutical properties and low toxicity. Targeted compounds 65b-d were derivatives with amino (alkylamino, amides, aminoxy, amino acid, guanidine) and azole functional groups.[99]

3.4. Endoperoxides

Yingzhaosu A 66 (Figure 7) is another active substance from the arsenal of traditional Chinese herbal medicine that has had a tremendous impact on the development of peroxidic antimalarial agents. Although it was isolated from a rare ornamental vine *Artabotrys uncinatus Lam.* and its structure determined in approximately the same time as that of artemisinin,[39,100] its biologically activity was only quantified recently.[101] One reason could be the scarcity of the herb and the difficulty in isolating the active compound. The total synthesis of yingzhaosu A consists of 14 steps and is economically unviable.[39,102] In 2005, however, a new total synthesis was reported consisting of only 8 steps starting with (S)-limonene and resulting in a in 7.3% overall yield of yingzhaosu A. This enabled the determination of its antimalarial activity and cytotoxicity.[101] Yingzhaosu A contains a 2,3-

dioxo[3.3.1]nonane structure which has become a unique bicyclic scaffold for various synthetic endoperoxide antimalarials.

3.4.1. Bicyclic Endoperoxides

Since yingzhaosu A 66 itself was not available, various approaches were taken to synthesize substrates that mimics its structure. The leading method for the preparation of 2,3-dioxo[3.3.1]nonanes was developed by Hoffmann-La Roche and consists of reacting an isomer of carvone or its analogue 67 by a singlet oxygen ene reaction, followed by cyclization of the intermediate hydroperoxide 68 into the desired bicyclic yingzhaosu A analogue 69 (Scheme 18).[103-105] The structure of 69 was then transformed by incorporation of various alkyl chains, aryl structures or functional groups. The cyclic structure by itself 69a is active *in vivo* (sc) and it is surprisingly non-sensitive to stereochemical factors (ED_{50} of stereoisomers is 51 and 61mg/kg, respectively). Lipophilic groups 69b enhance the activity as well as aryl groups with electron-withdrawing substitutents. The difference in the activities of these endoperoxides and artemisinin is smaller *in vivo* than *in vitro*, while the dioxane structure is more stable leading to longer half-lives in plasma. Arteflene 69c was selected as the most potent drug candidate and entered into Phase II clinical trials, before it was abandoned. However, indepth studies on the mechanism of activity has provided important insights into the interaction of the peroxidic antimalarial agent with Fe(II) and the formation of secondary carbon radicals.[106,107]

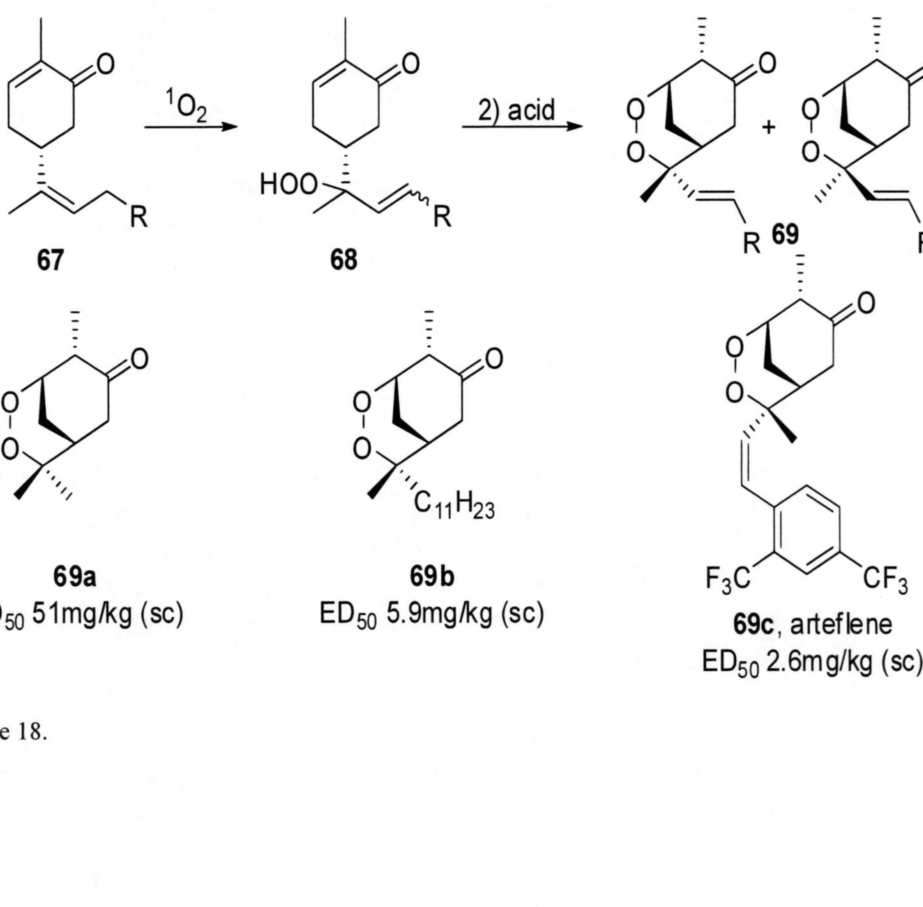

Scheme 18.

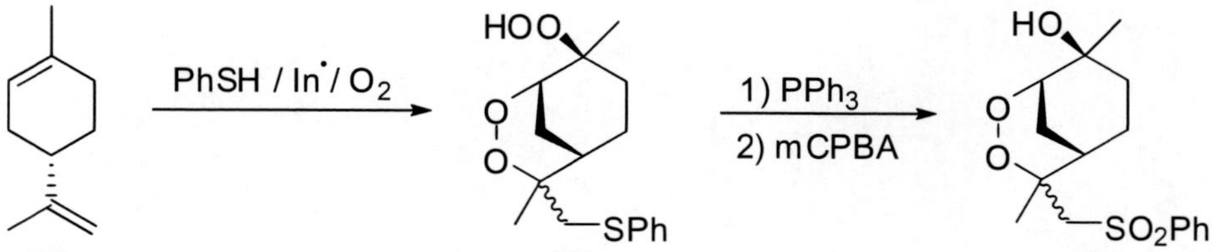

70 71 72

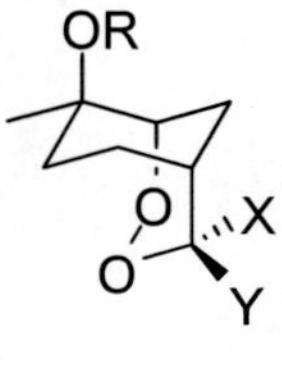

	R	X	Y	IC_{50} (nM)	ED_{50} (mg/kg)
72a	H	CH_2SO_2Ph	Me	55	>30
72b	Ac	CH_2SO_2Ph	Me	17	3.7
72c	Bn	CH_2SO_2Ph	Me	6.5	0.8
72d	Ac	Ph	CH_2SO_2Ph	42	

Scheme 19.

2,3-Dioxabicyclo[3.3.1]nonane was established as a pharmacophore and further synthetic strategies for its synthesis were initiated. An important group of bicyclic β-sulfonyl endoperoxides 72 was developed by thiol induced free radical cyclization of monoterpenes and oxygen (TOCO – Thiol Olefin Co-Oxygenation), where molecular oxygen is used to provide peroxide functionality as exemplified in the case of limonene 70 (Scheme 19).[108] Here, a free radical reaction is initiated by UV light, and AIBN or di-tert-butylperoxolate and an endoperoxide 71 is produced in a single step by forming five bonds simultaneously. The transformation into the sulfonyl derivative 72 involves the reduction of the hydroperoxy group into an hydroxy group followed by the oxidation of the sulfenyl group to a sulfonyl one. The hydroxy functional group in 72 presents an entry point for further transformations, while derivatives of monoterpenes, taken as starting substrates, can also broaden the structural scope. In this way, over fifty derivatives were synthesized and tested for their antimalarial activity.[109,110] Results were similar to arteflene derivatives regarding the insensitivity of their activity to stereoelectronic effects. Furthermore, the best endoperoxides have a better activity than the currently used artemisinin-based drugs, especially for in vivo values (sc). They also have a low toxicity.

Further indication of the importance of 2,3-dioxabicyclo[3.3.1]nonane pharmacophore emerged after the preparation of iodinated analogues of yingzhaosu A. Unsaturated hydroperoxides 73 were prepared by Co(II)-catalyzed autooxidation of alkenes, which is another method for introducing a peroxide functional group using molecular oxygen. Bis(collidine)iodine hexafluorophosphate (BCIH) was then used to construct the endoperoxide structure, where the reaction proceeds first by iodination of the double bond to form the cyclic iodonium ion that reacts with the hydroperoxy group as an internal nucleophile to form an endoperoxide bridge (Scheme 20).[111,112] The *in vitro* antimalarial activity of iodo-functionalized 2,3-dioxa[3.3.1]nonanes was high, however lower *in vivo* activity suggests that derivatives should be transformed to transfer this high activity from *in vitro* into *in vivo*.

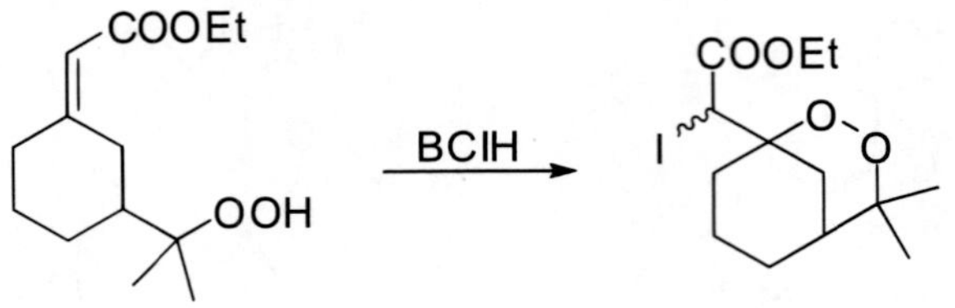

73 74

EC$_{50}$ 11nM
100mg/kg
20% supression on day 4
survival: 6.5 days

Scheme 20.

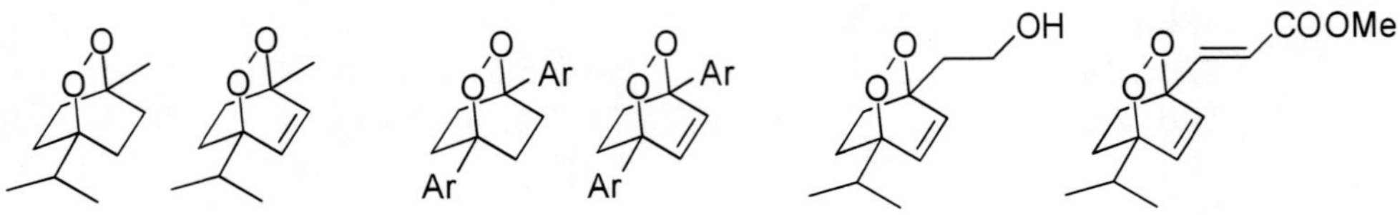

75 76 77 78 79 80

Scheme 21.

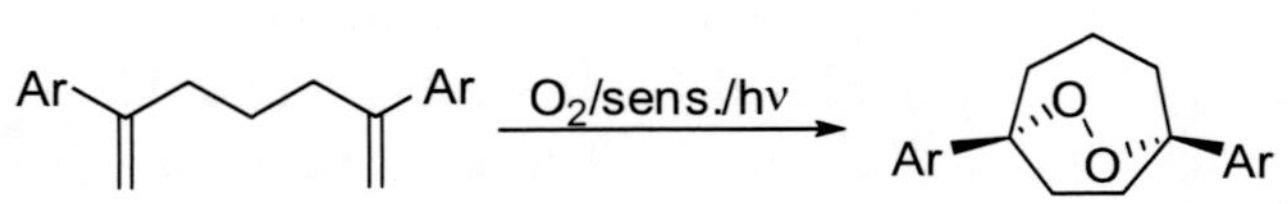

81

	EC$_{50}$ (nM)
82a: Ar= p-FC$_6$H$_4$	250
82b: Ar= C$_6$H$_5$	90
82c: Ar= p-MeC$_6$H$_4$	160
82d: Ar= p-MeOC$_6$H$_4$	160

Scheme 22.

Monoterpenes are interesting starting compounds for the formation of various bicyclic [2.2.2]endoperoxides by the addition of singlet oxygen. Examples of these compounds are found in nature like ascaridol 75 and dihydroascaridol 76 (Scheme 21). A disadvantage is their volatile nature and lipophilicity. Diaryl substituted bicyclic [2.2.2] endoperoxides 77, 78 were first synthesized by the same method to study their antimalarial properties.[113,114] While more polar analogues of bicyclic [2.2.2] endoperoxides 79 and 80 were prepared from terpenoids with polar functional groups like nopol or perillyl alcohol by the addition of singlet oxygen.[115]

Another type of antimalarial bicyclic endoperoxide was synthesized from 2,6-diaryl-1,6-heptadienes 81 by photo-electron transfer oxygenation to give the bicyclic [3.2.2] endoperoxides 82 shown in Scheme 22. *In vitro* antimalarial activities against *P. falciparum* were moderate and dependent on the substituents. Interestingly, fluorine in 82a did not enhance the activity of the bicyclic endoperoxidic [3.2.2]nonanes. The mechanism of decomposition of these endoperoxides with Fe(II) salt has been studied and besides a common electron transfer reaction leading to the generation of oxygen and carbon radicals a Lewis acid pathway is also possible by generating the carbocation.[116]

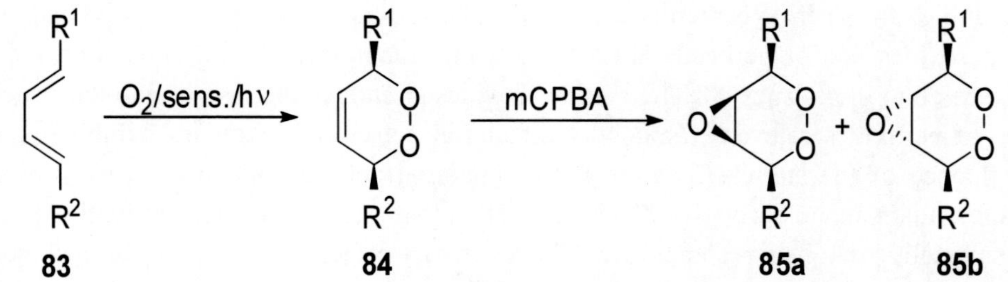

Scheme 23.

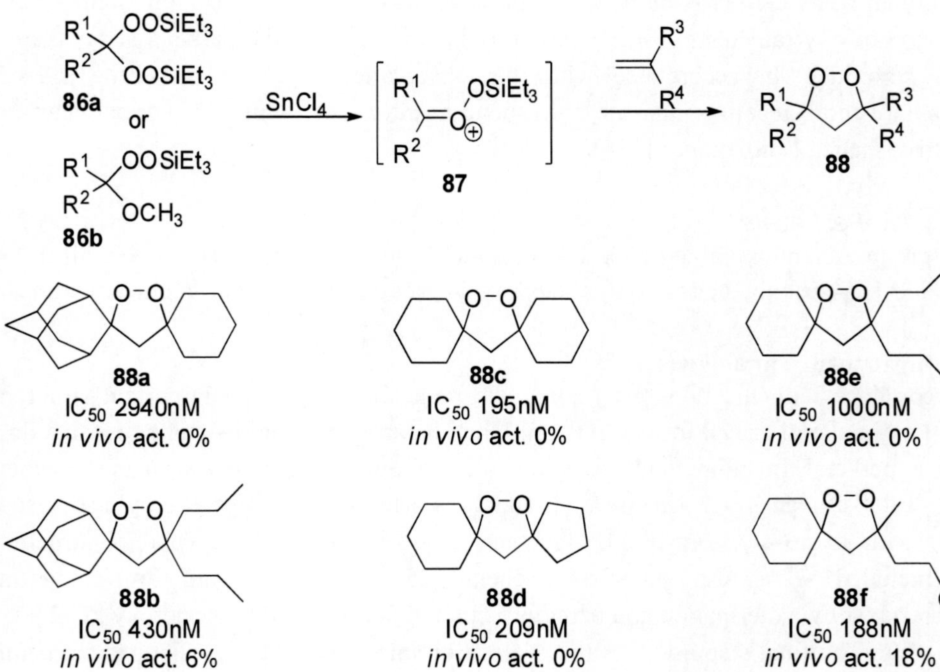

Scheme 24.

3.4.2. Dioxanes and Dioxolanes

There are only a few examples of simple dioxanes and dioxolanes as antimalarial agents. Unsaturated dioxanes 84 are produced by the cycloaddition of a singlet oxygen to 1,3-dienes 83 (Scheme 23). Another oxygen atom is introduced by epoxidation of the double bond to form an epoxy dioxane 85. This serves as a steric analogue to the cyclic oxygen atom in the 1,2,4-trioxane ring of artemisinin.[117] Although the reactivity of unsaturated and saturated dioxanes were moderate, research points to the importance of the interaction with Fe(II) atoms.

To better understand the effect that the peroxide bond has on the antimalarial action of organic peroxides Vennerstrom's group conducted research into the activity of various dioxolanes and compared their results with those obtained for trioxanes and tetraoxanes or trioxolanes, respectively.[118] They used a different synthetic strategy to prepare dioxolanes

88 involving the peroxycarbenium ion 87. This was formed from silylated *gem*-dihydroperoxides 86a or perketals 86b before being transformed by an annulation reaction with alkenes into dioxolanes 88. Their study provides an interesting insight into the structural features of peroxides relevant for good antimalarial activity. Dioxolanes exhibit a similar high influence of the steric effects on the antimalarial activity and in the case of dispiro dioxolanes, adamantane derivative 88a is less active than the cyclohexane derivative 88c and even less reactive that its spiro analogue 88b. A contrary effect was observed for cyclohexane analogues where dispiro dioxolanes 88c and 88d are more active than the spiro one 88e, while for *in vivo* activity a polar group is essential. The key element for good antimalarial activity of the cyclic peroxides is, according to the authors, the perketal structure. Therefore, the C-atom that bears the peroxide bond should have attached another oxygen atom because the β-scission of oxy radicals to form a carbon radical is faster in the perketal series than in the alkyl peroxides. In accordance with this observation 1,2,4-trioxanes and 1,2,4,5-tetraoxanes are more reactive than the corresponding dioxanes, while 1,2,4-trioxolanes are more reactive than 1,2-dioxolanes.[118]

3.4.3. Cyclic Perketals

This group of antimalarial peroxides share a common perketal structure with 1,2,4-trioxanes and 1,2,4-trioxolanes but only the peroxide group is a part of the cyclic structure.

3.4.3.1. Yingzhaosu A analogues

In accordance with the previous finding the perketal group is an important structural element of antimalarial drugs. In fact, it is only the yingzhaosu A and its analogues that does not have a perketal functional group, while all the others have this structural element included – 1,2,4-trioxanes, 1,2,4-trioxolanes and 1,2,4,5-tetraoxanes. However, yingzhaosu A analogues with a 2,3-dioxabicyclo[3.3.1]nonane scaffold and with a perketal structural element included were also prepared (Scheme 25). Synthesis starts by converting dihydrocarvone 89 via olefination and ozonolysis into an unsaturated hydroperoxy ketal 90 or hydroperoxide. The final step involves the cyclization into a bicyclic [3.3.1]nonane structure 91 by ozonolysis in 2,2,2-trifluoroethanol (TFE).[112,119]

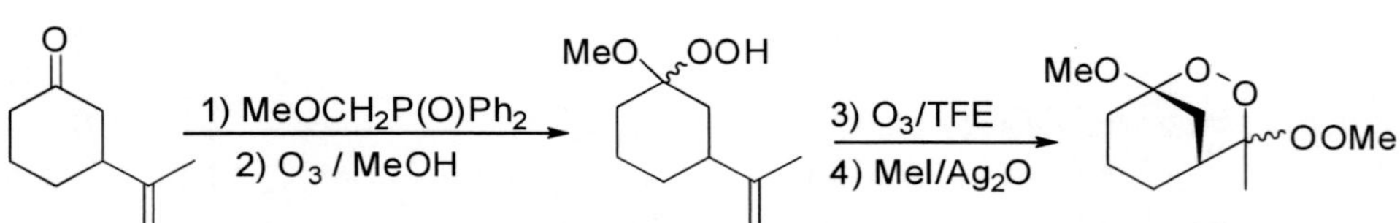

89 90 91

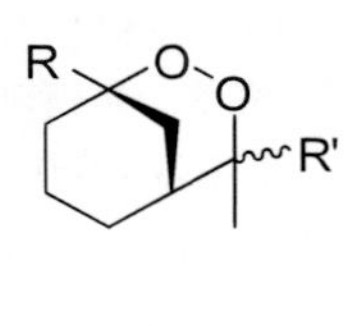

	R	R'	EC_{50} (M)
91a	Me	OOMe	2.9×10^{-5}
91b	OMe	OOMe	4.6×10^{-6}
91c endo	OOMe	OMe	1.7×10^{-5}
exo			1.8×10^{-6}
91d	OOMe	Me	7×10^{-5}

Scheme 25.

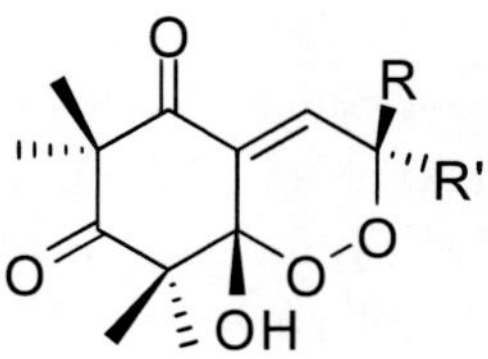

92
G1: R=Me, R'=Et
G2: R=Et, R'=Me
G3: R=Me, R'=Me

Figure 8.

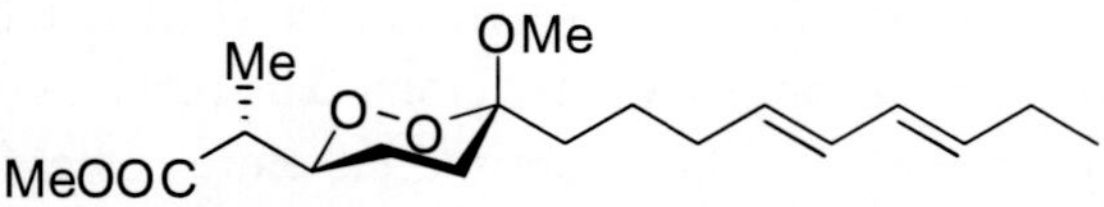

93a, Peroxyplacoric acid A3 methyl ester

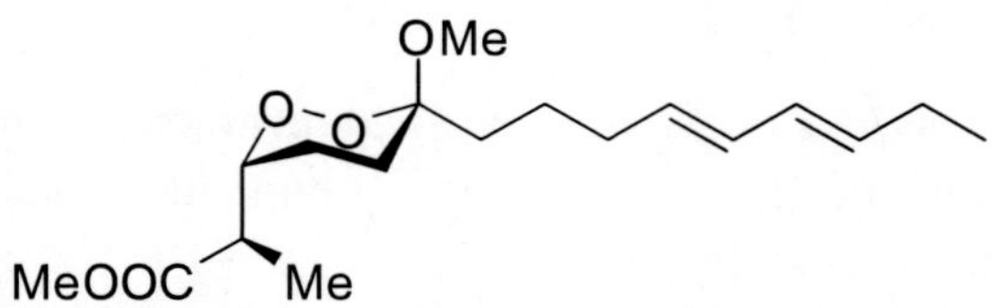

93b, Peroxyplacoric acid B3 methyl ester

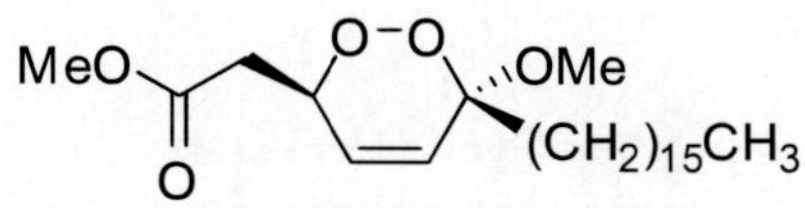

93c, Chondrillin

Figure 9.

3.4.3.2. G Factors

G factors 92 are phytohormones and growth regulators first isolated from *Eucalyptus grandis* (Figure 8). As they are toxic to the plant they are synthesized on demand. Synthesis for the preparation of G factor analogues begins with the syncarpic acid that is first transformed into ethylenic ketones that spontaneously react with oxygen to form a compound based on a G factor skeleton.[120,121] The G3 factor 92 does possess some antimalarial activity (IC_{50} 20μM) that can be improved by methylation of the hydroxy group to give a more active compound (IC_{50} 0.28μM). The activity still remains significantly lower than that of artemisinin, albeit they do have comparable electrochemical properties.[120]

The structure of G factors does allow some modification on the C-atom of the peroxide bond as well as through derivatization of the hydroxy group. It was shown that substitution of hydroxy group with fluorine, to produce a dioxane structure, completely inhibits activity. This is more evidence to the important role of the ketal structure. Alkylation of the hydroxy group in G3 increases its activity but the length of the alkyl chain does not have a big influence.[122-124]

3.4.3.3. Spongean Peroxides

Spongean metabolites have been investigated on account of their physiological activity. Two peroxidic metabolites were isolated: Plakorin 93a,b and Chondrillin 93c.[125,126] They share the same cyclic 3-methoxy-1,2-dioxane cyclic structure with a carbomethoxymethyl substituent in position 6 (Figure 9).

These natural derivatives possess some antimalarial activity with plakorins being more active than chondrillins. A simple method was developed to construct the basic 6-

carbomethoxymethly-3-methoxy-1,2-dioxane scaffold that is necessary for the activity. It consists of a peroxyhemiacetalization of ketoester 94 with a urea-hydrogen peroxide complex to give 95 that is converted by an intramolecular Michael addition in fluorinated alcohol to yield 96 (Scheme 26).[127] To fine tune the antimalarial activity, different 3-alkyl substituents were added to adjust lipophilicity.[128] However, the alkyl group does not influence only the lipophilicity but the stability of its radical also needs to be taken into account. The pentyl radical is unstable and the parent 96b is only moderately active. Alternatively, the alkenyl chain can form a radical that is stabilized and therefore longer-lived to react with the parasite's proteins.[129] Although reported activities were better, these substrates remain inactive *in vivo* due to the hydrolysis of the ester group. The methyl ester was transformed into amide that is not hydrolysed by the organism and therefore possess *in vivo* activity.[130]

3.4.3.4. Other Cyclic Perketals

A similar synthetic route was applied to various cyclic perketals with photooxygenation being replaced by intramolecular addition of an hydroperoxy group obtained by hydroperoxidation of the ketone using hydrogen peroxide.

Scheme 27 presents a typical synthesis of the simplified analogue of artemisinin 99 with a 7-membered endoperoxide structure and cyclic perketal oxygen atom incorporated into the tricyclic system.[131]

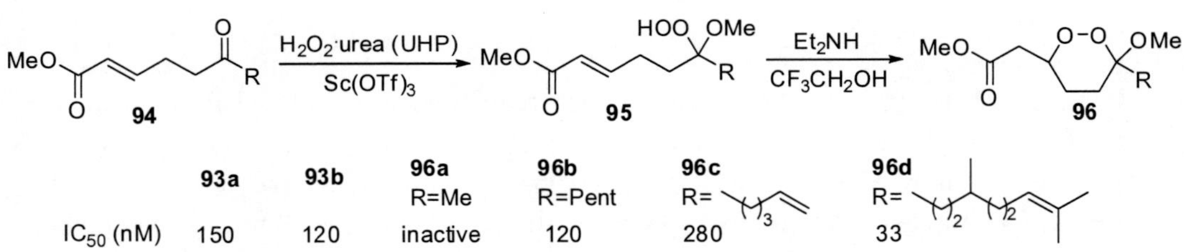

Scheme 26.

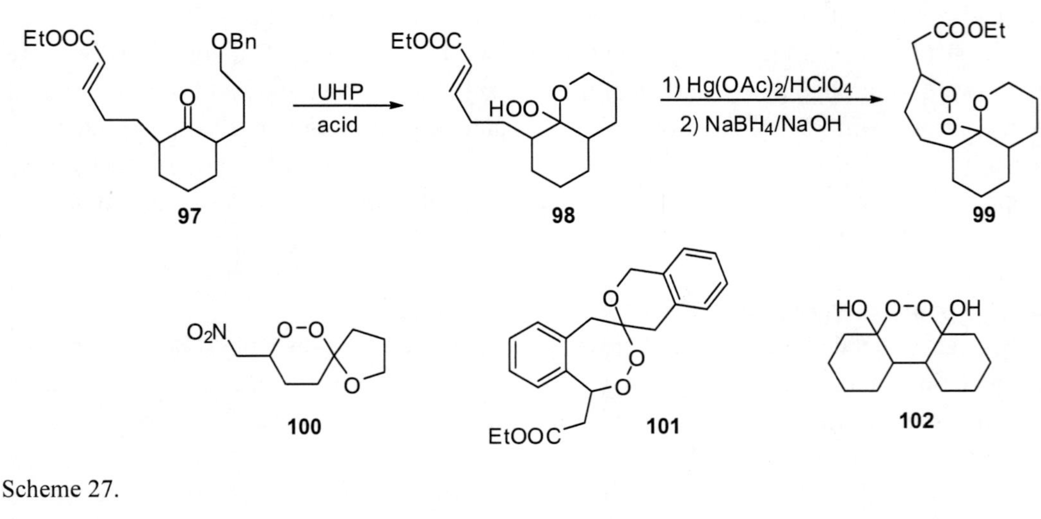

Scheme 27.

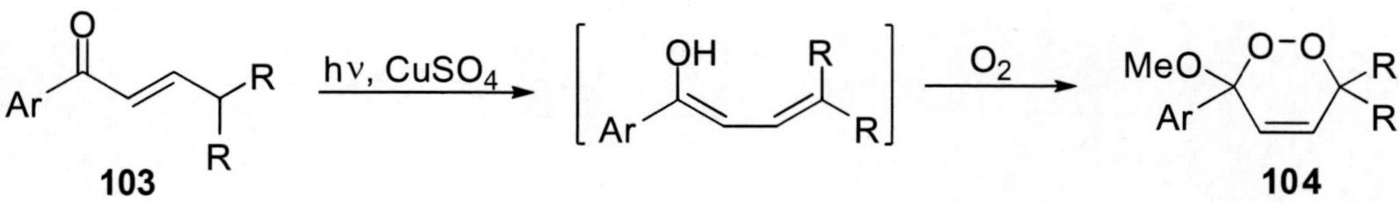

Ar =	R,R =	IC_{50} (nM)
4-$MeSO_2$-Ph	cyclohexane	56
	cycloheptane	31
4-MeS-Ph	cycloheptane	78

Scheme 28.

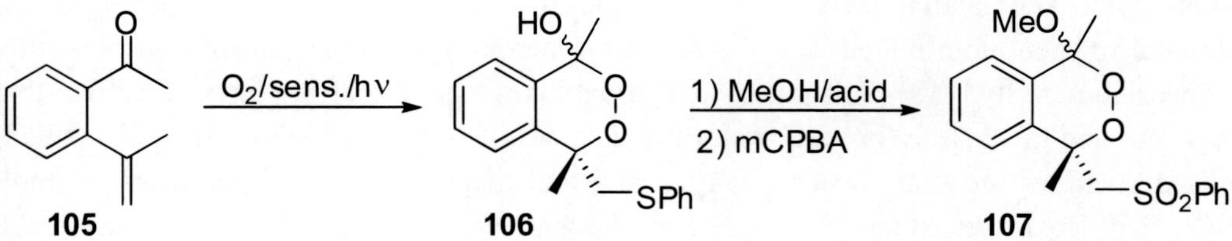

Scheme 29.

Spiroperoxides 100 and 101, analogues of 99 with an endoperoxide bond in the 6- or 7-membered cycle were also prepared. When a benzene ring was fused to the peroxy ring, formation of seven-membered derivatives is facilitated, while a nitro group can replace the carboethoxy one. Although in this case due to a possible interference of the nitro group in radical processes, the *in vitro* antimalarial activity is reduced. The activity of spiroperketals with the carboethoxy group is in the order of the peroxyplakoric acid derivatives.[132] The perketal 102, prepared from bis(cyclohexyl)-2,2'-dione and hydrogen peroxide, also shows an antimalarial activity.[133]

The majority of synthetic procedures still utilize the singlet oxygen as a source of peroxide functionality. Posner's group has synthesized 3-aryl-3-methoxy-1,2-dioxene derivatives 104 as a special case of cyclic peroxy ketals *via* the photooxygenation of unsaturated ketones 103 (Scheme 28).[134] Although mechanistic debates were focused on the possibility of a single oxygen addition or radical oxygenation[42] this does not effect their potent antimalarial activity with the most active substrates prepared having a quarter of artemisinin's activity. Interestingly, the activity of the spiro perketals is higher with the spiro cycloheptane ring than with the cyclohexane one.

The TOCO protocol (Scheme 19), used to construct 1,2-dioxanes, was modified to obtain the 3-alkoxy-1,2-dioxane scaffold.[135] The unsaturated ketone 105 (2'-isopropenyl acetophenone) was taken as the starting substrate and transformed by thiol-olefin-co-oxygenation into a cyclic benzo-fused peroxy hemiketal 106. Finally, the hydroxy group was methylated, while the thiol group was oxidized into a sulfonyl one (Scheme 29) to obtain the desired benzo-fused ketal 107, however it has a relatively weak antimalarial activity.

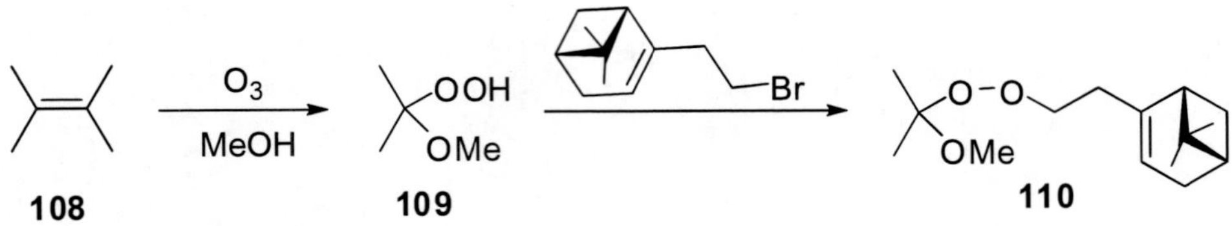

Scheme 30.

3.4. Perketals and Bis-Perethers

Even a simple peroxide compound like hydrogen peroxide and *tert*-butyl hydroperoxide possess some antimalarial activity. In the series of cyclic peroxides it is shown that an additional oxygen atom bound to a C-atom at the peroxide bond significantly increases the antimalarial activity.[118] Trioxanes and trioxolanes are therefore more reactive than dioxolanes and this is true for tetraoxanes *vs*. dioxanes. It is reasonable to believe that among acylic derivatives the same observation is valid and that perketals and perethers are more active than hydroperoxides or peroxides. Recent years have witnessed considerable development in the field of α-heteroatom substituted peroxides to allow the targeted preparation of perketals and perethers.[42]

The most common route to synthesize perketals is ozonolysis of the double bonds in the presence of alcohol to form a hydroperoxy ketal that is then transformed into a more stable perketal.[136] This method was used for the preparation of various 2-methoxyprop-2-yl peroxides 110 by the ozonolysis of 2,3-dimethyl-2-butene 108 in methanol followed by the alkylation of the hydroperoxy ketal 109 with the addition of desired alkyl bromide (Scheme 30).[137] However, their antimalarial activity remains moderate to weak with the highest *in vitro* IC_{50} activity of 370nM recorded for 110. Interestingly, the activity diminishes by introducing polar groups like ethers, ciano or esters, while a pinene structure augments the activity.

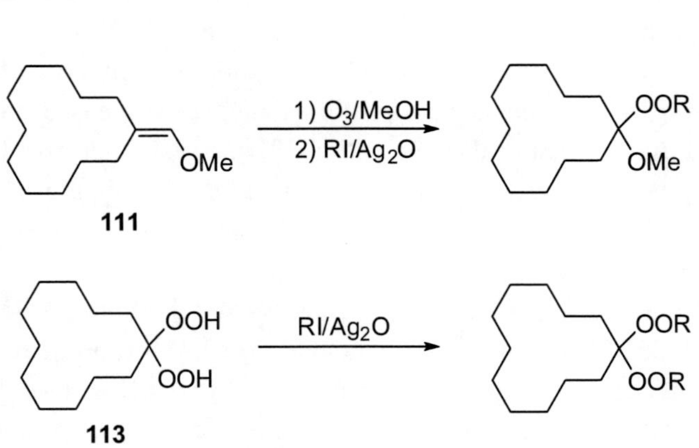

	R	IC_{50} (nM)	ED_{50} (mg/kg) *ip*
112a	Me	80	30
112b	Et	230	>100
112c	Pr	620	

	R	IC_{50} (nM)	ED_{50} (mg/kg) *ip*	ED_{50} (mg/kg) *po*
114a	Me	86	13	30
114b	Et	200	41	
114c	Pr	1800		

Scheme 31.

The research on 1,2,4,5-tetraoxacycloalkanes reveal that the cyclododecane ring is a potent structure for antimalarial agents. Therefore, the antimalarial activity of open analogues were studied, these included *gem*-bisperethers, together with the open analogues of 1,2,4-trioxanes and 1,2,4-trioxolanes, namely peroxy ketals.[138] The starting point for both products was cyclododecanone and for the synthesis of perketals it was first methoxymethylated into 111 before being converted into the hydroperoxy ketal by ozonolysis in methanol. The hydroperoxide group was then alkylated to obtain the targeted perketals 112. The *in vitro* antimalarial activity was tested on *P. falciparum* chloroquine sensitive FCR-3 strain. The compounds possess potent antimalarial activity that is sensitive to the structure of the alkyl groups and that of the organic core (Scheme 31). The highest activity belonged to a dimethylated cyclododecyl perketal 112a, while prolongation of alkyl chain on the peroxide oxygen rapidly reduces activity. Again, cyclic perketals 112 are more active than dialkyl analogues with the dibutyl derivative having an IC_{50} of 8600nM.

A similar relationship between activity and the peroxide structure is observed in the bis-perether series. The preparation of perethers includes the transformation of a ketone into the *gem*-dihydroperoxide 113 with hydrogen peroxide or ozonolysis followed by alkylation of the hydroperoxide groups (Scheme 31). Results from the *in vitro* screening of 114 produced results similar to those for perketals 112 *i.e.*, the methylated derivatives are the most active.

Four days *in vivo* studies against *P. berghei* revealed large differences between perketals and bis-perethers and the latter being more active. Surprisingly, 114a is also orally active and on *ip* administration of 20mg/kg dose 4 day suppressive test failed to show any parasites in the blood.

4. Chimeric Compounds

Peroxides are fast acting antimalarial agents but require an additional longer acting agent to clear the host of malaria parasites. Furthermore, during combination therapy parasites have more trouble in developing resistance. In chimeric compounds this approach of combination therapy is united in a single molecule in which two different pharmacophores are covalently joined.

The first such compound was published by the group led by Meunier who synthesized "trioxaquines" as agents for "covalent bitherapy".[139-141] The group was able to join a 4-aminoquinoline structure (facilitates the penetration of an agent) to a trioxane structural element (a potent alkylating agent essential for good antimalarial activity) to obtain trioxaquines *i.e.*, 115 (Figure 10). Research on the mechanism of action of peroxidic antimalarial suggests that the alkylating property might not be the only factor governing antimalarial activity, nevertheless trioxaquines are potent antimalarial drugs that act against the asexual and sexual (gametocytes) stages of the parasite cycle.[142] The most active among this group is di-citrate trioxaquine DU1302 115 having a potent oral *in vivo* activity against *P. yoelli nigeriensis* higher than artemisinin and artemether and similar to artesunate. Furthermore, with an oral dose of 50mg/kg/day trioxaquine 115 cured all infected mice without any recrudescence at 60 days. Another chimeric compound 116 was prepared from a spiro 1,2,4-trioxane ring and 4-aminoquinoline.[143] A comparison of the oral activity of each separate element of the hybrid molecule and that of 116 was made to determine the *in vivo* antimalarial activity against multidrug resistant *P. yoelii.* Some improvement was observed over the trioxane part or quinoline, however neither of the three drugs resulted in a cure after 28 days.

Following a similar approach, mefloquine and artemisinin were joined in two ways: directly or with a divisible linker that can be hydrolysed *in vivo*.[144] Chimera 117 proved potent *in vitro* against various strains of *P. falciparum* with an IC_{50} of 2.4 to 17.2nM, an activity comparable to artemether but better than mefloquine. Chimera 117 was more effective *in vivo* (ip, 30mg/kg) in controlling the parasitemia than the parent compounds, the CF_3-artemisinin and artemether, in completely inhibiting the growth of parasites. Another report presents the hybrid antimalarial agent 118 as a combination of quinine and dihydroartemisinin linked by an ester linkage.[145] Its potency has been compared to each individual component as well as to a mixture of both. Results show that the hybrid is more potent (IC_{50} against chloroquine resistant strain FcB1 was 9.6nM), while artemisinin and quinine have an IC_{50} of 50.0 and 96.8nM, respectively and the mixture of quinine and artemisinin had an IC_{50} of 27.9nM. Interesting is that the chimera 118 is more active than a mixture of both components and each component individually, which could indicate some kind of synergetic action when both constituents are covalently bound. This observation requires a more complete understanding of the exact mechanism of action of chimeras.

A masked combination therapy is an innovative approach based on a directly acting pharmacophore from the peroxide family and a latent pharmacophore of the chalcone family. Once inside the parasite, the peroxide pharmacophore damages the parasite either by alkylation or some other action. In this case the peroxide is reduced to the ketone function to form another pharmacophore in the form of a chalcone that is a cysteine protease inhibitor that further damages the parasite.[146] This approach is akin to a "Trojan horse". When composing such an agent 119, a yingzhaosu A analogue similar to arteflene is used as a peroxide pharmacophore, while substituents on position 4 of the endoperoxide ring were modulated to form a chalcone during decomposition. Indeed, the reaction of 119 with an Fe(II) salt reveals that the reaction with the heme should produce a secondary carbon radical 121 that is toxic to the parasite's proteins and the targeted chalcone 120 as a second agent for inhibiting cysteine protease (Scheme 32). Activities of these chimeras were determined only *in vitro* against *P. falciparum* chloroquine resistant strain K1 but show that substrates have an activity higher than that of the parent arteflene.

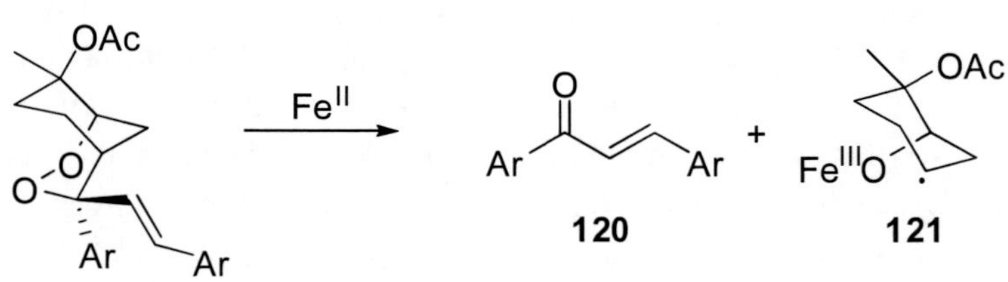

119

	IC_{50} (nM)
119a: R = C_6H_5	34
119b: R = *p*-FC_6H_4	29
119c: R = *p*-ClC_6H_4	23

Scheme 32.

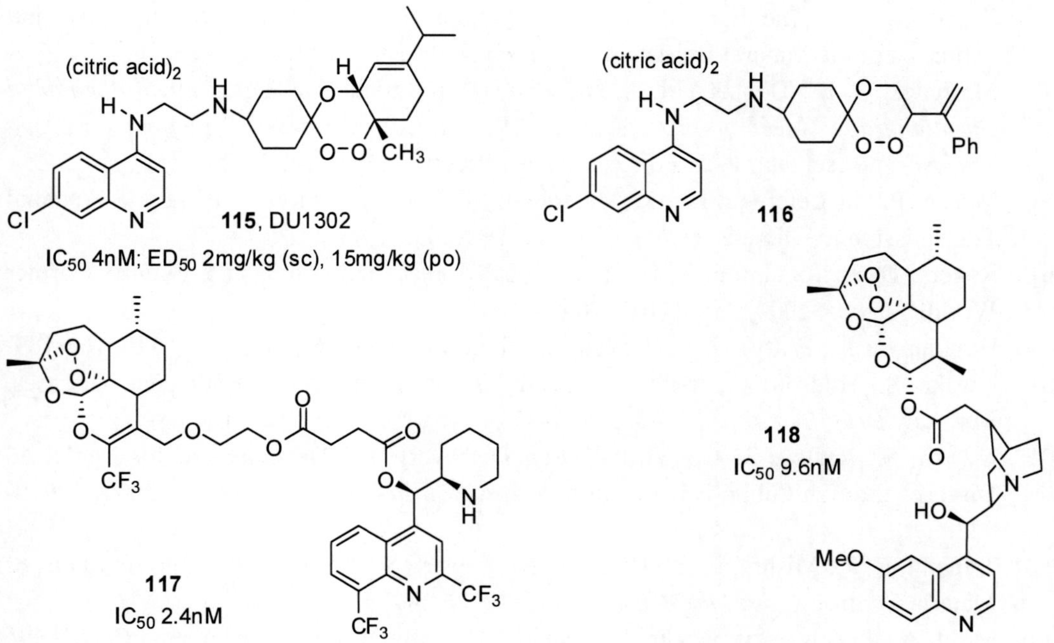

Figure 10.

5. Conclusion

The field of organic peroxides has witnessed immense progress after the recognition of the value of artemisinin in the current chemotherapy of malaria. New synthetic methods have been developed to incorporate a peroxide bond into an organic scaffold that enables the preparation of organic peroxides deemed to have antimalarial activity. Until recently, the main methods involved using singlet oxygen and ozone, however their use has drawbacks when the synthesis is scaled up. Alternative solutions proposed in recent years include radical reactions with molecular oxygen and the use of aqueous hydrogen peroxide, which is a much safer reagent. Improvement in the synthesis of organic peroxides has increased the spectrum of available organic peroxides that provide a greater understanding of the mechanism of action of antimalarial peroxides. With this knowledge it will be possible to define better antimalarial agents and transfer good ideas from theory to practice.

References

[1] Joy, D. A.; Feng, X.; Mu, J.; Furuya, T.; Chotivanich, K.; Krettli, A. U.; Ho, M.; Wang, A.; White, N. J.; Suh, E.; Beerli, P.; Su, X. Z.; Early Origin and Recent Expansion of *Plasmodium Falciparum*. *Science*, 2003, *300*, 318-321.

[2] Snow, R. W.; Guerra, C. A.; Noor, A. M.; Myint, H. Y.; Hay, S. I.; The Global Distribution of Clinical Episodes of *Plasmodium Falciparum* Malaria. *Nature*, 2005, *434*, 214-217.

[3] Breman, J. G.; The Ears of the Hippopotamus: Manifestations, Determinants, and Estimates of the Malaria Burden. *Am. J. Trop. Med. Hyg.*, 2001, *64*, 1-11.

[4] Meshnick, S. R.; Dobson, M. J. The History of Antimalarial Drugs. In *Antimalarial Chemotherapy. Mechanisms of Action, Resistance, and New Directions in Drug Discovery*; Rosenthal, P. J., Editor; Humana Press: Totowa, 2001; Chapter 2, pp 15-25.

[5] Martin, P. H.; Lefebvre, M. G.; Malaria and Climate: Sensitivity of Malaria Potential Transmission to Climate. *Ambio*, 1995, *24*, 200-207.

[6] Rogers, D. J.; Randolph, S. E.; The Global Spread of Malaria in a Future, Warmer World. *Science*, 2000, *289*, 1763-1766.

[7] Hopkins, A. L.; Witty, M. J.; Nwaka, S.; Mission Possible. *Nature*, 2007, *449*, 166-169.

[8] Nwaka, S.; Hudson, A.; Innovative Lead Discovery Strategies for Tropical Diseases. *Nat. Rev. Drug Discovery*, 2006, *5*, 941-955.

[9] Nwaka, S.; Ridley, R. G.; Virtual Drug Discovery and Development for Neglected Diseases through Public-Private Partnerships. *Nat. Rev. Drug Discovery*, 2003, *2*, 919-928.

[10] Tripathi, R. P.; Mishra, R. C.; Dwivedi, N.; Tewari, N.; Verma, S. S.; Current Status of Malaria Control. *Curr. Med. Chem.*, 2005, *12*, 2643-2659.

[11] Mital, A.; Recent Advances in Antimalarial Compounds and their Patents. *Curr. Med. Chem.*, 2007, *14*, 759-773.

[12] Jana, S.; Paliwal, J.; Novel Molecular Targets for Antimalarial Chemotherapy. *Int. J. Antimicrob. Agents*, 2007, *30*, 4-10.

[13] Padmanaban, G.; Nagaraj, V. A.; Rangarajan, P. N.; Drugs and Drug Targets against Malaria. *Curr. Sci.*, 2007, *92*, 1545-1555.

[14] O'Neill, P. M.; Ward, S. A.; Berry, N. G.; Jeyadevan, J. P.; Biagini, G. A.; Asadollaly, E.; Park, B. K.; Bray, P. G.; A Medicinal Chemistry Perspective on 4-Aminoquinoline Antimalarial Drugs. *Curr. Top. Med. Chem.*, 2006, *6*, 479-507.

[15] Biagini, G. A.; O'Neill, P. M.; Nzila, A.; Ward, S. A.; Bray, P. G.; Antimalarial Chemotherapy: Young Guns or Back to the Future? *Trends Parasitol.*, 2003, *19*, 479-487.

[16] Hsu, E.; Reflections on the 'Discovery' of the Antimalarial Qinghao. *Br. J. Clin. Pharmacol.*, 2006, *61*, 666-670.

[17] Mueller, M. S.; Runyambo, N.; Wagner, I.; Borrmann, S.; Dietz, K.; Heide, L.; Randomized Controlled Trial of a Traditional Preparation of Artemisia Annua L. (Annual Wormwood) in the Treatment of Malaria. *Trans. R. Soc. Trop. Med. Hyg.*, 2004, *98*, 318-321.

[18] Rath, K.; Taxis, K.; Walz, G.; Gleiter, C. H.; Li, S. M.; Heide, L.; Pharmacokinetic Study of Artemisinin after Oral Intake of a Traditional Preparation of *Artemisia Annua L.* (Annual Wormwood). *Am. J. Trop. Med. Hyg.*, 2004, *70*, 128-132.

[19] Jansen, F. H.; The Herbal Tea Approach for Artemisinin as a Therapy for Malaria? *Trans. R. Soc. Trop. Med. Hyg.*, 2006, *100*, 285-286.

[20] Heide, L.; Artemisinin in Traditional Tea Preparations of *Artemisia Annua*. *Trans. R. Soc. Trop. Med. Hyg.*, 2006, *100*, 802.

[21] http://www.who.int/mediacentre/news/releases/2006/pr02/en/

[22] Krishna, S.; Woodrow, C. J.; Staines, H. M.; Haynes, R. K.; Mercereau-Puijalon, O.; Re-Evaluation of How Artemisinins Work in Light of Emerging Evidence of *in Vitro* Resistance. *Trends Mol. Med.*, 2006, *12*, 200-205.

[23] Jefford, C. W.; New Developments in Synthetic Peroxidic Drugs as Artemisinin Mimics. *Drug Discovery Today*, 2007, *12*, 487-495.

[24] Haynes, R. K.; From Artemisinin to New Artemisinin Antimalarials: Biosynthesis, Extraction, Old and New Derivatives, Stereochemistry and Medicinal Chemistry Requirements. *Curr. Top. Med. Chem.*, 2006, *6*, 509-537.

[25] O'Neill, P. M.; The Therapeutic Potential of Semi-Synthetic Artemisinin and Synthetic Endoperoxide Antimalarial Agents. *Expert Opin. Investig. Drugs*, 2005, *14*, 1117-1128.

[26] Begue, J.-P.; Bonnet-Delpon, D.; The Future of Antimalarials: Artemisinins and Synthetic Endoperoxides. *Drugs Fut.*, 2005, *30*, 509-518.

[27] O'Neill, P. M.; Posner, G. H.; A Medicinal Chemistry Perspective on Artemisinin and Related Endoperoxides. *J. Med. Chem.*, 2004, *47*, 2945-2964.

[28] Borstnik, K.; Paik, I. H.; Posner, G. H.; Malaria: New Chemotherapeutic Peroxide Drugs. *Mini-Rev. Med. Chem.*, 2002, *2*, 573-583.

[29] Singh, C.; Chaudhary, S.; Puri, S. K.; New Orally Active Derivatives of Artemisinin With High Efficacy against Multidrug-Resistant Malaria in Mice. *J. Med. Chem.*, 2006, *49*, 7227-7233.

[30] Posner, G. H.; Paik, I. H.; Chang, W.; Borstnik, K.; Sinishtaj, S.; Rosenthal, A. S.; Shapiro, T. A.; Malaria-Infected Mice are Cured by a Single Dose of Novel Artemisinin Derivatives. *J. Med. Chem.*, 2007, *50*, 2516-2519.

[31] Paik, I. H.; Xie, S.; Shapiro, T. A.; Labonte, T.; Narducci Sarjeant, A. A.; Baege, A. C.; Posner, G. H.; Second Generation, Orally Active, Antimalarial, Artemisinin-Derived Trioxane Dimers with High Stability, Efficacy, and Anticancer Activity. *J. Med. Chem.*, 2006, *49*, 2731-2734.

[32] Haynes, R. K.; Fugmann, B.; Stetter, J.; Rieckmann, K.; Heilmann, H. D.; Chan, H. W.; Cheung, M. K.; Lam, W. L.; Wong, H. N.; Croft, S. L.; Vivas, L.; Rattray, L.; Stewart, L.; Peters, W.; Robinson, B. L.; Edstein, M. D.; Kotecka, B.; Kyle, D. E.; Beckermann, B.; Gerisch, M.; Radtke, M.; Schmuck, G.; Steinke, W.; Wollborn, U.; Schmeer, K.; Romer, A.; Artemisone - A Highly Active Antimalarial Drug of the Artemisinin Class. *Angew. Chem., Int. Ed.*, 2006, *45*, 2082-2088.

[33] Magueur, G.; Crousse, B.; Ourevitch, M.; Bonnet-Delpon, D.; Begue, J.-P.; Fluoro-Artemisinins: When a Gem-Difluoroethylene Replaces a Carbonyl Group. *J. Fluorine Chem.*, 2006, *127*, 637-642.

[34] http://www.rbm.who.int/wmr2005/html/3-2.htm#3_2_3

[35] Ferreira, J. F. S.; Laughlin, J. C.; Delabays, N.; de Magalhaes, P. M.; Cultivation and Genetics of *Artemisia Annua L.* for Increased Production of the Antimalarial Artemisinin. *Plant Genet. Resour.*, 2005, *3*, 206-229.

[36] Ro, D. K.; Paradise, E. M.; Ouellet, M.; Fisher, K. J.; Newman, K. L.; Ndungu, J. M.; Ho, K. A.; Eachus, R. A.; Ham, T. S.; Kirby, J.; Chang, M. C. Y.; Withers, S. T.; Shiba, Y.; Sarpong, R.; Keasling, J. D.; Production of the Antimalarial Drug Precursor Artemisinic Acid in Engineered Yeast. *Nature*, 2006, *440*, 940-943.

[37] Avery, M. A.; Jennings-White, C.; Chong, W. K. M.; The Total Synthesis of (+)-Artemesinin and (+)-9-Desmethylartemesinin. *Tetrahedron Lett.*, 1987, *28*, 4629-4632.

[38] Avery, M. A.; Chong, W. K. M.; Jennings-White, C.; Stereoselective Total Synthesis of (+)-Artemisinin, the Antimalarial Constituent of *Artemisia Annua L. J. Am. Chem. Soc.*, 1992, *114*, 974-979.

[39] Zhou, W. S.; Xu, X. X.; Total Synthesis of the Antimalarial Sesquiterpene Peroxide *Qinghaosu* and *Yingzhaosu A*. *Acc. Chem. Res.*, 1994, *27*, 211-216.

[40] Tang, Y.; Dong, Y.; Vennerstrom, J. L.; Synthetic Peroxides as Antimalarials. *Med. Res. Rev.*, 2004, *24*, 425-448.

[41] Masuyama, A.; Wu, J. M.; Nojima, M.; Kim, H. S.; Wataya, Y.; 1,2,4,5-Tetraoxacycloalkanes: Synthesis and Antimalarial Activity. *Mini-Rev. Med. Chem.*, 2005, *5*, 1035-1043.

[42] Zmitek, K.; Zupan, M.; Iskra, J.; Alpha-Substituted Organic Peroxides: Synthetic Strategies for a Biologically Important Class of Gem-Dihydroperoxide and Perketal Derivatives. *Org. Biomol. Chem.*, 2007, *5*, 3895-3908.

[43] Eckstein-Ludwig, U.; Webb, R. J.; Van Goethem, I. D. A.; East, J. M.; Lee, A. G.; Kimura, M.; O'Neill, P. M.; Bray, P. G.; Ward, S. A.; Krishna, S.; Artemisinins Target the SERCA of *Plasmodium Falciparum*. *Nature*, 2003, *424*, 957-961.

[44] Krishna, S.; Uhlemann, A. C.; Haynes, R. K.; Artemisinins: Mechanisms of Action and Potential for Resistance. *Drug Resist. Updates*, 2004, *7*, 233-244.

[45] Dockrell, H. M.; Playfair, J. H. L.; Killing of Blood-Stage Murine Malaria Parasites by Hydrogen-Peroxide. *Infect. Immun.*, 1983, *39*, 456-459.

[46] Clark, I. A.; Cowden, W. B.; Butcher, G. A.; Free Oxygen Radical Generators as Anti-Malarial Drugs. *Lancet*, 1983, *1*, 234.

[47] Jefford, C. W.; Velarde, J. A.; Bernardinelli, G.; Bray, D. H.; Warhurst, D. C.; Milhous, W. K.; Synthesis, Structure, and Antimalarial Activity of Tricyclic 1,2,4-Trioxanes Related to Artemisinin. *Helv. Chim. Acta*, 1993, *76*, 2775-2788.

[48] Cazelles, J.; Camuzat-Dedenis, B.; Provot, O.; Robert, A.; Mayrargue, J.; Meunier, B.; Alkylating Properties of Synthetic Trioxanes Related to Artemisinin. *J. Chem. Soc. Perkin Trans. 1*, 2000, 1265-1270.

[49] Posner, G. H.; Cumming, J. N.; Woo, S. H.; Ploypradith, P.; Xie, S.; Shapiro, T. A.; Orally Active Antimalarial 3-Substituted Trioxanes: New Synthetic Methodology and Biological Evaluation. *J. Med. Chem.*, 1998, *41*, 940-951.

[50] Posner, G. H.; Oh, C. H.; Wang, D.; Gerena, L.; Milhous, W. K.; Meshnick, S. R.; Asawamahasadka, W.; Mechanism-Based Design, Synthesis, and *in Vitro* Antimalarial Testing of New 4-Methylated Trioxanes Structurally Related to Artemisinin: The Importance of a Carbon-Centered Radical for Antimalarial Activity. *J. Med. Chem.*, 1994, *37*, 1256-1258.

[51] Posner, G. H.; Oh, C. H.; Gerena, L.; Milhous, W. K.; Extraordinarily Potent Antimalarial Compounds: New, Structurally Simple, Easily Synthesized, Tricyclic 1,2,4-Trioxanes. *J. Med. Chem.*, 1992, *35*, 2459-2467.

[52] Posner, G. H.; Jeon, H. B.; Ploypradith, P.; Paik, I. H.; Borstnik, K.; Xie, S.; Shapiro, T. A.; Orally Active, Water-Soluble Antimalarial 3-Aryltrioxanes: Short Synthesis and Preclinical Efficacy Testing in Rodents. *J. Med. Chem.*, 2002, *45*, 3824-3828.

[53] Posner, G. H.; Jeon, H. B.; Parker, M. H.; Krasavin, M.; Paik, I. H.; Shapiro, T. A.; Antimalarial Simplified 3-Aryltrioxanes: Synthesis and Preclinical Efficacy/Toxicity Testing in Rodents. *J. Med. Chem.*, 2001, *44*, 3054-3058.

[54] Water-Soluble Trioxanes as Potent and Safe Antimalarial Agents. *Expert Opin. Ther. Patents*, 2001, *11*, 1351-1354.

[55] O'Neill, P. M.; Rawe, S. L.; Borstnik, K.; Miller, A.; Ward, S. A.; Bray, P. G.; Davies, J.; Oh, C. H.; Posner, G. H.; Enantiomeric 1,2,4-Trioxanes Display Equivalent *in Vitro* Antimalarial Activity versus *Plasmodium Falciparum* Malaria Parasites: Implications for the Molecular Mechanism of Action of the Artemisinins. *ChemBioChem*, 2005, *6*, 2048-2054.

[56] Posner, G. H.; Maxwell, J. P.; O'Dowd, H.; Krasavin, M.; Xie, S.; Shapiro, T. A.; Antimalarial Sulfide, Sulfone, and Sulfonamide Trioxanes. *Bioorg. Med. Chem.*, 2000, *8*, 1361-1370.

[57] Jefford, C. W.; Rossier, J. C.; Milhous, W. K.; The Structure and Antimalarial Activity of Some 1,2,4-Trioxanes, 1,2,4,5-Tetroxanes, and Bicyclic Endoperoxides. Implications for the Mode of Action. *Heterocycles*, 2000, *52*, 1345-1352.

[58] Jefford, C. W.; Kohmoto, S.; Jaggi, D.; Timari, G.; Rossier, J. C.; Rudaz, M.; Barbuzzi, O.; Gerard, D.; Burger, U.; Kamalaprija, P.; Mareda, J.; Bernardinelli, G.; Manzanares, I.; Canfield, C. J.; Fleck, S. L.; Robinson, B. L.; Peters, W.; Synthesis, Structure, and Antimalarial Activity of Some Enantiomerically Pure, *Cis*-Fused Cyclopenteno-1,2,4-trioxanes. *Helv. Chim. Acta*, 1995, *78*, 647-662.

[59] Peters, W.; Robinson, B. L.; Rossier, J. C.; Jefford, C. W.; The Chemotherapy of Rodent Malaria. XLVIII. The Activities of Some Synthetic 1,2,4-Trioxanes against Chloroquine-Sensitive and Chloroquine-Resistant Parasites. Part 1: Studies Leading to the Development of Novel *Cis*-Fused Cyclopenteno Derivatives. *Ann. Trop. Med. Parasitol.*, 1993, *87*, 1-7.

[60] Griesbeck, A. G.; Blunk, D.; El-Idreesy, T. T.; Raabe, A.; Bicyclic Peroxides and Perorthoesters with 1,2,4-Trioxane Structures. *Angew. Chem., Int. Ed.*, 2007, *46*, 8883-8886.

[61] O'Neill, P. M.; Pugh, M.; Davies, J.; Ward, S. A.; Park, B. K.; Regioselective Mukaiyama Hydroperoxysilylation of 2-Alkyl- or 2-Aryl-prop-2-en-1-ols: Application to a New Synthesis of 1,2,4-Trioxanes. *Tetrahedron Lett.*, 2001, *42*, 4569-4571.

[62] Griesbeck, A. G.; Bartoschek, A.; El-Idreesy, T. T.; Hoinck, L.-O.; Miara, C.; Type II Photooxygenation in Polymer Matrices for the Synthesis of New Antimalarial Peroxides. *J. Mol. Catal. A - Chem.*, 2006, *251*, 41-48.

[63] Griesbeck, A. G.; El-Idreesy, T. T.; Hoinck, L. O.; Lex, J.; Brun, R.; Novel Spiroanellated 1,2,4-Trioxanes with High *in Vitro* Antimalarial Activities. *Bioorg. Med. Chem. Lett.*, 2005, *15*, 595-597.

[64] Griesbeck, A. G.; El-Idreesy, T. T.; Fiege, M.; Brun, R.; Synthesis of Antimalarial 1,2,4-Trioxanes *via* Photooxygenation of a Chiral Allylic Alcohol. *Org. Lett.*, 2002, *4*, 4193-4195.

[65] Singh, C.; Gupta, N.; Puri, S. K.; Geraniol-Derived 1,2,4-Trioxanes with Potent *in-Vivo* Antimalarial Activity. *Bioorg. Med. Chem. Lett.*, 2003, *13*, 3447-3450.

[66] Singh, C.; Gupta, N.; Puri, S. K.; Photo-Oxygenation of Geraniol: Synthesis of a Novel Series of Hydroxy-Functionalized Anti-malarial 1,2,4-Trioxanes. *Bioorg. Med. Chem. Lett.*, 2002, *12*, 1913-1916.

[67] Singh, C.; Sharma, U.; Saxena, G.; Puri, S.; Orally Active Antimalarials: Synthesis and Bioevaluation of a New Series of Steroid-Based 1,2,4-Trioxanes Against Multi-Drug Resistant Malaria in Mice. *Bioorg. Med. Chem. Lett.*, 2007, *17*, 4097-4101.

[68] Singh, C.; Malik, H.; Puri, S. K.; Orally Active 1,2,4-Trioxanes: Synthesis and Antimalarial Assessment of a New Series of 9-Functionalized 3-(1-Arylvinyl)-1,2,5-trioxaspiro[5.5]undecanes against Multi-drug-resistant *Plasmodium Yoelii Nigeriensis* in Mice. *J. Med. Chem.*, 2006, *49*, 2794-2803.

[69] Vennerstrom, J. L.; Dong, Y.; Andersen, S. L.; Ager, A. L. Jr.; Fu, H. N.; Miller, R. E.; Wesche, D. L.; Kyle, D. E.; Gerena, L.; Walters, S. M.; Wood, J. K.; Edwards, G.; Holme, A. D.; McLean, W. G.; Milhous, W. K.; Synthesis and Antimalarial Activity of Sixteen Dispiro-1,2,4,5-Tetraoxanes: Alkyl-Substituted 7,8,15,16- Tetraoxadispiro [5.2.5.2]hexadecanes. *J. Med. Chem.*, 2000, *43*, 2753-2758.

[70] McCullough, K. J.; Wood, J. K.; Bhattacharjee, A. K.; Dong, Y.; Kyle, D. E.; Milhous, W. K.; Vennerstrom, J. L.; Methyl-Substituted Dispiro-1,2,4,5-tetraoxanes: Correlations of Structural Studies with Antimalarial Activity. *J. Med. Chem.*, 2000, *43*, 1246-1249.

[71] Dong, Y.; Matile, H.; Chollet, J.; Kaminsky, R.; Wood, J. K.; Vennerstrom, J. L.; Synthesis and Antimalarial Activity of 11 Dispiro-1,2,4,5-tetraoxane Analogues of WR 148999. 7,8,15,16-Tetraoxadispiro[5.2.5.2]hexadecanes Substituted at the 1 and 10 Positions With Unsaturated and Polar Functional Groups. *J. Med. Chem.*, 1999, *42*, 1477-1480.

[72] Vennerstrom, J. L.; Fu, H. N.; Ellis, W. Y.; Ager, A. L. Jr.; Wood, J. K.; Andersen, S. L.; Gerena, L.; Milhous, W. K.; Dispiro-1,2,4,5-tetraoxanes: a New Class of Antimalarial Peroxides. *J. Med. Chem.*, 1992, *35*, 3023-3027.

[73] Vennerstrom, J. L.; Ager, A. L. Jr.; Andersen, S. L.; Grace, J. M.; Wongpanich, V.; Angerhofer, C. K.; Hu, J. K.; Wesche, D. L.; Assessment of the Antimalarial Potential of Tetraoxane WR 148999. *Am. J. Trop. Med. Hyg.*, 2000, *62*, 573-578.

[74] Zmitek, K.; Stavber, S.; Zupan, M.; Bonnet-Delpon, D.; Iskra, J.; Fluorinated Alcohol Directed Formation of Dispiro-1,2,4,5-tetraoxanes by Hydrogen Peroxide under Acid Conditions. *Tetrahedron*, 2006, *62*, 1479-1484.

[75] Dong, Y.; Vennerstrom, J. L.; Differentiation Between 1,2,4,5-Tetraoxanes and 1,2,4,5,7,8-Hexaoxonanes Using H-1 and C-13 NMR Analyses. *J. Heterocycl. Chem.*, 2001, *38*, 463-466.

[76] Dong, Y.; Vennerstrom, J. L.; Dispiro-1,2,4,5-tetraoxanes *via* Ozonolysis of Cycloalkanone O-Methyl Oximes: A Comparison with the Peroxidation of Cycloalkanones in Acetonitrile-Sulfuric Acid Media. *J. Org. Chem.*, 1998, *63*, 8582-8585.

[77] Iskra, J.; Bonnet-Delpon, D.; Begue, J. P.; One-Pot Synthesis of Non-Symmetric Tetraoxanes with the H_2O_2/MTO/Fluorous Alcohol System. *Tetrahedron Lett.*, 2003, *44*, 6309-6312.

[78] Zmitek, K.; Stavber, S.; Zupan, M.; Bonnet-Delpon, D.; Charneau, S.; Grellier, P.; Iskra, J.; Synthesis and Antimalarial Activities of Novel 3,3,6,6-Tetraalkyl-1,2,4,5-tetraoxanes. *Bioorg. Med. Chem.*, 2006, *14*, 7790-7795.
[79] Amewu, R.; Stachulski, A. V.; Ward, S. A.; Berry, N. G.; Bray, P. G.; Davies, J.; Labat, G.; Vivas, L.; O'Neill, P. M.; Design and Synthesis of Orally Active Dispiro 1,2,4,5-tetraoxanes; Synthetic Antimalarials with Superior Activity to Artemisinin. *Org. Biomol. Chem.*, 2006, *4*, 4431-4436.
[80] Kim, H. S.; Tsuchiya, K.; Shibata, Y.; Wataya, Y.; Ushigoe, Y.; Masuyama, A.; Nojima, M.; McCullough, K. J.; Synthetic Methods for Unsymmetrically-Substituted 1,2,4,5-Tetroxanes and of 1,2,4,5,7-Pentoxocanes. *J. Chem. Soc., Perkin Trans. 1*, 1999, 1867-1870.
[81] Opsenica, I.; Terzic, N.; Opsenica, D.; Milhous, W. K.; Solaja, B. A.; 7,8,15,16-Tetraoxa-dispiro[5.2.5.2]hexadecane-3-carboxylic Acid Derivatives and their Antimalarial Activity. *J. Serb. Chem. Soc.*, 2004, *69*, 919-922.
[82] Terent'ev, A. O.; Kutkin, A. V.; Starikova, Z. A.; Antipin, M. Y.; Ogibin, Y. N.; Nikishina, G. I.; New Preparation of 1,2,4,5-Tetraoxanes. *Synthesis*, 2004, 2356-2366.
[83] Solaja, B. A.; Terzic, N.; Pocsfalvi, G.; Gerena, L.; Tinant, B.; Opsenica, D.; Milhous, W. K.; Mixed Steroidal 1,2,4,5-Tetraoxanes: Antimalarial and Antimycobacterial Activity. *J. Med. Chem.*, 2002, *45*, 3331-3336.
[84] Opsenica, D.; Angelovski, G.; Pocsfalvi, G.; Juranic, Z.; Zizak, Z.; Kyle, D.; Milhous, W. K.; Solaja, B. A.; Antimalarial and Antiproliferative Evaluation of Bis-Steroidal Tetraoxanes. *Bioorg. Med. Chem.*, 2003, *11*, 2761-2768.
[85] Opsenica, D.; Pocsfalvi, G.; Juranic, Z.; Tinant, B.; Declercq, J. P.; Kyle, D. E.; Milhous, W. K.; Solaja, B. A.; Cholic Acid Derivatives as 1,2,4,5-Tetraoxane Carriers: Structure and Antimalarial and Antiproliferative Activity. *J. Med. Chem.*, 2000, *43*, 3274-3282.
[86] Opsenica, I.; Terzic, N.; Opsenica, D.; Angelovski, G.; Lehnig, M.; Eilbracht, P.; Tinant, B.; Juranic, Z.; Smith, K. S.; Yang, Y. S.; Diaz, D. S.; Smith, P. L.; Milhous, W. K.; Dokovic, D.; Solaja, B. A.; Tetraoxane Antimalarials and their Reaction with Fe(II). *J. Med. Chem.*, 2006, *49*, 3790-3799.
[87] Terzic, N.; Opsenica, D.; Milic, D.; Tinant, B.; Smith, K. S.; Milhous, W. K.; Solaja, B. A.; Deoxycholic Acid-Derived Tetraoxane Antimalarials and Antiproliferatives. *J. Med. Chem.*, 2007, *50*, 5118-5127.
[88] Kim, H. S.; Nagai, Y.; Ono, K.; Begum, K.; Wataya, Y.; Hamada, Y.; Tsuchiya, K.; Masuyama, A.; Nojima, M.; McCullough, K. J.; Synthesis and Antimalarial Activity of Novel Medium-Sized 1,2,4,5-Tetraoxacycloalkanes. *J. Med. Chem.*, 2001, *44*, 2357-2361.
[89] Kim, H. S.; Begum, K.; Ogura, N.; Wataya, Y.; Nonami, Y.; Ito, T.; Masuyama, A.; Nojima, M.; McCullough, K. J.; Antimalarial Activity of Novel 1,2,5,6-Tetraoxacycloalkanes and 1,2,5-Trioxacycloalkanes. *J. Med. Chem.*, 2003, *46*, 1957-1961.
[90] Griesbaum, K.; Liu, X.; Kassiaris, A.; Scherer, M.; Ozonolyses of O-Alkylated Ketoximes in the Presence of Carbonyl Groups: a Facile Access to Ozonides. *Liebigs Ann. Recl.*, 1997, 1381-1390.

[91] Vennerstrom, J. L.; Arbe-Barnes, S.; Brun, R.; Charman, S. A.; Chiu, F. C. K.; Chollet, J.; Dong, Y.; Dorn, A.; Hunziker, D.; Matile, H.; McIntosh, K.; Padmanilayam, M.; Santo Tomas, J.; Scheurer, C.; Scorneaux, B.; Tang, Y.; Urwyler, H.; Wittlin, S.; Charman, W. H.; Identification of an Antimalarial Synthetic Trioxolane Drug Development Candidate. *Nature*, 2004, *430*, 900-904.

[92] http://www.ranbaxyusa.com/newsdisp12132005.aspx

[93] Tang, Y.; Dong, Y.; Karle, J. M.; DiTusa, C. A.; Vennerstrom, J. L.; Synthesis of Tetrasubstituted Ozonides by the Griesbaum Coozonolysis Reaction: Diastereoselectivity and Functional Group Transformations by Post-Ozonolysis Reactions. *J. Org. Chem.*, 2004, *69*, 6470-6473.

[94] Dong, Y.; Chollet, J.; Matile, H.; Charman, S. A.; Chiu, F. C. K.; Charman, W. N.; Scorneaux, B.; Urwyler, H.; Santo Tomas, J.; Scheurer, C.; Snyder, C.; Dorn, A.; Wang, X.; Karle, J. M.; Tang, Y.; Wittlin, S.; Brun, R.; Vennerstrom, J. L.; Spiro and Dispiro-1,2,4-trioxolanes as Antimalarial Peroxides: Charting a Workable Structure-Activity Relationship Using Simple Prototypes. *J. Med. Chem.*, 2005, *48*, 4953-4961.

[95] Tang, Y.; Dong, Y.; Wang, X.; Sriraghavan, K.; Wood, J. K.; Vennerstrom, J. L.; Dispiro-1,2,4-trioxane Analogues of a Prototype Dispiro-1,2,4-trioxolane: Mechanistic Comparators for Artemisinin in the Context of Reaction Pathways with Iron(II). *J. Org. Chem.*, 2005, *70*, 5103-5110.

[96] Osorio, L.; Murillo, C.; Aponte, S.; Mayagaya, V.; Scheurer, C.; Brun, R.; Matile, H.; Wittlin, S.; *In Vitro* Susceptibility of *P. Falciparum* Populations from Colombia and Tanzania to a New Synthetic Peroxide (OZ277). *Am. J. Trop. Med. Hyg.*, 2007, *76*, 1024-1026.

[97] Padmanilayam, M.; Scorneaux, B.; Dong, Y.; Chollet, J.; Matile, H.; Charman, S. A.; Creek, D. J.; Charman, W. N.; Santo Tomas, J.; Scheurer, C.; Wittlin, S.; Brun, R.; Vennerstrom, J. L.; Antimalarial Activity of N-Alkyl Amine, Carboxamide, Sulfonamide, and Urea Derivatives of a Dispiro-1,2,4-trioxolane Piperidine. *Bioorg. Med. Chem. Lett.*, 2006, *16*, 5542-5545.

[98] Dong, Y.; Tang, Y.; Chollet, J.; Matile, H.; Wittlin, S.; Charman, S. A.; Charman, W. N.; Santo Tomas, J.; Scheurer, C.; Snyder, C.; Scorneaux, B.; Bajpai, S.; Alexander, S. A.; Wang, X.; Padmanilayam, M.; Cheruku, S. R.; Brun, R.; Vennerstrom, J. L.; Effect of Functional Group Polarity on the Antimalarial Activity of Spiro and Dispiro-1,2,4-trioxolanes. *Bioorg. Med. Chem.*, 2006, *14*, 6368-6382.

[99] Tang, Y.; Dong, Y.; Wittlin, S.; Charman, S. A.; Chollet, J.; Chiu, F. C. K.; Charman, W. N.; Matile, H.; Urwyler, H.; Dorn, A.; Bajpai, S.; Wang, X.; Padmanilayam, M.; Karle, J. M.; Brun, R.; Vennerstrom, J. L.; Weak Base Dispiro-1,2,4-trioxolanes: Potent Antimalarial Ozonides. *Bioorg. Med. Chem. Lett.*, 2007, *17*, 1260-1265.

[100] Liang, X. T.; Yu, D. Q.; Wu, W. L.; Deng, H. C.; *Huaxue Xuebao (Acta Chimica Sinica)*, 1979, *37*, 215.

[101] Szpilman, A. M.; Korshin, E. E.; Rozenberg, H.; Bachi, M. D.; Total Syntheses of Yingzhaosu A and of its C(14)-Epimer Including the First Evaluation of their Antimalarial and Cytotoxic Activities. *J. Org. Chem.*, 2005, *70*, 3618-3632.

[102] Xu, X. X.; Zhu, J.; Huang, D. Z.; Zhou, W. S.; Total Synthesis of (+)-Yingzhaosu-A. *Tetrahedron Lett.*, 1991, *32*, 5785-5788.

[103]Hofheinz, W.; Burgin, H.; Gocke, E.; Jaquet, C.; Masciadri, R.; Schmid, G.; Stohler, H.; Urwyler, H.; Ro42-1611 (Arteflene), a New Effective Antimalarial: Chemical Structure and Biological Activity. *Trop. Med. Parasitol.*, 1994, *45*, 261-265.

[104]Jaquet, C.; Stohler, H. R.; Chollet, J.; Peters, W.; Antimalarial Activity of the Bicyclic Peroxide Ro42-1611 (Arteflene) in Experimental Models. *Trop. Med. Parasitol.*, 1994, *45*, 266-271.

[105]Weidekamm, E.; Dumont, E.; Jaquet, C.; Tolerability and Pharmacokinetics of Ro42-1611 (Arteflene) in Man. *Trop. Med. Parasitol.*, 1994, *45*, 278-283.

[106]O'Neill, P. M.; Bishop, L. P. D.; Searle, N. L.; Maggs, J. L.; Storr, R. C.; Ward, S. A.; Park, B. K.; Mabbs, F.; Biomimetic Fe(II)-Mediated Degradation of Arteflene (Ro-42-1611). The First EPR Spin-Trapping Evidence for the Previously Postulated Secondary Carbon-Centered Cyclohexyl Radical. *J. Org. Chem.*, 2000, *65*, 1578-1582.

[107]Cazelles, J.; Robert, A.; Meunier, B.; Characterization of the Main Radical and Products Resulting From a Reductive Activation of the Antimalarial Arteflene (Ro 42-1611). *J. Org. Chem.*, 1999, *64*, 6776-6781.

[108]Korshin, E. E.; Hoos, R.; Szpilman, A. M.; Konstantinovski, L.; Posner, G. H.; Bachi, M. D.; An Efficient Synthesis of Bridged-Bicyclic Peroxides Structurally Related to Antimalarial Yingzhaosu A Based on Radical Co-Oxygenation of Thiols and Monoterpenes. *Tetrahedron*, 2002, *58*, 2449-2469.

[109]O'Neill, P. M.; Verissimo, E.; Ward, S. A.; Davies, J.; Korshin, E. E.; Araujo, N.; Pugh, M. D.; Cristiano, M. L. S.; Stocks, P. A.; Bachi, M. D.; Diels-Alder/Thiol-Olefin Co-Oxygenation Approach to Antimalarials Incorporating the 2,3-Dioxabicyclo[3.3.1]nonane Pharmacophore. *Bioorg. Med. Chem. Lett.*, 2006, *16*, 2991-2995.

[110]Bachi, M. D.; Korshin, E. E.; Hoos, R.; Szpilman, A. M.; Ploypradith, P.; Xie, S.; Shapiro, T. A.; Posner, G. H.; A Short Synthesis and Biological Evaluation of Potent and Nontoxic Antimalarial Bridged Bicyclic Beta-Sulfonyl-Endoperoxides. *J. Med. Chem.*, 2003, *46*, 2516-2533.

[111]Kim, H. S.; Begum, K.; Ogura, N.; Wataya, Y.; Tokuyasu, T.; Masuyama, A.; Nojima, M.; McCullough, K. J.; Antimalarial Activity of Yingzhaosu A Analogues. *J. Med. Chem.*, 2002, *45*, 4732-4736.

[112]Tokuyasu, T.; Masuyama, A.; Nojima, M.; McCullough, K. J.; Kim, H. S.; Wataya, Y.; Yingzhaosu A Analogues: Synthesis by the Ozonolysis of Unsaturated Hydroperoxides, Structural Analysis and Determination of Anti-Malarial Activity. *Tetrahedron*, 2001, *57*, 5979-5989.

[113]Kamata, M.; Satoh, C.; Kim, H. S.; Wataya, Y.; Iron(II)-Promoted Rearrangement of 1,4-Diaryl-2,3-dioxabicyclo[2.2.2]oct-5-enes: A Mechanism Distinct from that Postulated Previously. *Tetrahedron Lett.*, 2002, *43*, 8313-8317.

[114]Posner, G. H.; Tao, X.; Cumming, J. N.; Klinedinst, D.; Shapiro, T. A.; Antimalarially Potent, Easily Prepared, Fluorinated Endoperoxides. *Tetrahedron Lett.*, 1996, *37*, 7225-7228.

[115]Hatzakis, E.; Opsenica, I.; Solaja, B. A.; Stratakis, M.; Synthesis of Novel Polar Derivatives of the Antimalarial Endoperoxides Ascaridole and Dihydroascaridole. *Arkivoc*, 2007, *2007*, 124-135.

[116]Kamata, M.; Ohta, M.; Komatsu, K. I.; Kim, H. S.; Wataya, Y.; Synthesis, Fe(II)-Induced Degradation, and Antimalarial Activities of 1,5-Diaryl-6,7-dioxabicyclo[3.2.2]nonanes: Direct Evidence for Nucleophilic O-1,2-Aryl Shifts. *Tetrahedron Lett.*, 2002, *43*, 2063-2067.

[117]Taylor, D. K.; Avery, T. D.; Greatrex, B. W.; Tiekink, E. R. T.; Macreadie, I. G.; Macreadie, P. I.; Humphries, A. D.; Kalkanidis, M.; Fox, E. N.; Klonis, N.; Tilley, L.; Novel Endoperoxide Antimalarials: Synthesis, Heme Binding, and Antimalarial Activity. *J. Med. Chem.*, 2004, *47*, 1833-1839.

[118]Wang, X.; Dong, Y.; Wittlin, S.; Creek, D.; Chollet, J.; Charman, S. A.; Santo Tomas, J.; Scheurer, C.; Snyder, C.; Vennerstrom, J. L.; Spiro- and Dispiro-1,2-dioxolanes: Contribution of Iron(II)-Mediated One-Electron *vs* Two-Electron Reduction to the Activity of Antimalarial Peroxides. *J. Med. Chem.*, 2007, *50*, 5840-5847.

[119]Tokuyasu, T.; Masuyama, A.; Nojima, M.; Kim, H. S.; Wataya, Y.; Synthesis and Anti-Malarial Activity of Yingzhaosu A Analogues From Unsaturated Hydroperoxy Acetals. *Tetrahedron Lett.*, 2000, *41*, 3145-3148.

[120]Najjar, F.; Baltas, M.; Gorrichon, L.; Moreno, Y.; Tzedakis, T.; Vial, H.; Andre-Barres, C.; Synthesis and Electrochemical Studies of New Antimalarial Endoperoxides. *Eur. J. Org. Chem.*, 2003, 3335-3343.

[121]Gavrilan, M.; Andre-Barres, C.; Baltas, M.; Tzedakis, T.; Gorrichon, L.; Bicyclic Peroxides in the G Factors Series: Synthesis and Electrochemical Studies. *Tetrahedron Lett.*, 2001, *42*, 2465-2468.

[122]Najjar, F.; Andre-Barres, C.; Baltas, M.; Lacaze-Dufaure, C.; Magri, D. C.; Workentin, M. S.; Tzedakis, T.; Electrochemical Reduction of G3-Factor Endoperoxide and its Methyl Ether: Evidence for a Competition Between Concerted and Stepwise Dissociative Electron Transfer. *Chem. Eur. J.*, 2007, *13*, 1174-1179.

[123]Najjar, F.; Gorrichon, L.; Baltas, M.; Andre-Barres, C.; Vial, H.; Alkylation of Natural Endoperoxide G3-Factor. Synthesis and Antimalarial Activity Studies. *Org. Biomol. Chem.*, 2005, *3*, 1612-1614.

[124]Najjar, F.; Gorrichon, L.; Baltas, M.; Vial, H.; Tzedakis, T.; Andre-Barres, C.; Crucial Role of the Peroxyketal Function for Antimalarial Activity in the G-Factor Series. *Bioorg. Med. Chem. Lett.*, 2004, *14*, 1433-1436.

[125]Kobayashi, M.; Kondo, K.; Kitagawa, I.; Antifungal Peroxyketal Acids from an Okinawan Marine Sponge of *Plakortis Sp. Chem. Pharm. Bull.*, 1993, *41*, 1324-1326.

[126]Quinoa, E.; Kho, E.; Manes, L. V.; Crews, P.; Bakus, G. J.; Heterocycles from the Marine Sponge *Xestospongia Sp. J. Org. Chem.*, 1986, *51*, 4260-4264.

[127]Murakami, N.; Kawanishi, M.; Itagaki, S.; Horii, T.; Kobayashi, M.; Facile Construction of 6-Carbomethoxymethyl-3-methoxy-1,2-dioxane, a Core Structure of Spongean Anti-Malarial Peroxides. *Tetrahedron Lett.*, 2001, *42*, 7281-7285.

[128]Murakami, N.; Kawanishi, M.; Itagaki, S.; Horii, T.; Kobayashi, M.; New Readily Accessible Peroxides with High Anti-Malarial Potency. *Bioorg. Med. Chem. Lett.*, 2002, *12*, 69-72.

[129]Kawanishi, M.; Kotoku, N.; Itagaki, S.; Horii, T.; Kobayashi, M.; Structure-Activity Relationship of Anti-Malarial Spongean Peroxides Having a 3-Methoxy-1,2-dioxane Structure. *Bioorg. Med. Chem.*, 2004, *12*, 5297-5307.

[130]Murakami, N.; Kawanishi, M.; Mostaqul, H. M.; Li, J.; Itagaki, S.; Horii, T.; Kobayashi, M.; New Anti-Malarial Peroxides with *in Vivo* Potency Derived from Spongean Metabolites. *Bioorg. Med. Chem. Lett.*, 2003, *13*, 4081-4084.

[131]Zhang, Q.; Wu, Y.; Simplified Analogues of Qinghaosu (Artemisinin). *Tetrahedron*, 2007, *63*, 10407-10414.

[132]Jin, H. X.; Zhang, Q.; Kim, H. S.; Wataya, Y.; Liu, H. H.; Wu, Y.; Design, Synthesis and *in Vitro* Antimalarial Activity of Spiroperoxides. *Tetrahedron*, 2006, *62*, 7699-7711.

[133]Howarth, J.; Wilson, D.; 1,4-Dihydroxy-2,3-dioxatricyclo[8.4.0.0]tetradecane and Derivatives with *in Vitro* Activity against *Plasmodium Falciparum*, *Trypanasoma b Brucei*, *Trypanasoma Cruzi*, and *Leishmaniasis Infantum*. *Bioorg. Med. Chem. Lett.*, 2003, *13*, 2013-2015.

[134]Posner, G. H.; O'Dowd, H.; Ploypradith, P.; Cumming, J. N.; Xie, S.; Shapiro, T. A.; Antimalarial Cyclic Peroxy Ketals. *J. Med. Chem.*, 1998, *41*, 2164-2167.

[135]Kim, J.; Li, H. B.; Rosenthal, A. S.; Sang, D.; Shapiro, T. A.; Bachi, M. D.; Posner, G. H.; Ground State Oxygen in Synthesis of Cyclic Peroxides. Part 1: Benzo Fused Ketals. *Tetrahedron*, 2006, *62*, 4120-4127.

[136]Dussault, P.; Sahli, A.; 2-Methoxyprop-2-yl Hydroperoxide - A Convenient Reagent for the Synthesis of Hydroperoxides and Peracids. *J. Org. Chem.*, 1992, *57*, 1009-1012.

[137]Cointeaux, L.; Berrien, J. F.; Peyrou, V.; Provot, O.; Ciceron, L.; Danis, M.; Robert, A.; Meunier, B.; Mayrargue, J.; Synthesis and Antimalarial Activity of 2-Methoxyprop-2-yl Peroxides Derivatives. *Bioorg. Med. Chem. Lett.*, 2003, *13*, 75-77.

[138]Hamada, Y.; Tokuhara, H.; Masuyama, A.; Nojima, M.; Kim, H. S.; Ono, K.; Ogura, N.; Wataya, Y.; Synthesis and Notable Antimalarial Activity of Acyclic Peroxides, 1-(Alkyldioxy)-1-(methyldioxy)cyclododecanes. *J. Med. Chem.*, 2002, *45*, 1374-1378.

[139]Dechy-Cabaret, O.; Benoit-Vical, F.; Loup, C.; Robert, A.; Gornitzka, H.; Bonhoure, A.; Vial, H.; Magnaval, J. F.; Seguela, J. P.; Meunier, B.; Synthesis and Antimalarial Activity of Trioxaquine Derivatives. *Chem. Eur. J.*, 2004, *10*, 1625-1636.

[140]Basco, L. K.; Dechy-Cabaret, O.; Ndounga, M.; Meche, F. S.; Robert, A.; Meunier, B.; *In Vitro* Activities of DU-1102, a New Trioxaquine Derivative, against *Plasmodium Falciparum* Isolates. *Antimicrob. Agents Chemother.*, 2001, *45*, 1886-1888.

[141]Dechy-Cabaret, O.; Benoit-Vical, F.; Robert, A.; Meunier, B.; Preparation and Antimalarial Activities of "Trioxaquines", New Modular Molecules with a Trioxane Skeleton Linked to a 4-Aminoquinoline. *ChemBioChem*, 2000, *1*, 281-283.

[142]Benoit-Vical, F.; Lelievre, J.; Berry, A.; Deymier, C.; Dechy-Cabaret, O.; Cazelles, J.; Loup, C.; Robert, A.; Magnaval, J. F.; Meunier, B.; Trioxaquines are New Antimalarial Agents Active on all Erythrocytic Forms, Including Gametocytes. *Antimicrob. Agents Chemother.*, 2007, *51*, 1463-1472.

[143]Singh, C.; Malik, H.; Puri, S. K.; Synthesis and Antimalarial Activity of a New Series of Trioxaquines. *Bioorg. Med. Chem.*, 2004, *12*, 1177-1182.

[144]Grellepois, F.; Grellier, P.; Bonnet-Delpon, D.; Begue, J.-P.; Design, Synthesis and Antimalarial Activity of Trifluoromethylartemisinin- Mefloquine Dual Molecules. *ChemBioChem*, 2005, *6*, 648-652.

[145] Walsh, J. J.; Coughlan, D.; Heneghan, N.; Gaynor, C.; Bell, A.; A Novel Artemisinin-Quinine Hybrid with Potent Antimalarial Activity. *Bioorg. Med. Chem. Lett.*, 2007, *17*, 3599-3602.

[146] O'Neill, P. M.; Stocks, P. A.; Pugh, M. D.; Araujo, N. C.; Korshin, E. E.; Bickley, J. F.; Ward, S. A.; Bray, P. G.; Pasini, E.; Davies, J.; Verissimo, E.; Bachi, M. D.; Design and Synthesis of Endoperoxide Antimalarial Prodrug Models. *Angew. Chem., Int. Ed.*, 2004, *43*, 4193-4197.

In: Antimalarial Drugs: Costs, Safety and Efficacy
Editors: Emanuel Csizmadia and Istvan Kalnoky
ISBN: 978-1-60741-432-2

Chapter IX

Antimalarial Resistance and Treatment of Malaria in Clinical Practice in Thailand: An Update

Viroj Wiwanitkit
Wiwanitkit House, Bangkhae, Bangkok Thailand

Abstract

The problem of drug resistance is the main problem affecting the success of malarial treatment worldwide. Southeast Asian countries including Thailand face up with the problem of antimalarial resistance at present. The details ranging from the molecular to social aspects of malarial resistance will be reviewed and presented. Also, the treatment of malaria in clinical practice in Thailand covering standard as well as alternative therapy for malaria to cope with the problem of high antimalarial resistance will be summarized in this article. New data were summarized and presented in this chapter.

Introduction to Malaria Treatment

The concept of treatment is similar to other infections: getting rid of the pathogen or control of the infection and supportive or symptomatic treatment. In malaria, many antimalarial drugs (Table 1) are available for a long time. The selection of antimalarial drugs depends on various factors including the species and the reported resistance pattern in each setting [1]. Randomized controlled trials have not revealed any significant benefit of the artemisinin derivatives over quinine in quinine sensitive areas [2]. Also, if quinine is administered in the recommended way, the side effects are no greater than artemisinins [2]. Drug resistant is a very important problem in using of antimalrial drug, Historically, first case of chloroquine resistance was along the Thai-Combodian border in the late 1950s then Southeast Asia has played an important role as a focus for the development of drug resistance in *Plasmodium falciparum* [2]. The foci led the attention to the society of malariology. In addition, the onset of chloroquine resistance marked the beginning of a new chapter in the history of malaria in Southeast Asia and by 1973 chloroquine finally had to be replaced by the combination of sulphadoxine and pyrimethamine (SP) as first line drug for the treatment of uncomplicated malaria in Thailand and more than 10 African countries have also switched their first line drug to other newly alternative drugs [3]. Farooq and Mahajan said that many molecular markers for antimalarial resistance had been identified, including pfmdr-1 and pfcrt polymorphisms related to chloroquine resistance and dhfr and dhps polymorphisms associated with SP resistance [3]. They noted that polymorphisms in pfmdr-1 might also be relating to resistance to chloroquine, mefloquine and artemisinin [3]. An important precaution of using antimalarial drug is drug - induced hemolysis in the patients with glucose-6-phosphate dehydrogenase (G-6-PD) deficiency, which is endemic in the same area as that of malaria. It should be noted that G6PD status is recommended before primaquine or tafenoquine is prescribed in this specific endemic area [4]. However, the G6PD deficiency, on the other hand, is a protective factor for malaria [4]. Wajcman and Galacteros noted that red blood cells with low G6PD activity can be a good environment to parasite growth and thus an advantage to G6PD deficiency carriers [4].

Table 1 Summary on recommended dosage and side effects of common antimalarial drugs

Drug	Group	Dosage
Quinine sulphate	Quinoline derivative	10 mg salt/kg 8 hourly for seven days (plus doxycycline 100 mg daily for 7 days)
Quinine Dihydrochloride	Quinoline derivative	20 mg salt/kg base given intravenously in 5% normal saline as a once-only 4 hour infusion followed, 4 hours later, 10 mg salt/kg base 4-hour infusions, 8 hourly.
Chloroquine	Quinoline derivative	4 tablets (600mg base) or 10 mg/kg first dose then 2 tablets (300mg base) or 5 mg/kg 6-8 hours later for 3 days (continue with primaquine 3.5mg/kg given as a divided daily dose over 14 days)
Artesunate	Artemesin derivative	120mg intravenously stat. 60 mg at 4, 24 and 48 hours, 50-60 mg on days 3-5
Artemeter	Artemesin Derivative	2 mg/kg intramuscularly stat then 1.6mg twice daily for 3-7 days

In additional to specific treatment, the supportive and symptomatic treatment is also important in taking care of malarial patients. Since several associated systemic complications like hypoglycemia, hypovolemia, hyperpyrexia, renal failure, bleeding disorders, anemia, lactic acidosis and pulmonary oedema may contribute in the pathogenesis of coma, and are responsible for high mortality, the meticulous supportive care along with intravenous administration of antimalarial drugs are corner-stone of the treatment [5]. Pamba and Maitland noted that reduction in case fatality could only come through the wider appreciation of the requirement for and application of supportive therapies to treat the life-threatening complications of malaria [6]. In severe malarial infection, fluid management is very important. Pamba and Maitland said that hypovolaemia had emerged as a common feature of children presenting with severe malaria complicated by acidosis [6]. They noted that early recognition and prompt treatment might bring improvements in outcome [6]. As soon as the patient is clinically stable and able to swallow, oral treatment should be given and the intravascular volume should be replaced at the maintaining lowest level sufficient for adequate systemic perfusion to prevent development of acute respiratory distress syndrome [7]. In addition, renal replacement therapy should be initiated early [7]. Therapeutic red cell-exchange (TREX) has been used with much interest over the years to correct severe anemia [7 - 8]. Singhal said that the role of exchange blood transfusion in the management of severe malaria was still a controversy issue and it might be considered in the presence of high parasites counts, more than10%, with multiorgan dysfunction if adequate quantities of safe blood were available [2].

Drug Resistance in Malaria

The problem of drug resistance is the main problem affecting the success of malarial treatment worldwide. The details ranging from the molecular to social aspects of malarial resistance will be reviewed and presented.

A. Molecular Aspect of Malarial Drug Resistance

The malarial drug resistance is believed to be owing to the natural selection process of the parasite. A modest increase in the range of antimalarial drugs approved for clinical use has been complemented by a more impressive expansion in the analysis and understanding of the molecular mechanisms underlying resistance to these agents [9]. It is widely assumed in genetics that most mutations disrupt metabolism to some extent, and are consequently likely to be disadvantageous for the organisms that inherit them [10]. This may lead to mutations encoding drug resistance in malaria, where the mutation may be disadvantageous in the absence of the drug, imposing a genetic “cost” of resistance [10]. Many resistance mutations have rather few independent origins [11]. Although several genetic mechanisms have been shown, the major source of drug resistance appears to be point mutations in protein target genes [12]. Clinically significant resistance to these agents requires the accumulation of multiple mutations, which genetic studies of parasite populations suggest increase focally and sweep through the population [12]. De novo mutation appears to be less important than migration for introducing resistance alleles into parasite populations [11]. Attempts to manage drug resistance will be of limited effectiveness unless this is considered into account [11].

Antifolate antimalarial drugs interfere with folate metabolism, a pathway essential to malaria parasite survival [13]. This class of drugs includes effective causal prophylactic and therapeutic agents, some of which act synergistically when used in combination [13]. Unfortunately, the antifolates have proven to be already resisted drug in the malaria parasite. Resistance is caused by point mutations in dihydrofolate reductase and dihydropteroate synthase, the two key enzymes in the folate biosynthetic pathway that are tagged by the antifolates [13]. Mechanisms of resistance other than reduced binding of inhibitors to mutant enzymes may be possible and need to be further explored [14]. New synergistic combinations of drugs targeting dihydrofolate reductase and dihydropteroate synthase may be employed, with new provisions against development of resistance [14].

At present, there are many advances on identification of molecular markers that can be employed and useful in predicting in vitro and in vivo resistance in southeast Asia. Recent achievements include the successful expression of the *Plasmodium falciparum* chloroquine resistance transporter gene, pfcrt, in yeast, the identification of polymorphisms on the gamma-glutamylcysteine synthetase gene, ggcs, as potential determinants of chloroquine and mefloquine resistance, and the usefulness of a combined Plasmodium falciparum dihydrofolate reductase gene, pfdhfr, 59ARG and Plasmodium falciparum dihydropteroate synthase gene, pfdhps, 540GLU marker in reliably representing resistance to antifolates [15]. Moreover, treatment with sulfadoxine-pyrimethamine in the presence of pfdhfr 108ASP alone delayed parasite clearance and increased [15 - 16].

B. Biochemical Aspect of Malarial Drug Resistance

Ever increasing drug resistance by *P. falciparum*, the most virulent of human malaria parasites, is introducing new challenges in malaria chemotherapy [17]. Applied to Plasmodium, proteomics combines high-resolution protein or peptide separation with mass spectrometry and computer software to rapidly identify large numbers of proteins expressed from various stages of parasite development [17]. Proteomic methods can be used to study sub-cellular localization, cell function, organelle composition, changes in protein expression patterns in response to drug exposure, drug-protein binding and validation of data from genomic annotation and transcript expression studies [17]. Recent high-throughput proteomic approaches have yielded a wealth of protein expression data on *P. falciparum*, while smaller-scale studies examining specific drug-related hypotheses are also appearing [17]. For new drug development, Aspects of the parasite glycolytic pathway, nucleotide metabolism, proteases, redox metabolism and organelle function have been used to highlight possible targets and molecules that could inhibit their function [18].

C. Clinical Aspect of Malarial Drug Resistance

Malarial drug resistance becomes an important problem in treatment of malaria at present. The factors which identify patients at risk of treatment failure were characterized in infected children and adults with uncomplicated falciparum malaria treated with 15 or 25 mg/kg of mefloquine on the borders of Thailand [19]. In this work, 6 independent predictors of failure were visible using multiple logistic regression. Age < or = 2 years, 3-15 years, vomiting < 30 min after a single dose of 25 mg/kg (despite re-administration of the dose) and diarrhoea after treatment were the strongest predictors of failure by day 7 [19]. Parasitaemias > 10 000/mm^3, and fever with a history of recent vomiting (OR 1.6) were specific risk factors for recrudescence of the infection between days 10 and 28 [19]. At present, the distribution of antimalrial resistant malaria from Southeast Asia to other regions of the world can be detected. Recently, et al studied Chloroquine resistant malaria in neonates [20]. According to this research [20], intrauterine growth retardation, hemolytic jaundice and history of fever in the mother in the last trimester of pregnancy in the congenital while fever, history of blood transfusion in the neonates in acquired malaria but pallor in both congenital and acquired malaria groups, were important clinical presentations [20]. However, pattern of chloroquine resistance and mortality in congenital and acquired malaria groups was statistically similar [20].

As previously described, the genetic adaptation to the antimalarial drug of parasite as the natural selection process is considered to be the root cause of drug resistant malaria. Indeed, self-medication with anti-malarial drugs is widespread, and chloroquine resistance is increasing. In 2005, Evans et al reported the extensive prior chloroquine use in the patients presenting with severe malaria, and a high prevalence of parasites with the chloroquine - resistance genotype [21]. They noted that chloroquine resistance in *P. falciparum* might lead to the development of severe but otherwise uncomplicated anemia [21].

D. Social Aspect of Malarial Drug Resistance

Despite more than 100 years since Laveran described plasmodium species and Ross confirmed that they were transmitted by female anopheline mosquitoes, malaria remains a leading etiology of morbidity and mortality worldwide [22]. Although the areas where transmission takes place have reduced, and they are by now limited to the inter tropical areas, the number of people living at risk has grown to about 3 billions, and is expected to go on increasin [22]. With the malpractice in using of insecticide as well as self-prescribed antimalarial drug use, the specific problem of malarial drug resistance is widely distributed. Of interest, most of the endemic sites with the problem are the far distance rural area with limited resources. This can affect the success in treatment and control of drug resistant malaria.

Problems of Malarial Drug Resistance in Thailand

Southeast Asian countries including Thailand face up with the problem of antimalarial resistance at present. Here, the treatment of malaria in clinical practice in Thailand covering standard as well as alternative therapy for malaria to cope with the problem of high antimalarial resistance will be summarized.

A. Clinical Practice for Treatment of Drug Resistant Malaria in Thailand

For standard treatment of drug resistant malaria in Thailand, the summarized recommendation is presented in Table 2. This recommendation is proved to be useful for managing the problem of high prevalence of drug resistant malaria in Thailand.

Table 2 Simplified guideline for selection of antimalarial drugs

Species	Recommendation
Vivax	Chloroquine (Increased Dose) And Primaquine
Falciparum	Quinine dihydrochloride (intravenous)
Ovale	Similar To Vivax
Malariae	Chloroquine

- dosage of each drug is adjusted according to the recommendation of each setting

In additional to standard treatment, there are a number of researches on alternative medicine for treatment of malaria. Several herbs are tested for the possibility in development of new antimalarial drug. However, there is no herb that can be successful processed to be the real antimalarial drug for clinical use.

B. Epidemiology of Antimalarial Resistance in Thailand

Drug-resistant falciparum continues to be an increasing problem in Thailand. The high endemicity of drug resistant malaria can be seen in Western and Northern Region of Thailand , next to Myanmar. *P. falciparum* has rapidly developed resistance to new synthetic antimalarial drugs and rapidly spread by uncontrolled population movement in country and inter country. National Malaria Control Program has enforced the different strategies to overcome malaria such as disease management, drug control, in vivo and in vitro monitoring, vector control and collaboration with neighboring country. However, all of these efforts will be successful, only with community participation [23].

For update on this topic, Wongsrichanalai et al studied on the historical evidence on drug resistant malaria on the Thai-Myanmar and Thai-Cambodian borders [24]. In this historical research, the introduction of artesunate-mefloquine combination in selected areas along the two borders in 1995 was identified to be one of the multiple factors responsible for stabilizing the multidrug resistance problems in Thailand today [24]. Vijaykadga et al also reported that the markedly reduced efficacy of the artesunate-mefloquine combination used in the southeastern border of Thailand with Cambodia led questions about the future of this therapy on because no new practical and affordable alternative was yet available [25]. Barends et al reported another important finding from the setting of Thai-Myanmar border that new ferroquine compound SSR97193, a new compound, had high anti-malarial activity in vitro against multi-drug resistant *P. falciparum* [26]. Singhasivanon also studied on mekong malaria focusing multi-drug resistance and economic development in the greater Mekong subregion of Southeast Asia, which include Thailand [27]. Singhasivanon concluded that malaria control should involve consideration of microeconomic capacity and operates in the broader context of macroeconomic policy including economic and social profiles [27].

References

[1] Farooq U, Mahajan RC. Drug resistance in malaria. *J Vector Borne Dis*. 2004 Sep-Dec;41(3-4):45-53.

[2] Singhal T. Management of severe malaria. *Indian J Pediatr*. 2004 Jan;71(1):81-8.

[3] Indonesian Society of Medicine. Consensus of Malaria Management 2003 (part 2). *Acta Med Indones*. 2004 Jul-Sep;36(3):187-93

[4] Wajcman H, Galacteros F. Glucose 6-phosphate dehydrogenase deficiency: a protection against malaria and a risk for hemolytic accidents. *C R Biol*. 2004 Aug;327(8):711-20

[5] Garg RK. Cerebral malaria. *J Assoc Physicians India*. 2000 Oct;48(10):1004-13.

[6] Pamba A, Maitland K. Fluid management of severe falciparum malaria in African children. *Trop Doct*. 2004 Apr;34(2):67-70.

[7] Trampuz A, Jereb M, Muzlovic I, Prabhu RM. Clinical review: Severe malaria. *Crit Care*. 2003 Aug;7(4):315-23.

[8] Valbonesi M, Bruni R. Clinical application of therapeutic erythrocytapheresis (TEA). *Transfus Sci*. 2000 Jun;22(3):183-94.

[9] Hyde JE. Drug-resistant malaria. *Trends Parasitol*. 2005 Nov;21(11):494-8.

[10] Hastings IM, Donnelly MJ. The impact of antimalarial drug resistance mutations on parasite fitness, and its implications for the evolution of resistance. *Drug Resist Updat*. 2005 Feb-Apr;8(1-2):43-50

[11] Anderson TJ, Roper C. The origins and spread of antimalarial drug resistance: lessons for policy makers. *Acta Trop*. 2005 Jun;94(3):269-80.

[12] Arav-Boger R, Shapiro TA. Molecular mechanisms of resistance in antimalarial chemotherapy: the unmet challenge. *Annu Rev Pharmacol Toxicol*. 2005;45:565-85.

[13] Gregson A, Plowe CV. Mechanisms of resistance of malaria parasites to antifolates. *Pharmacol Rev*. 2005 Mar;57(1):117-45.

[14] Yuthavong Y. Basis for antifolate action and resistance in malaria. *Microbes Infect*. 2002 Feb;4(2):175-82.

[15] Wernsdorfer WH, Noedl H. Molecular markers for drug resistance in malaria: use in treatment, diagnosis and epidemiology. *Curr Opin Infect Dis*. 2003 Dec;16(6):553-8.

[16] Uhlemann AC, Krishna S. Antimalarial multi-drug resistance in Asia: mechanisms and assessment. *Curr Top Microbiol Immunol*. 2005;295:39-53.

[17] Cooper RA, Carucci DJ. Proteomic approaches to studying drug targets and resistance in Plasmodium. *Curr Drug Targets Infect Disord*. 2004 Mar;4(1):41-51.

[18] Pattanaik P, Raman J, Balaram H. Perspectives in drug design against malaria. *Curr Top Med Chem*. 2002 May;2(5):483-505.

[19] Kuile FO, Luxemburger C, Nosten F, Thwai KL, Chongsuphajaisiddhi T, White NJ. Predictors of mefloquine treatment failure: a prospective study of 1590 patients with uncomplicated falciparum malaria. *Trans R Soc Trop Med Hyg*. 1995 Nov-Dec;89(6):660-4.

[20] Khichi QK, Channar MS, Wairraich MI, Butt A. Chloroquine resistant malaria in neonates. *J Coll Physicians Surg Pak*. 2005 Jan;15(1):34-6.

[21] Evans JA, May J, Tominski D, Eggelte T, Marks F, Abruquah HH, Meyer CG, Timmann C, Agbenyega T, Horstmann RD. Pre-treatment with chloroquine and parasite chloroquine resistance in Ghanaian children with severe malaria. *QJM*. 2005 Nov;98(11):789-96.

[22] Guinovart C, Navia MM, Tanner M, Alonso PL. Malaria: burden of disease. *Curr Mol Med*. 2006 Mar;6(2):137-40.

[23] Vichaikatthaka S. The spread or drug-resistant malaria in Thailand and strategy to control. *Thai J Health Res* 1997; 13(1): 39-49.

[24] Wongsrichanalai C, Sirichaisinthop J, Karwacki JJ, Congpuong K, Miller RS, Pang L, Thimasarn K. Drug resistant malaria on the Thai-Myanmar and Thai-Cambodian borders. *Southeast Asian J Trop Med Public Health*. 2001 Mar;32(1):41-9.

[25] Vijaykadga S, Rojanawatsirivej C, Cholpol S, Phoungmanee D, Nakavej A, Wongsrichanalai C. In vivo sensitivity monitoring of mefloquine monotherapy and artesunate-mefloquine combinations for the treatment of uncomplicated falciparum malaria in Thailand in 2003. *Trop Med Int Health*. 2006 Feb;11(2):211-9.

[26] Barends M, Jaidee A, Khaohirun N, Singhasivanon P, Nosten F. In vitro activity of ferroquine (SSR 97193) against Plasmodium falciparum isolates from the Thai-Burmese border. *Malar J*. 2007 Jun 27;6:81.

[27] Singhasivanon P. Mekong malaria. Malaria, multi-drug resistance and economic development in the greater Mekong subregion of Southeast Asia. *Southeast Asian J Trop Med Public Health*. 1999;30 Suppl 4:i-iv, 1-101.

In: Antimalarial Drugs: Costs, Safety and Efficacy
Editors: Emanuel Csizmadia and Istvan Kalnoky
ISBN: 978-1-60741-432-2

Chapter X

Biochemoinformatics Technology and Antimalarial Drug: A Useful of "Omics" Technology

Viroj Wiwanitkit
Wiwanitkit House, Bangkhae, Bangkok Thailand

Abstract

Biochemoinformatics is a new science that can lead several advantages in medicine. New drug development can be easily performed with the new advancements in bioinformatics. Advanced biochemoinformatics technologies for drug search can be applied for new antimalarial drug search. This is useful for case of antimalarial drug resistance.

Application of Biochemoinformatics for Drug Search

A. Brief History

Clinical bioinformatics provides biological and medical information to help real usage for individualized healthcare [1 – 2]. In the past 10 years, the field of bioinformatics has been revealed by the mapping of many genomes [1]. These efforts have stimulated explosive development of novel bioinformatics and experimental approaches to predict the functions and metabolic role of the new proteins [1]. The main application of the work is to search, validate, and prioritize new targets for designing new drugs [1]. Proteomics strategy tools usually focus on similarity searches, structure prediction, and protein modeling [2]. In clinical bioinformatics, the proteomic data only have meaning if they are coperated with clinical data. In pharmacogenomics, clinical bioinformatics includes elaborate studies of bioinformatics tools and various facets of proteomics related to drug target identification and clinical validation [2]. In the genome era upon us, researchers want rapid, easy-to-use, reliable instruments for functional characterisation of newly determined sequences [3]. For the pharmaceutical industry in particular, the bioinformatics provides an information-rich nugget, ripe with potential drug targets and possible new routes for the development of therapeutic agents [3].

B. Bioinformatics and Drug search

Bioinformatics can be applied for new drug search. Advances in genomics, proteomics, and structural genomics have detected a large number of protein targets [4]. Virtual screening has gained popularity in identifying drug leads by computationally screening large numbers of specific chemicals against experimentally determined protein targets [4]. Bioinformatics is widely used for new antibiotic search. Current research in bioinformatics relating to new antibiotic drug search can be divided into: (i) genomics--sequencing and comparative study of genomes to identify gene and genome functionality, (ii) proteomics--identification and characterization of protein related properties and reconstruction of metabolic and regulatory pathways, (iii) cell visualization and simulation to study and model cell behavior, and (iv) application to the development of new drugs and new anti-microbial agents [5].

For genomics, comparative genomics technique can be useful in identification of the common sequence within the genome of human and microorganism. This can help identify the possible toxicity of the new drug. For example, Wiwanitkit performed a database searching to detect the recorded complete genes with complete sequences of *Mycobacterium leprae* and studied their homology to human genomes by BLAST method [6]. From a total of 35 genes, the potential candidates for further target-based drug development were determined [6]. Functional genomics can also be applied for new drug search. Functional genomics can be defined as the finding for the physiological role of a gene for which only its primary sequence is known [7]. A good example of a successful functional genomics adventure is the search for the natural ligands of orphan G protein-coupled receptors (GPCRs) [7]. GPCRs are proteins containing 7 hydrophobic domains that are the recognition sites of neurotransmitters and neuropeptides [7]. Although many of these have been shown to interact with known natural ligands, several bind ligands that have not been thus far isolated [7]. Structural genomics can also be applied for new drug search. For example, the use of comparative and structural genomics for the search and characterization of new *Mycobacterium tuberculosis* genes, whose products may prove to be important antigens for the development of vaccines or target proteins for remedies against tuberculosis, is considered [8]. In past, long discovery and development times were needed to bring launch drugs to market and the bottlenecks at the stages of identifying good lead compounds and optimizing these leads into new drug candidates [9]. Structural genomics will hopefully yield opportunities to overcome these bottlenecks and populate the antimicrobial pipeline [9].

C. Chemoinformatics and Drug Search

Sequencing of the human genome along with developments in combinatorial synthesis and high-throughput biological screening provide unparallel opportunities to drug discovery [10]. It has been noted that the increased number of synthesized and annotated compounds did not yield the expected increase in number of new drug candidates [10]. There are several applications of new computational technologies in chemoinformatics to help drug searching. For example, the identification of three-dimensional pharmacophores from large, heterogeneous data sets is still a persisted problem [11]. Fortunately, Chen et al developed a novel program, SCAMPI (statistical classification of activities of molecules for pharmacophore identification), for this purpose by combining a fast conformation search with recursive partitioning, a data-mining technique, which can easily manage large data sets [11]. Oloff et al developed a novel structure-based chemoinformatics approach to search for Complimentary Ligands Based on Receptor Information (CoLiBRI) [12]. CoLiBRI is relied on the representation of both receptor binding sites and their respective ligands in view of universal chemical descriptors [12]. The binding site atoms involved in the specific interaction with ligands are detected by the means of a computational geometry technique known as Delaunay tessellation as applied to X-ray characterized ligand-receptor complexes [12].

Bioinformatics for Antimalarial Drug Search

1. Bioinformatics Research for Antimalarial Drug Search

1.1 Genomics Research for Antimalarial Drug Search

Quantitative trait loci (QTL) mapping is an effective tool for tracking multi-gene traits by partitioning genetic effects that influence these traits into specific genomic regions [13]. The specific allele forms and their combinations contributed by each parent are specific genetic signatures of their unique evolutionary histories [13]. When alleles conferring drug resistance spread through a population of malaria parasites, they let characteristic markers in the parasite genome [14]. In addition to resistance genes, per se, a drug resistant parasite carries co-evolved gene combinations comprising a genetic background of drug resistance [13]. Quinine remains effective against *Plasmodium falciparum*, but its decreasing efficacy is documented from different continents. Multiple genes are likely to bring the evolution of quinine resistance [15]. Chloroquine-resistant strains of *Plasmodium falciparum* counter the drug by expelling it rapidly via a questioned mechanism [16]. Inheritance data from 16 independent recombinant progeny show that the rapid efflux, chloroquine-resistant phenotype is governed by a single locus within an approximately 400-kilobase region of chromosome [16]. In the absence of explicit biochemical basic knowledge of this efflux mechanism, reverse genetics provides a powerful approach to the molecular basis of chloroquine resistance [16]. QTL mapping, by superimposing real biological phenotypes on genome sequence, structural polymorphisms, and gene expression data, can give an alternative, unbiased view of the network of gene actions that build a complex phenotype [13]. To locate genes contributing to QN response variation, Ferdig et al searched a *Plasmodium falciparum* genetic cross for QTL [15]. The mapped segments of Chrs 7 and 5 contain pfcrt, the determinant of chloroquine resistance, and pfmdr1, a gene known to affect QN responses [15]. Association of pfcrt with a QTL of chloroquine resistance points to anecdotal evidence for an evolutionary relationship between chloroquine resistance and reduced quinine sensitivity [15]. The reconstruction of the evolutionary and molecular presentations underlying chloroquine resistance is important at several levels, including: (i) its potential to assist in the development of rational approaches to thwart future drug resistances; (ii) the stimulation of the use of chloroquine -like compounds in drug combinations for new therapeutic approaches; and (iii) the consideration of how the chloroquine -selected genome will function as the context in which current and future drugs will act, particularly in light of the many reports of multidrug resistance [17]. Through an integrated approach, studies can move excess the present search for markers of resistance to instead characterize the predisposition of parasites to develop new resistances and cross-resistances [13].

Functional genomics can be helpful for antimalarial drug search. Combinatorial use of data analysis tools enables powerful data mining queries, such as combining gene and protein expression data to monitor changes through various life-cycle stages [18]. Functional predictions can be used to explore potential targets for antimalarial drug development [18]. The complete annotated genomes of the human parasite *Plasmodium falciparum* and the rodent model *Plasmodium yoelii* is now available thus providing a good prediction of their possible gene products [18]. This makes probably the application of functional genomics to malaria research with the final goal of providing a complete survey of Plasmodium life cycle [19]. Genome-wide approaches to the study of transcriptome or proteome were successfully applied to malaria parasite with the promise for new drug and vaccine candidates in the next future [19]. Another interesting application of functional genomics is specific for functional study of mitochrondrion of Plasmodium spp. One of the functional roles of the mitochondrion in the parasite is the coordination of pyrimidine biosynthesis, the electron transport system and oxygen utilization via dihydroorotate dehydrogenase and coenzyme Q [20]. Complete sets of genes encoding enzymes of the tricarboxylic acid cycle and the ATP synthase complex are already predicted from *Plasmodium falciparum* genomics information [20]. Other metabolic roles of this organelle include membrane potential maintenance, heme and coenzyme Q biosynthesis, and oxidative phosphorylation [20]. Furthermore, the mitochondrion might be a chemotherapeutic target for antimalarial drug development. The antimalarial drug atovaquone targets the mitochondrion [20].

Structural genomics can also be applied for antimalarial drug search. The crystal structure of Pfal009167AAA, a putative ribulose 5-phosphate 3-epimerase (PfalRPE) from *Plasmodium falciparum*, has been detected to 2 A resolution [21]. RPE represents an exciting potential drug target for developing antimalarials because it is involved in the shikimate and the pentose phosphate pathways [21]. This structure is already clarified in the framework of the Structural Genomics of Pathogenic Protozoa (SGPP) consortium [21]. Although the conformation of the bound analogue resembles those of ligands bound in the active sites of OMPDC and KGPDC, the identities of the active site residues that coordinate the essential $Zn(2+)$ and participate as acid/base catalysts are not conserved [22]. Akana et al concluded that only the phosphate binding motif located at the end points of the seventh and eighth beta-strands of the (beta/alpha)(8)-barrel is functionally conserved among RPE, OMPDC, and KGPDC, consistent with the hypothesis that the members of the "ribulose phosphate binding" (beta/alpha)(8)-barrel "superfamily" as determined by SCOP have not evolved by evolutionary processes involving the intact (beta/alpha)(8)-barrel [22]. Akana et al proposed that this "superfamily" might be got from assembly from smaller modules, including the conserved phosphate binding motif associated with the C-terminal (beta/alpha)(2)-quarter barrel [22].

1.2 Proteomics Research for Antimalarial Drug Search

The search for novel antimalarial drug targets is urgent owing to the growing resistance of Plasmodium falciparum parasites to available drugs [23]. The ability to measure accurately comparative levels of protein expression after drug challenge, metabolic stress, developmental programming or other perturbation represents one of the most important aims in post-genomics malaria research [24]. Applied to Plasmodium, proteomics combines high-resolution protein or peptide separation with mass spectrometry and computer software to rapidly identify large numbers of proteins expressed from various stages of parasite development [25]. Proteomic methods can be helpful to study sub-cellular localization, cell function, organelle composition, changes in protein expression patterns in response to drug exposure, drug-protein binding and validation of data from genomic annotation and transcript expression studies [25]. Proteases are attractive antimalarial targets because of their indispensable roles in parasite infection and development, especially in the processes of host erythrocyte rupture/invasion and hemoglobin degradation [23]. Wu et al represents an initial effort to identify a set of expressed, active, and essential proteases as aims for inhibitor-based drug design based on proteomics techniques [23]. Recently, Nirmalan et al described a simple and robust quantitative methodology that was ideally suited to in vitro experiments designed to assess changes in the proteome of the most important of the human parasites, the lethal species *Plasmodium falciparum* [24]. According to this work, the metabolic labeling technique makes use of parasite uptake of heavy isotope-containing isoleucine during normal growth followed by two-dimensional separation of individual proteins and mass spectrometry [24]. Recent high-throughput proteomic approaches have provided a wealth of protein expression data on *Plasmodium falciparum*, while smaller-scale studies examining specific drug-related hypotheses are also appearing [25].

2. Chemoinformatics Research Antimalarial drug Search

New antimalarial targets are required to let the discovery of chemically diverse, effective drugs. The search for such new targets and new drug chemotypes will likely be helped by the advent of functional genomics and structure-based drug design [26]. After validation of the putative targets as those capable of providing effective and safe drugs, targets can be used as the basis for screening compounds in order to identify new leads, which, in turn, will qualify for bring optimization work [26]. The combined use of combinatorial chemistry to generate large numbers of structurally diverse compounds and of high throughput screening systems to increase speed of the testing of compounds will help to optimize the process [26]. For example, the 4-aminoquinolines have provided a number of useful antimalarials, and *Plasmodium falciparum*, the causative organism for the most deadly form of human malaria, is generally slow to develop resistance to these mentioned drugs [27]. Therefore, diverse screening libraries of quinolines continue to be useful for antimalarial drug discovery [27]. The effects of these substitutions were tested by screening this library for activity against *Plasmodium falciparum*, revealing four potent compounds active against drug-resistant strains [27].

A consideration on molecular mechanics of antimalarial drug is also helpful for further development of new antimalarial drug. The selection of antimalarial drugs is based on the species and the reported resistance pattern in each setting. The mechanism of action of artemisinin compounds consists of two important steps: (a) activation and (b) alkylation. In the activation step by iron, there are two possible pathways for developing C-4 free radical: (a) 1.5 H-shift and (b) C-C cleavage. Recently, Wiwanitkit performed a specific quantum chemical analysis of the activation reaction of artemisinin by the two alternative pathways [28]. According to this study, the required energy for compound formation in C-C cleavage is more than that for C-O cleavage [28]. It can be noted that the C-C cleavage pathway is less preferable in nature, implying that the 1.5 H-shift should be the more common phenomenon [28]. However, compounds that can easily proceed along the pathway 1 have high activity [29]. Therefore, both pathways are important for antimalarial activity. Moreover, effective discrimination between high and low activity compounds using EA1, deltaE1, and deltaE(1A-2A) was shown [29].

Finally, reconstructing synthetic metabolic pathways in microbes has great promise for the production of pharmaceuticals in large-scale fermentations [30]. By recreating biosynthetic pathways in bacteria, complex molecules traditionally harvested from scarce natural resources can be generated in microbial cultures [30]. Recently, Newman et al reported on a strain of *Escherichia coli* having a heterologous, nine-gene biosynthetic pathway for the production of the terpene amorpha-4,11-diene, a precursor to the anti-malarial drug artemisinin [30]. Computational screening of molecular targets in Plasmodium for novel non resistant anti-malarial drugs is also another new application of chemoinformatics [31]. Singh and Mishra tested several combinations including combination of artemisinin and diarylheptanoids based on this procedure and identified that such combinations were useful in treatment of drug resistant malaria [31]. As a conclusion, chemoinformatics have several advantages in rational drug design [32]. Molecular modelling studies based on database, docking, pharmacophore mapping, homology modelling, and quantum chemical studies are all useful in searching for new drug [33 - 34].

References

[1] Ivanov AS, Veselovsky AV, Dubanov AV, Skvortsov VS. Bioinformatics platform development: from gene to lead compound. *Methods Mol Biol.* 2006;316:389-431.

[2] Chang PL. Clinical bioinformatics. *Chang Gung Med J.* 2005;28:201-11.

[3] Attwood PK. The quest to deduce protein function from sequence: the role of pattern databases. *Int J Biochem Cell Biol*. 2000;32:139-55.

[4] Pany YP. In silico drug discovery: solving the "target-rich and lead-poor" imbalance using the genome-to-drug-lead paradigm. *Clin Pharmacol Ther*. 2007;81:30-4.

[5] Bansal AK. Bioinformatics in microbial biotechnology--a mini review. *Microb Cell Fact*. 2005;4:19.

[6] Wiwanitkit V. Analysis of Mycobacterium leprae genome: in silico searching for drug targets. *Southeast Asian J Trop Med Public Health*. 2005;36 Suppl 4:225-7.

[7] Civelli O, Nothacker HP. Functional genomics and the discovery of new drug targets. *Diabetes Technol Ther*. 1999;1:71-6.

[8] Kariagina AS, Naroditskii BS, Apt AS, Gintsburg AL. Genomics and gene engineering: rationale to the development of new means of tuberculosis control. *Zh Mikrobiol Epidemiol Immunobiol*. 2004;(4):94-101.

[9] Schmid MB. Seeing is believing: the impact of structural genomics on antimicrobial drug discovery. *Nat Rev Microbiol*. 2004;2:739-46.

[10] Balakin KV, Kozintsev AV, Kiselyov AS, Savchuk NP.Rational design approaches to chemical libraries for hit identification. *Curr Drug Discov Technol*. 2006;3:49-65.

[11] Chen X, Rusinko A 3rd, Tropsha A, Young SS. Automated pharmacophore identification for large chemical data sets. *J Chem Inf Comput Sci*. 1999;39:887-96.

[12] Oloff S, Zhang S, Sukumar N, Breneman C, Tropsha A. Chemometric analysis of ligand receptor complementarity: identifying Complementary Ligands Based on Receptor Information (CoLiBRI). *J Chem Inf Model*. 2006;46:844-51.

[13] Sen S, Ferdig M. QTL analysis for discovery of genes involved in drug responses. *Curr Drug Targets Infect Disord*. 2004;4:53-63.

[14] Anderson TJ. Mapping drug resistance genes in Plasmodium falciparum by genome-wide association. *Curr Drug Targets Infect Disord*. 2004;4:65-78.

[15] Ferdig MT, Cooper RA, Mu J, Deng B, Joy DA, Su XZ, Wellems TE. Dissecting the loci of low-level quinine resistance in malaria parasites. *Mol Microbiol*. 2004;52:985-97.

[16] Wellems TE, Walker-Jonah A, Panton LJ. Genetic mapping of the chloroquine-resistance locus on Plasmodium falciparum chromosome 7. *Proc Natl Acad Sci U S A*. 1991;88:3382-6.

[17] Cooper RA, Hartwig CL, Ferdig MT. pfcrt is more than the Plasmodium falciparum chloroquine resistance gene: a functional and evolutionary perspective. *Acta Trop*. 2005;94:170-80.

[18] Di Girolamo F, Raggi C, Bultrini E, Lanfrancotti A, Silvestrini F, Sargiacomo M, Birago C, Pizzi E, Alano P, Ponzi M. Functional genomics, new tools in malaria research. *Ann Ist Super Sanita*. 2005;41:469-77.

[19] Fraunholz MJ, Roos DS. PlasmoDB: exploring genomics and post-genomics data of the malaria parasite, Plasmodium falciparum. *Redox Rep*. 2003;8:317-20.

[20] Krungkrai J. The multiple roles of the mitochondrion of the malarial parasite. *Parasitology*. 2004;129:511-24.

[21] Caruthers J, Bosch J, Buckner F, Van Voorhis W, Myler P, Worthey E, Mehlin C, Boni E, DeTitta G, Luft J, Lauricella A, Kalyuzhniy O, Anderson L, Zucker F, Soltis M, Hol

WG.Structure of a ribulose 5-phosphate 3-epimerase from Plasmodium falciparum. *Proteins*. 2006;62:338-42.

[22] Akana J, Fedorov AA, Fedorov E, Novak WR, Babbitt PC, Almo SC, Gerlt JA. D-Ribulose 5-phosphate 3-epimerase: functional and structural relationships to members of the ribulose-phosphate binding (beta/alpha)8-barrel superfamily. *Biochemistry*. 2006;45:2493-503.

[23] Wu Y, Wang X, Liu X, Wang Y. Data-mining approaches reveal hidden families of proteases in the genome of malaria parasite. *Genome Res*. 2003;13:601-16.

[24] Nirmalan N, Sims PF, Hyde JE. Quantitative proteomics of the human malaria parasite Plasmodium falciparum and its application to studies of development and inhibition. *Mol Microbiol*. 2004;52:1187-99.

[25] Cooper RA, Carucci DJ. Proteomic approaches to studying drug targets and resistance in Plasmodium. *Curr Drug Targets Infect Disord*. 2004;4:41-51.

[26] Olliaro PL, Yuthavong Y. An overview of chemotherapeutic targets for antimalarial drug discovery. *Pharmacol Ther*. 1999;81:91-110.

[27] Madrid PB, Wilson NT, DeRisi JL, Guy RK. Parallel synthesis and antimalarial screening of a 4-aminoquinoline library. *J Comb Chem*. 2004;6:437-42.

[28] Wiwanitkit V. Quantum chemical analysis of alternative pathways for iron activation step for artemisinin, a new antimalarial drug. *J Infect*. 2006;53:148-51.

[29] Tonmunphean S, Parasuk V, Kokpol S. Effective discrimination of antimalarial potency of artemisinin compounds based on quantum chemical calculations of their reaction mechanism. *Bioorg Med Chem*. 2006;14:2082-8.

[30] Newman JD, Marshall J, Chang M, Nowroozi F, Paradise E, Pitera D, Newman KL, Keasling JD.High-level production of amorpha-4,11-diene in a two-phase partitioning bioreactor of metabolically engineered Escherichia coli. *Biotechnol Bioeng*. 2006;95:684-91.

[31] Singh N, Misra K. Computational screening of molecular targets in Plasmodium for novel non resistant anti-malarial drugs. *Bioinformation*. 2009;3(6):255-62. Epub 2009 Jan 12.

[32] de Beer TA, Wells GA, Burger PB, Joubert F, Marechal E, Birkholtz L, Louw AI. Antimalarial drug discovery: in silico structural biology and rational drug design. *Infect Disord Drug Targets*. 2009 Jun;9(3):304-18.

[33] Adane L, Bharatam PV. Modelling and informatics in the analysis of P. falciparum DHFR enzyme inhibitors. *Curr Med Chem*. 2008;15(16):1552-69.

[34] Joubert Y, Joubert F. A structural annotation resource for the selection of putative target proteins in the malaria parasite. *Malar J*. 2008 May 23;7:90.

Chapter Sources

The following chapters have been previously published:

Chapter 8 was also published in *New Developments in Medicinal Chemistry,* edited by Marta P. Ortega and Irene C. Gil, published by Nova Science Publishers, Inc. It was submitted for appropriate modifications in an effort to encourage wider dissemination of research.

Chapter 9 was also published in *Malaria Research in Southeast Asia,* by Viroj Wiwanitkit, published by Nova Science Publishers, Inc. It was submitted for appropriate modifications in an effort to encourage wider dissemination of research.

Chapter 10 was also published in *Malaria Research in Southeast Asia,* by Viroj Wiwanitkit, published by Nova Science Publishers, Inc. It was submitted for appropriate modifications in an effort to encourage wider dissemination of research.

Index

A

B

C

D

I

J

K

L

M

Q

R

S

T

U

V